Algebraic Structures and Graph Theory, 2nd Edition

Algebraic Structures and Graph Theory, 2nd Edition

Guest Editors

Irina Cristea
Alessandro Linzi

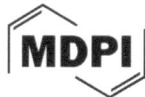

Basel • Beijing • Wuhan • Barcelona • Belgrade • Novi Sad • Cluj • Manchester

Guest Editors

Irina Cristea
Centre for Information
Technologies and Applied
Mathematics
University of Nova Gorica
Nova Gorica
Slovenia

Alessandro Linzi
Centre for Information
Technologies and Applied
Mathematics
University of Nova Gorica
Nova Gorica
Slovenia

Editorial Office
MDPI AG
Grosspeteranlage 5
4052 Basel, Switzerland

This is a reprint of the Special Issue, published open access by the journal *Mathematics* (ISSN 2227-7390), freely accessible at: https://www.mdpi.com/journal/mathematics/special_issues/1RKT503SSL.

For citation purposes, cite each article independently as indicated on the article page online and as indicated below:

Lastname, A.A.; Lastname, B.B. Article Title. *Journal Name* **Year**, *Volume Number*, Page Range.

ISBN 978-3-7258-3355-9 (Hbk)
ISBN 978-3-7258-3356-6 (PDF)
https://doi.org/10.3390/books978-3-7258-3356-6

© 2025 by the authors. Articles in this book are Open Access and distributed under the Creative Commons Attribution (CC BY) license. The book as a whole is distributed by MDPI under the terms and conditions of the Creative Commons Attribution-NonCommercial-NoDerivs (CC BY-NC-ND) license (https://creativecommons.org/licenses/by-nc-nd/4.0/).

Contents

About the Editors vii

Irina Cristea and Alessandro Linzi
Preface to the Special Issue "Algebraic Structures and Graph Theory, 2nd Edition"
Reprinted from: *Mathematics* **2025**, *13*, 577, https://doi.org/10.3390/math13040577 1

T. Asir, K. Mano, Jehan A. Al-Bar and Wafaa M. Fakieh
Class of Crosscap Two Graphs Arising from Lattices–I
Reprinted from: *Mathematics* **2023**, *11*, 1553, https://doi.org/10.3390/math11061553 3

Yongsheng Rao, Muhammad Ahsan Binyamin, Adnan Aslam, Maria Mehtab and Shazia Fazal
On the Planarity of Graphs Associated with Symmetric and Pseudo Symmetric Numerical Semigroups
Reprinted from: *Mathematics* **2023**, *11*, 1681, https://doi.org/10.3390/math11071681 29

Krittawit Limkul and Sayan Panma
On the Independence Number of Cayley Digraphs of Clifford Semigroups
Reprinted from: *Mathematics* **2023**, *11*, 3445, https://doi.org/10.3390/math11163445 40

Renbing Xiao, Xiaojiao Zhang and Hua Zhang
On Edge-Primitive Graphs of Order as a Product of Two Distinct Primes
Reprinted from: *Mathematics* **2023**, *11*, 3896, https://doi.org/10.3390/math11183896 58

Ahmad H. Alkasasbeh, Elsayed Badr, Hala Attiya and Hanan M. Shabana
Radio Number for Friendship Communication Networks
Reprinted from: *Mathematics* **2023**, *11*, 4232, https://doi.org/10.3390/math11204232 68

Wei Chen
The Structure of Semiconic Idempotent Commutative Residuated Lattices
Reprinted from: *Mathematics* **2024**, *12*, 179, https://doi.org/10.3390/math12020179 82

Yingbi Jiang, Bo Ling, Jinlong Yang and Yun Zhao
Classifying Seven-Valent Symmetric Graphs of Order $8pq$
Reprinted from: *Mathematics* **2024**, *12*, 787, https://doi.org/10.3390/math12060787 98

Alaa Altassan, Anwar Saleh, Marwa Hamed and Najat Muthana
Characterizing Finite Groups through Equitable Graphs: A Graph-Theoretic Approach
Reprinted from: *Mathematics* **2024**, *12*, 2126, https://doi.org/10.3390/math12132126 108

Kaique M. A. Roberto, Kaique R. P. Santos and Hugo Luiz Mariano
On Non-Commutative Multi-Rings with Involution
Reprinted from: *Mathematics* **2024**, *12*, 2931, https://doi.org/10.3390/math12182931 131

Andromeda Pătrașcu Sonea and Ciprian Chiruță
Optimizing HX-Group Compositions Using $C++$: A Computational Approach to Dihedral Group Hyperstructures
Reprinted from: *Mathematics* **2024**, *12*, 3492, https://doi.org/10.3390/math12223492 148

Nicolò Cangiotti
Feynman Diagrams beyond Physics: From Biology to Economy
Reprinted from: *Mathematics* **2024**, *12*, 1295, https://doi.org/10.3390/math12091295 162

About the Editors

Irina Cristea

Irina Cristea received her PhD degree in Mathematics from the University Ovidius of Constanta, Romania. She concluded her postdoctoral studies at the University of Udine, Italy. She currently works as an Associate Professor at the University of Nova Gorica, Slovenia, where she leads the Centre of Information Technologies and Applied Mathematics. Her research interests are mainly related to the theory of hypercompositional algebra, having published more than 80 articles in journals indexed by Scopus or the Web of Science and co-authored one book, entitled "Fuzzy Algebraic Hyperstructures: An Introduction", published by Springer in 2015. Over the past 4 years, she has acted as the Chief Editor for the *Italian Journal of Pure and Applied Mathematics*, the Associate Editor of *Mathematics* (published by MDPI), *Heliyon Mathematics* (published by Cell press), and seven other international journals. She is also a Guest Editor for several Special Issues related to algebraic structures and graph theory.

Alessandro Linzi

Alessandro Linzi received his PhD degree in Mathematics in 2022. His research involves various areas of the discipline such as mathematical logic and the foundations of mathematics, category theory, valuation theory, and hypercompositional algebra. He has several publications indexed by the WoS and Scopus, some of which also appear in MDPI journals. Furthermore, Dr. Linzi is an active reviewer for MDPI, as well as several other esteemed publishing companies.

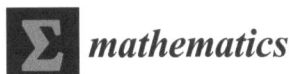

Editorial

Preface to the Special Issue "Algebraic Structures and Graph Theory, 2nd Edition"

Irina Cristea * and Alessandro Linzi

Centre for Information Technologies and Applied Mathematics, University of Nova Gorica, Vipavska Cesta 13, 5000 Nova Gorica, Slovenia; alessandro.linzi@ung.si
* Correspondence: irina.cristea@ung.si

This is a continuation of the work initiated in [1], representing a reprint of the second edition of the Special Issue "Algebraic Structures and Graph Theory", which was published in the MDPI journal *Mathematics*. Among the 36 submissions received for this Special Issue, the editors selected ten articles and one review paper that successfully passed the peer-review process, and were then published in the journal in the period from March 2023 to November 2024. They contain original research ideas that have made a significant advancements in the theory of algebraic structures and graph theory. In particular, the topics discussed in these 11 papers are related to graphs constructed from lattices, semigroups, or groups, to particular types of graphs (as edge-primitive, friendship, or equitable graphs), and to hypercompositional algebras (HX-groups and multi-rings).

Contribution 1 proposes a characterization of the crosscap two annihilating ideals graphs of lattices with at most four atoms. As a consequence, a large class of r-partite graphs that can be embedded in the Klein bottle has been introduced. Contribution 2 discusses the planarity of $S(m,e)$-graphs associated with some irreducible numerical semigroups with multiplicity m and embedding dimension e. In Contribution 3, the authors characterize the maximal connected subdigraphs of the Cayley digraph of a Clifford semigroup related to one of its subsets. This study helps to investigate on the independence numbers of the Cayley digraphs of Clifford semigroups. Based on the properties of non-abelian simple groups having at least one subgroup of order pq, where p and q are two distinct odd primes, the authors of Contribution 4 completely determined the edge-primitive graphs of order pq. In Contribution 5 we can find a model for calculating the upper bounds of the radio numbers of the so-called friendship graphs having k cycles, each of length m, with $3 \leq m \leq 6$, and having one common vertex. The study conducted in Contribution 6 leads to a structure theorem for semiconic idempotent commutative residuated lattices. This theorem is the key element to prove that the variety of strongly semiconic idempotent commutative residuated lattices has the amalgamation property. A classification of the seven-valent symmetric graphs of order $8pq$, where p and q are distinct primes, is presented in Contribution 7. The main idea used by the authors of this paper is the reduction of the automorphism groups of the considered graphs to some non-commutative simple groups. Another interesting connection between graphs and groups arises in Contribution 8. In this paper, the authors study some topological indices and graph-theoretic properties (such as connectedness, diameter, girth, clique number, and radius) of equitable graphs of type I constructed from various groups. The last two original articles within this Special Issue deal with algebraic multistructures. In Contribution 9, the concept of Marshall's quotient of a non-commutative multi-ring with involution is studied, leading to new examples of multialgebras with involution. Contribution 10 presents an algorithm for computing the HX-groups that have support equal to the dihedral group D_n. We conclude this Special

Received: 6 February 2025
Accepted: 7 February 2025
Published: 10 February 2025

Citation: Cristea, I.; Linzi, A. Preface to the Special Issue "Algebraic Structures and Graph Theory, 2nd Edition". *Mathematics* **2025**, *13*, 577. https://doi.org/10.3390/math13040577

Copyright: © 2025 by the authors. Licensee MDPI, Basel, Switzerland. This article is an open access article distributed under the terms and conditions of the Creative Commons Attribution (CC BY) license (https://creativecommons.org/licenses/by/4.0/).

Issue with Contribution 11, which is a review paper on Feynam diagrams, introduced in quantum electrodynamics and also used in biology and economy nowadays. The main analytical and algebraic properties of these diagrams are summarized, with examples related to wave propagation, information field theory, and medicine.

The Guest Editors extend their sincere appreciation to all of the authors for their valuable contributions to this Special Issue. We are also deeply grateful to the anonymous reviewers for their insightful and professional evaluation reports, which have significantly enhanced the quality of the submitted manuscripts. Furthermore, we acknowledge the excellent collaboration with the publisher, the constant assistance provided by the MDPI associate editors in bringing this project to the end, and the great support of the Managing Editor of this Special Issue, Ms. Ursula Tian.

Conflicts of Interest: The authors declare no conflicts of interest.

List of Contributions:

1. Asir, T.; Mano, K.; Al-Bar, J.A.; Fakieh, W.M. Class of Crosscap Two Graphs Arising from Lattices–I. *Mathematics* **2023**, *11*, 1553. https://doi.org/10.3390/math11061553.
2. Rao, Y.; Binyamin, M.A.; Aslam, A.; Mehtab, M.; Fazal, S. On the Planarity of Graphs Associated with Symmetric and Pseudo Symmetric Numerical Semigroups. *Mathematics* **2023**, *11*, 1681. https://doi.org/10.3390/math11071681.
3. Limkul, K.; Panma, S. On the Independence Number of Cayley Digraphs of Clifford Semigroups. *Mathematics* **2023**, *11*, 3445. https://doi.org/10.3390/math11163445.
4. Xiao, R.; Zhang, X.; Zhang, H. On Edge-Primitive Graphs of Order as a Product of Two Distinct Primes. *Mathematics* **2023**, *11*, 3896. https://doi.org/10.3390/math11183896.
5. Alkasasbeh, A.H.; Badr, E.; Attiya, H.; Shabana, H.M. Radio Number for Friendship Communication Networks. *Mathematics* **2023**, *11*, 4232. https://doi.org/10.3390/math11204232.
6. Chen, W. The Structure of Semiconic Idempotent Commutative Residuated Lattices. *Mathematics* **2024**, *12*, 179. https://doi.org/10.3390/math12020179.
7. Jiang, Y.; Ling, B.; Yang, J.; Zhao, Y. Classifying Seven-Valent Symmetric Graphs of Order 8pq. *Mathematics* **2024**, *12*, 787. https://doi.org/10.3390/math12060787.
8. Altassan, A.; Saleh, A.; Hamed, M.; Muthana, N. Characterizing Finite Groups through Equitable Graphs: A Graph-Theoretic Approach. *Mathematics* **2024**, *12*, 2126. https://doi.org/10.3390/math12132126.
9. Roberto, K.M.A.; Santos, K.R.P.; Mariano, H.L. On Non-Commutative Multi-Rings with Involution. *Mathematics* **2024**, *12*, 2931. https://doi.org/10.3390/math12182931.
10. Sonea, A.P.; Chiruta, C. Optimizing HX-Group Compositions Using C++: A Computational Approach to Dihedral Group Hyperstructures. *Mathematics* **2024**, *12*, 3492. https://doi.org/10.3390/math12223492.
11. Cangiotti, N. Feynman Diagrams beyond Physics: From Biology to Economy. *Mathematics* **2024**, *12*, 1295. https://doi.org/10.3390/math12091295.

Reference

1. Cristea, I.; Bordbar, H. (Eds.) *Algebraic Structures and Graph Theory*; MDPI Books: Basel, Switzerland, 2023.

Disclaimer/Publisher's Note: The statements, opinions and data contained in all publications are solely those of the individual author(s) and contributor(s) and not of MDPI and/or the editor(s). MDPI and/or the editor(s) disclaim responsibility for any injury to people or property resulting from any ideas, methods, instructions or products referred to in the content.

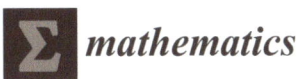

Article

Class of Crosscap Two Graphs Arising from Lattices–I

T. Asir [1],*, K. Mano [2], Jehan A. Al-Bar [3] and Wafaa M. Fakieh [3]

[1] Department of Mathematics, Pondicherry University, Pondicherry 605 014, Tamil Nadu, India
[2] Department of Mathematics, Fatima College, Madurai 625 018, Tamil Nadu, India
[3] Department of Mathematics, Faculty of Science, King Abdulaziz University, Jeddah 21461, Saudi Arabia
* Correspondence: asirjacob75@gmail.com

Abstract: Let $\mathcal{L}$ be a lattice. The annihilating-ideal graph of $\mathcal{L}$ is a simple graph whose vertex set is the set of all nontrivial ideals of $\mathcal{L}$ and whose two distinct vertices I and J are adjacent if and only if $I \wedge J = 0$. In this paper, crosscap two annihilating-ideal graphs of lattices with at most four atoms are characterized. These characterizations provide the classes of multipartite graphs, which are embedded in the Klein bottle.

Keywords: crosscap; Klein bottle; lattice; annihilating-ideal graph

MSC: 05C75; 05C25; 05C10; 06A07; 06B99

1. Introduction

According to the well-known theorem of Kuratowski and Wagner, a graph is planar if and only if it does not contain either of the two forbidden graphs K_5 and $K_{3,3}$. The Graph Minor Theorem of Robertson and Seymour [1] can be considered a powerful generalization of Kuratowski's Theorem. In particular, their theorem, which is the "deepest" and "most important" result in the arena of graph theory [2], implies that each graph property, *no matter what*, is characterized by a corresponding finite list of graphs. Thus, for surfaces (both orientable and non-orientable) in general, it is known that the set of forbidden minors is finite [3]. An analogous characterization for the embedding of graphs on surfaces is known for the crosscap one surface (Möbius strip) where 103 forbidden subgraphs (equivalently 35 forbidden minors) are characterized [4,5]. So, an open problem is to determine the several forbidden subgraphs for crosscap two surfaces (the Klein bottle). In this sequel, finding a family of graphs that has a crosscap two is an interesting one. Note that most of the 103 graphs contain a subgraph that is homeomorphic to $K_{3,3}$, and multipartite graphs play a vital role in finding these 103 forbidden subgraphs for the projective plane. It is worth mentioning that the crosscap value of bipartite and tripartite graphs are well known (refer to Proposition 1). The main goal of this paper is to identify a large class of crosscap two r-partite graphs where $r \geq 4$.

Let us introduce the concept of the *annihilating-ideal graph of a lattice*, a type of multipartite graph. Note that the annihilating-ideal graph is an extension of the concept of the zero-divisor graph. The idea of the zero-divisor graph of a ring structure is due to Beck [6]. In 2009, Halaš et al. [7] introduced the zero-divisor graph for a partially ordered set, and, in 2012, Estaji et al. [8] extended the concept of the zero-divisor graph to an arbitrary finite bounded lattice. For a clear exposition of the work completed in the area of zero-divisor graphs and their related areas, the reader is referred to the book by Anderson et al. [9]. In 2011, Behboodi et al. [10] defined and investigated the ideal theoretic version of the zero-divisor graph, called the *annihilating-ideal graph of a ring*, and, thereafter, many facts about zero-divisors were expressed in the language of ideals. The concept of an annihilating-ideal graph of a ring was extended to an arbitrary lattice by Afkhami et al. [11] in 2015. The *annihilating-ideal graph of a lattice* $\mathcal{L}$, denoted by $\mathbb{AG}(\mathcal{L})$, is defined to be a simple graph whose vertex set is the set of all non-trivial ideals of $\mathcal{L}$, and whose two distinct vertices I and J are adjacent if and only if $I \wedge J = 0$. The hope when studying the annihilating-ideal graph of a lattice is that the graph theoretic properties of the graph from the lattice will help us to better understand the lattice theoretic properties of the lattice.

One of the most important topological properties of a graph is its genus, which can be orientable or non-orientable (crosscap). The genus of graphs associated with algebraic structures has been studied by many authors (see [12–17]). The planar zero-divisor graph was first explicitly characterized by Smith [18], and the characterization of commutative rings with projective zero-divisor graphs was obtained by Chiang-Hsieh [15]. In 2019, Asir et al. [12] enumerated all commutative rings whose zero-divisor graph has a crosscap two. The planar and crosscap one annihilating-ideal graph of lattices were characterized by Shahsavar [19] and Parsapour et al. [20], respectively. Additionally, whether the line graph associated with the annihilating-ideal graph of a lattice is planar or projective was characterized by Parsapour et al. [21]. Moreover, the authors of [22] characterized all lattices $\mathcal{L}$ whose line graph of $\mathbb{AG}(\mathcal{L})$ is toroidal.

Now, this paper aims to classify lattices with a number of atoms less than or equal to four whose annihilating-ideal graph can be embedded in the non-orientable surfaces of crosscap two. The main results of this paper are Theorems 2, 3, and 5, in which we have obtained our classifications. As a result, this classification provides a large class of r-partite graphs that can be embedded in the Klein bottle. Further, in the proof of the main theorems, we have shown several minimal r-partite graphs that cannot be embedded in the Klein bottle. Possibly, these graphs may be realized as forbidden subgraphs for crosscap two surfaces (refer to Example 1). Further, in order to cover the missing cases in the proof of Theorem 2.6 [20], which affects the statement of the corresponding theorem, the modified version is included as Theorem 4.

2. Preliminaries

In this section, we present the definitions and results needed to prove the main results in the subsequent sections. First, we recall some definitions and notations on lattices. A *lattice* is an algebra $\mathcal{L} = (\mathcal{L}, \wedge, \vee)$, where $\wedge$ and $\vee$ are the binary operations, satisfying the following conditions: for all $a, b, c \in \mathcal{L}$

1. $a \wedge a = a, a \vee a = a$;
2. $a \wedge b = b \wedge a, a \vee b = b \vee a$;
3. $(a \wedge b) \wedge c = a \wedge (b \wedge c); a \vee (b \vee c) = (a \vee b) \vee c$;
4. $a \vee (a \wedge b) = a \wedge (a \vee b) = a$.

According to [23] (Theorem 2.1), we can define an order $\leq$ on $\mathcal{L}$ as follows: for any $a, b \in \mathcal{L}$, we set $a \leq b$ if and only if $a \wedge b = a$. Then $(\mathcal{L}, \leq)$ is an ordered set in which every pair of elements has the greatest lower bound (glb) and the least upper bound (lub). Conversely, let P be an ordered set such that, for every pair $a, b \in P$, $glb(a, b)$ and $lub(a, b)$ belong to P. For each a and b in P, we define $a \wedge b = glb(a, b)$ and $a \vee b = lub(a, b)$. Then $(P, \wedge, \vee)$ is a lattice. A lattice $\mathcal{L}$ is said to be *bounded* if there are the elements 0 and 1 in $\mathcal{L}$ such that $0 \wedge a = 0$ and $a \vee 1 = 1$, for all $a \in \mathcal{L}$. Clearly, every finite lattice is bounded. Let $(\mathcal{L}, \wedge, \vee)$ be a lattice with a least element 0 and I be a non-empty subset of $\mathcal{L}$. Then I is said to be the *ideal* of $\mathcal{L}$, denoted by $I \trianglelefteq \mathcal{L}$,

1. For all $a, b \in I, a \vee b \in I$.
2. If $0 \leq a \leq b$ and $b \in I$, then $a \in I$.

In a lattice $(\mathcal{L}, \wedge, \vee)$ with a least element 0, an element a is called an *atom* if $a \neq 0$, and, for an element $x \in \mathcal{L}$, the relation $0 \leq x \leq a$ implies that either $x = 0$ or $x = a$. We denote the set of all atoms of $\mathcal{L}$ by $A(\mathcal{L})$. For basic facts about lattices, we refer the reader to [24].

Next, we recall the following terms regarding graph embedding. For the non-negative integers ℓ and k, let S_ℓ denote the sphere with ℓ handles, and N_k denote a sphere with k crosscaps attached to it. Note that every connected compact surface is homeomorphic to S_ℓ or N_k for some non-negative integers ℓ and k. The *genus* $\gamma(G)$ of a simple graph G is the minimum ℓ such that G can be embedded in S_ℓ. Similarly, *crosscap number (non-orientable genus)* $\tilde{\gamma}(G)$ is the minimum k such that G can be embedded in N_k. Note that the projective space is of crosscap one and the Klein bottle is of crosscap two. If $e = xy \in E(G)$, then the *contraction* of e in G, denoted as $[x, y]$ is the graph obtained from $G - xy$ by identifying vertices x and y to create a new vertex z incident with all edges of G that were incident with either x or y. We say H is a *minor* of G, if H can be obtained from G by deleting vertices, edges, and/or contracting edges. For a graph G, we denote $\tilde{G}$ for the subgraph $G - V'$ where $V' = \{v \in V | \deg(v) = 1\}$, and we call this graph the *reduction* of G. For details on the notion of the embedding of graphs in a surface, we recommend reading [25].

The following three results on the non-orientable embedding of graphs are used frequently in this paper. In what follows, we denote the complete graph with p vertices by K_p, the complete bipartite graph with parts of sizes p and q by $K_{p,q}$, the complete tripartite graph with parts of sizes p, q, and r by $K_{p,q,r}$, and the complete four-partite graph with parts of sizes p, q, r, and s by $K_{p,q,r,s}$.

Proposition 1 ([25,26]). *Let p, q, r, and s be positive integers greater than or equal to two. Then*

(a) $\tilde{\gamma}(K_p) = \begin{cases} \left\lceil \frac{(p-3)(p-4)}{6} \right\rceil & \text{if } p \geq 3 \\ 3 & \text{if } p = 7. \end{cases}$

(b) $\tilde{\gamma}(K_{p,q}) = \left\lceil \frac{(p-2)(q-2)}{2} \right\rceil$.

(c) $\tilde{\gamma}(K_{p,q,r}) = \left\lceil \frac{(p-2)(q+r-2)}{2} \right\rceil$ *except for* $K_{3,3,3}$, $K_{4,4,1}$ *and* $K_{4,4,3}$. *Further,* $\tilde{\gamma}(K_{3,3,3}) = 3, \tilde{\gamma}(K_{4,4,1}) = 4$ *and* $\tilde{\gamma}(K_{4,4,3}) = 6$.

(d). *If $p \geq q + r$, then $\tilde{\gamma}(K_{p,q,r,s}) \geq \left\lceil \frac{(p-2)(q+r+s-2)}{2} \right\rceil$. If $p \leq q + r$, then $\tilde{\gamma}(K_{p,q,r,s}) \geq \left\lceil \frac{(p+s-2)(q+r-2)}{2} \right\rceil$.*

Proposition 2 (([16] Theorem 1.3) (Euler formula)). *Let $\phi : G \to N_k$ be a two-cell embedding of a connected graph G to the non-orientable surface N_k. Then $|V| - |E| + |F| = 2 - k$, where $|V|, |E|$, and $|F|$ are the number of vertices, edges, and faces that $\phi(G)$ has, respectively, and k is the crosscap of N_k.*

The following is an easy observation that will be used in the proof of the main theorem.

Observation 1. *Let G be a simple graph with $|E|$ edges embedded with $|F|$ faces. Then $\frac{2|E|}{|F|} \geq gr(G)$ where $gr(G)$ denotes the length of the shortest cycle in G.*

3. Basic Results and Notations

Before going into the classifications, we need to be familiar with the following notations and observations given by Parsapour and Javaheri in [20].

Notation: ([20]) Let $\mathcal{L}$ be a lattice and $A(\mathcal{L}) = \{a_1, a_2, \ldots, a_n\}$ be the set of all atoms. Let $i_1, i_2, \ldots, i_k$ be integers with $1 \leq i_1 < i_2 < \ldots < i_k \leq n$. The notation $U_{i_1 i_2 \ldots i_k}$ stands for the following set:

$$\left\{ I \trianglelefteq \mathcal{L} : \{a_{i_1}, a_{i_2}, \ldots, a_{i_k}\} \subseteq I \text{ and } a_{i_j} \notin I \text{ for } i_j \in \{1, 2, \ldots, n\} \setminus \{i_1, i_2, \ldots, i_k\} \right\}.$$

The next result provides the structure of $\mathbb{AG}(\mathcal{L})$.

Proposition 3. *Let $\mathcal{L}$ be a lattice with n atoms. Then $\mathbb{AG}(\mathcal{L})$ is a $2^n - 2$-partite graph.*

Proof. Let $|A(\mathcal{L})| = n$. For $1 \leq i_1 < i_2 < \ldots < i_k \leq n$ and $1 \leq j_1 < j_2 < \ldots < j_{k'} \leq n$, if the index sets $\{i_1, i_2, \ldots, i_k\}$ and $\{j_1, j_2, \ldots, j_{k'}\}$ of $U_{i_1 i_2 \ldots i_k}$ and $U_{j_1 j_2 \ldots j_{k'}}$ respectively, are distinct, then $U_{i_1 i_2 \ldots i_k} \cap U_{j_1 j_2 \ldots j_{k'}} = \emptyset$. Clearly, $V(\mathbb{AG}(\mathcal{L})) = \bigcup_{1 \leq i_1 < i_2 < \ldots < i_k \leq n} U_{i_1 i_2 \ldots i_k}$.

Therefore, for $1 \leq i_1 < i_2 < \ldots < i_k \leq n$, the set $U_{i_1i_2\ldots i_k}$ forms a partition of $V(\mathbb{AG}(\mathcal{L}))$. Since $0 \neq a_{i_1}$ belongs to every ideal in $U_{i_1i_2\ldots i_k}$, no pair of distinct vertices in $U_{i_1i_2\ldots i_k}$ are adjacent in $\mathbb{AG}(\mathcal{L})$. Note that the number of distinct $U_{i_1i_2\ldots i_k}$s is $2^n - 1$. This, together with the fact that every vertex in $U_{12\ldots n}$ is isolated in $\mathbb{AG}(\mathcal{L})$, implies that $\mathbb{AG}(\mathcal{L})$ is a $2^n - 2$-partite graph. □

According to the abovementioned result regarding the structure of $\mathbb{AG}(\mathcal{L})$, in order to identify the crosscap two r-partite graph or to classify the forbidden r-partite graphs of a non-orientable surface of order two for some $3 \leq r \in \mathbb{N}$, one may be interested in finding all crosscap two annihilating-ideal graphs. This is the main objective of this paper.

We shall also need the following notations:

Notations: Before proving our main results, the following points are assumed for convenience in notations and clarity in proofs. Let us take $|A(\mathcal{L})| = n$.

- To avoid repetition, we assume $|U_1| \geq |U_2| \geq \ldots \geq |U_n|$.
- We denote the vertices of the set $U_{i_1i_2\ldots i_k}$ by $\{I_{i_1i_2\ldots i_k}, I'_{i_1i_2\ldots i_k}, I''_{i_1i_2\ldots i_k}, \ldots\}$.
- For an integer p, an integer different from p will be denoted by p'.
- For the sake of convenience, we shall denote $U_{(i_1i_2\ldots i_k)^c} = U_{j_1j_2\ldots j_\ell}$ where $j_1, j_2, \ldots, j_\ell = \{1, 2, \ldots, n\} \setminus \{i_1, i_2, \ldots, i_k\}$ and the notation $U_{(i_1i_2\ldots i_k)^c}$ exists only when $U_{i_1i_2\ldots i_k} \neq \emptyset$.
- The edge between the two vertices I and J is denoted by (I, J).
- The notations $|F|$ and f_i denote the number of faces and number of i-gons in an embedding of G in N_k, respectively.
- There may be sets $U_{i_1i_2\ldots i_k}$ such that each vertex of $U_{i_1i_2\ldots i_k}$ is isolated, ends, or is adjacent to exactly two ends of an edge in $\mathbb{AG}(\mathcal{L})$. In such places, the vertices of $U_{i_1i_2\ldots i_k}$ do not affect the crosscap number of $\mathbb{AG}(\mathcal{L})$, which leads to ignoring the set $U_{i_1i_2\ldots i_k}$ from the corresponding embedding. This fact is used throughout the article and is sometimes not explicitly pointed out.
- For convenience in any drawing, we provide a particular type of N_2-embedding of $\mathbb{AG}(\mathcal{L})$. This means that instead of drawing graphs for the case U_{ij} with $1 \leq i \leq j \leq 3$, we assume $i = 1$ and $j = 2$ in figures. Additionally, the notation $\cdots$ is used to denote the possibility of embedding any number of vertices.

We show a few simple, but useful, properties of a crosscap on $\mathbb{AG}(\mathcal{L})$. We now state and prove the following lemma, which provides a subgraph and super-graph structure of $\mathbb{AG}(\mathcal{L})$.

Lemma 1. *Let $\mathcal{L}$ be a lattice, $|A(\mathcal{L})| = n$, and $n \geq k \in \mathbb{N}$. Let $\alpha_{i_1i_2\ldots i_k} = |U_{i_1i_2\ldots i_k}|$, $\lambda = \max\{\alpha_{i_1i_2\ldots i_k}\}$ for all $1 \leq i_1 < i_2 < \ldots < i_k \leq n$. Then*

(a). *$K_{\alpha_1,\alpha_2,\ldots,\alpha_n}$ is a subgraph of $\mathbb{AG}(\mathcal{L})$.*

(b). *$K_{(2^n-2)(\lambda)}$ is a super-graph of $\mathbb{AG}(\mathcal{L})$.*

Proof. Let H be the induced subgraph of $\mathbb{AG}(\mathcal{L})$, induced by the vertex subset $\bigcup_{i=1}^n U_i$. It is clear that no two distinct vertices in U_i are adjacent, and every vertex in U_i is adjacent to all of the vertices of U_j for $i \neq j$ in $\mathbb{AG}(\mathcal{L})$. Thus $H = K_{\alpha_1,\alpha_2,\ldots,\alpha_n}$.

The second part follows from the facts that $V(\mathbb{AG}(\mathcal{L})) = \bigcup U_{i_1i_2\ldots i_k}$; the number of vertex subsets $U_{i_1i_2\ldots i_k}$, except $U_{12\ldots n}$, in $V(\mathbb{AG}(\mathcal{L}))$ is $\binom{n}{1} + \binom{n}{2} + \ldots + \binom{n}{n-1} = 2^n - 2$; and $\lambda = \max\{\alpha_{i_1i_2\ldots i_k}\}$. □

We are now in the position to provide a lower bound for the crosscap of $\mathbb{AG}(\mathcal{L})$. Applying Proposition 1c,d in the first part of the above lemma, we obtain the following result.

Theorem 1. *Let $\mathcal{L}$ be a lattice, $|A(\mathcal{L})| = n \geq 3$, and $|U_1| \geq |U_2| \geq \ldots \geq |U_n|$.*

(a). If $n = 3$, then $\tilde{\gamma}(\mathbb{AG}(\mathcal{L})) \geq \left\lceil \frac{(|U_1|-2)(|U_2|+|U_3|-2)}{2} \right\rceil$. Moreover, the equality holds whenever $U_{ij} = \emptyset$ for all $1 \leq i \leq j \leq 3$.

(b). If $n \geq 4$, then $\tilde{\gamma}(\mathbb{AG}(\mathcal{L})) \geq \begin{cases} \left\lceil \frac{(|U_1|-2)(|U_2|+|U_3|+|U_4|-2)}{2} \right\rceil & \text{if } |U_1| \geq |U_2|+|U_3| \\ \left\lceil \frac{(|U_1|+|U_4|-2)(|U_2|+|U_3|-2)}{2} \right\rceil & \text{if } |U_1| < |U_2|+|U_3|. \end{cases}$

We now enter into the core part of the paper. We first observe that $\mathbb{AG}(\mathcal{L})$ is totally disconnected when $|A(\mathcal{L})| = 1$, and $\mathbb{AG}(\mathcal{L})$ contains K_7 as a subgraph when $|A(\mathcal{L})| \geq 7$. Further, according to Proposition 1a, the crosscap of K_7 is three. Thus, one obtains the following result, which provides a bound for the number of atoms in lattice $\mathcal{L}$ with $\tilde{\gamma}(\mathbb{AG}(\mathcal{L})) = 2$.

Proposition 4. *Let $\mathcal{L}$ be a lattice. If the crosscap of the annihilating-ideal graph $\mathbb{AG}(\mathcal{L})$ is two, then $2 \leq |A(\mathcal{L})| \leq 6$.*

We start the characterization by analyzing the simple case that $|A(\mathcal{L})| = 2$. If $|A(\mathcal{L})| = 2$, then Theorem 2.6 [20] implies that $\mathbb{AG}(\mathcal{L}) \cong K_{|U_1|,|U_2|}$, and so

$$\tilde{\gamma}(\mathbb{AG}(\mathcal{L})) = \left\lceil \frac{(|U_1|-2)(|U_2|-2)}{2} \right\rceil$$

whenever $|U_1|, |U_2| \geq 2$. Now, a simple calculation has yielded the following result, which characterized lattice $\mathcal{L}$ with a crosscap two $\mathbb{AG}(\mathcal{L})$ in the case of $|A(\mathcal{L})| = 2$.

Theorem 2. *Let $\mathcal{L}$ be a lattice and $|A(\mathcal{L})| = 2$. Then $\tilde{\gamma}(\mathbb{AG}(\mathcal{L})) = 2$ if and only if $|U_1| = |U_2| = 4$ or $|U_i| = 3$ and $|U_j| \in \{5, 6\}$ where $i, j \in \{1, 2\}$ with $i \neq j$.*

To finish this section we show two results that will be used to prove the main results. The graphs given in Figures 1 and 2 play a vital role in characterizing a lattice with crosscap two annihilating-ideal graphs, and, therefore, we draw the graph with its embedding in the first result.

Lemma 2. *For the graphs H_1 and H_2, as shown in Figures 1 and 2, we have $\tilde{\gamma}(H_1) = \tilde{\gamma}(H_2) = 2$.*

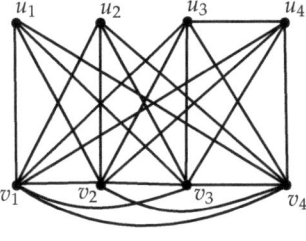
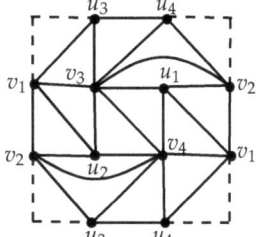

(a). The graph H_1 (b). An N_2-embedding of H_1

Figure 1. The graph H_1 and its N_2-embedding.

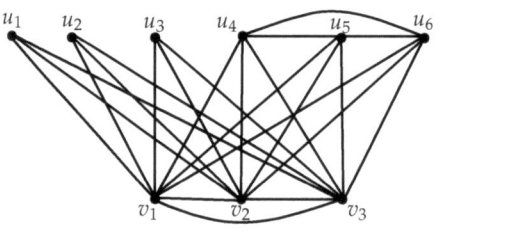
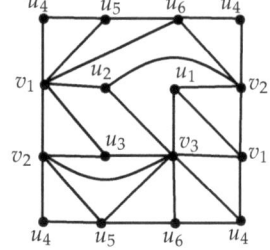

(**a**). The graph H_2
(**b**). An N_2-embedding of H_2

Figure 2. The graph H_2 and its N_2-embedding.

The graphs H_3 and H_4 given in Figure 3 play a vital role in our main theorems.

Lemma 3. *For the graphs H_3 and H_4, as shown in Figure 3, we have $\tilde{\gamma}(H_3) \geq 3$ and $\tilde{\gamma}(H_4) \geq 3$.*

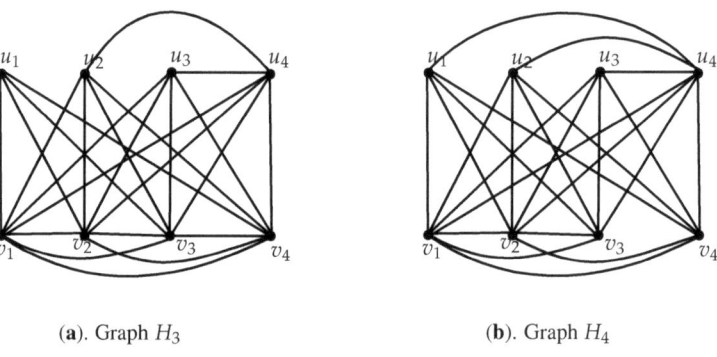

(**a**). Graph H_3
(**b**). Graph H_4

Figure 3. The graphs H_3 and H_4.

Proof. (a). Consider the subgraph $H'_3 = H_3 - \{u_1\}$. Clearly $H'_3 \cong K_7 - e$ where $e = (u_2, u_3)$, and there are 13 faces in any N_2-embedding of H'_3 of which 12 are triangular, and 1 is rectangular. Now, we try to recover an N_2-embedding of H_3 by inserting u_1 with its edges. Since u_1 is adjacent to four vertices of H'_3, u_1 should be inserted into the rectangular face of H'_3. However, all vertices of H'_3 are adjacent to each other, except for u_2 and u_3, so the rectangular face of H'_3 must contain either u_2 or u_3, which is in contradiction to u_2 and u_3 not belonging to the neighborhood set of u_1. Therefore, $\tilde{\gamma}(H_3) \geq 3$.

(b). Apply a similar argument as in (a) for the subgraph $H'_4 = H_4 - \{u_1\} \cong K_7 - 2e$. Here, notice that the largest face in any N_2-embedding of H'_4 is a unique pentagon, and u_1 is adjacent to the five vertices v_1, v_2, v_3, v_4, and u_4. □

4. The Case When $|A(\mathcal{L})| = 3$

Let us start the classification result with a lattice containing exactly three atoms. Note that the following theorem provides a class of multipartite graphs, which are embedded in the Klein bottle (refer to Example 1 for an illustration).

Theorem 3. *Let $\mathcal{L}$ be a lattice with $|A(\mathcal{L})| = 3$, and let $1 \leq i \neq j \neq k \leq 3$. Then $\tilde{\gamma}(\mathbb{AG}(\mathcal{L})) = 2$ if and only if one of the following conditions hold:*

(i). $|\bigcup_{n=1}^{3} U_n| = 9$; *there is U_i with $|U_i| = 6$ and $U_{jk} = \emptyset$.*

(ii). $|\bigcup_{n=1}^{3} U_n| = 8$, *and one of the following cases is satisfied:*
  [a] *There is U_i with $|U_i| = 6$ and $|U_{jk}| = 1$.*

[b] *There exist U_i and U_j such that $|U_i| \in \{5,4\}$ and $|U_j| = 2$ with $U_{jk} = \emptyset$.*
[c] *There exist U_i and U_j such that $|U_i| = 4$ and $|U_j| = 3$ with $U_{ik} = U_{jk} = \emptyset$.*
[d] *There exist U_i and U_j such that $|U_i| = |U_j| = 3$ with $U_{ij} = U_{ik} = U_{jk} = \emptyset$.*

(iii). $|\bigcup_{n=1}^{3} U_n| = 7$, and one of the following cases is satisfied:
[a] *There is U_i with $|U_i| \in \{5,4\}$ and $|U_{jk}| = 1$.*
[b] *There exist U_i and U_j such that $|U_i| = |U_j| = 3$ with either $|U_{ik}| \in \{1,2\}$ and $U_{jk} = \emptyset$ or $U_{ik} = \emptyset$ and $|U_{jk}| \in \{1,2\}$.*
[c] *There exist U_i and U_j such that $|U_i| = 3$, $|U_j| = 2$ with $|U_{jk}| \in \{1,2\}$. Further, if $|U_{jk}| = 1$, then either $U_{ij} = \emptyset$ or $U_{ik} = \emptyset$ and, if $|U_{jk}| = 2$, then $U_{ij} = U_{ik} = \emptyset$.*

(iv). $|\bigcup_{n=1}^{3} U_n| = 6$, and one of the following cases is satisfied:
[a] *There is U_i with $|U_i| = 4$ and $|U_{jk}| = 2$.*
[b] *There is U_i with $|U_i| = 3$ and $|U_{jk}| \in \{2,3\}$.*

(v). $|\bigcup_{n=1}^{3} U_n| = 5$; there is U_i with $|U_i| = 3$ and $|U_{jk}| \in \{3,4\}$.

Proof. Assume that $\tilde{\gamma}(\mathbb{AG}(\mathcal{L})) = 2$. First of all, if $|\bigcup_{n=1}^{3} U_n| \leq 4$, then $\mathbb{AG}(\mathcal{L})$ is planar (see [19]). Suppose $|\bigcup_{n=1}^{3} U_n| \geq 10$. If $|U_2| \geq 2$, then by Theorem 1 we have $\tilde{\gamma}(\mathbb{AG}(\mathcal{L})) \geq \lceil \frac{(|U_1|-2)(|U_2|+|U_3|-2)}{2} \rceil \geq 3$, which is a contradiction. Suppose $|U_2| = 1$. Then $|U_3| = 1$. Note that every vertex in U_{12}, U_{13}, and U_{23} is adjacent to all of the vertices of U_3, U_2, and U_1, respectively. So, if $U_{23} = \emptyset$, then clearly $\mathbb{AG}(\mathcal{L})$ is planar. If not, the vertices in U_1 are adjacent to all of the vertices of $U_2 \cup U_3 \cup U_{23}$. Since $|U_1| \geq 8$, $K_{8,3}$ is a subgraph of $\mathbb{AG}(\mathcal{L})$ that has a crosscap of more than three, refer to Proposition 1a. Thus, $5 \leq |\bigcup_{n=1}^{3} U_n| \leq 9$.

Case 1 Let $|\bigcup_{n=1}^{3} U_n| = 9$. Then, clearly, $|U_1| \leq 7$. If $|U_1| = 7$, then a slight modification to the discussion made in the above paragraph would show that $\mathbb{AG}(\mathcal{L})$ is planar whenever $U_{23} = \emptyset$ and the graph $\mathbb{AG}(\mathcal{L})$ contains $K_{7,3}$ as a subgraph when $U_{23} \neq \emptyset$. If $|U_1| = 6$, then $|U_2| = 2$ and $|U_3| = 1$. Now, if $U_{23} \neq \emptyset$, then $\mathbb{AG}(\mathcal{L})$ contains $K_{6,4}$ as a subgraph, which is a contradiction. So, $U_{23} = \emptyset$. Here, all of the vertices in U_{12} are adjacent to a single vertex of U_3, and, therefore, the vertices in U_{12} do not affect the crosscap. In Figure 4a, we provide the canonical representation of the embedding of the resulting graph in N_2 so that, in this case, $\tilde{\gamma}(\mathbb{AG}(\mathcal{L})) = 2$. Next, if $|U_1| = 5$ or 4, then $|U_2| + |U_3| \geq 4$, and so, by Theorem 1a, we obtain $\tilde{\gamma}(\mathbb{AG}(\mathcal{L})) \geq 3$. Thus, $|U_1| = 3$, and, therefore, $|U_2| = |U_3| = 3$. Here, $K_{3,3,3}$ is a subgraph of $\mathbb{AG}(\mathcal{L})$, and, therefore, according to Proposition 1c, we have $\tilde{\gamma}(\mathbb{AG}(\mathcal{L})) \geq 3$.

Case 2 Let $|\bigcup_{n=1}^{3} U_n| = 8$.

If $|U_1| = 6$, then $|U_2| = |U_3| = 1$. Clearly, by [19], $\mathbb{AG}(\mathcal{L})$ is planar in the case that U_{23} is empty. If $|U_{23}| \geq 2$, then the partite sets $X = U_1$ and $Y = U_2 \cup U_3 \cup U_{23}$ form $K_{6,4}$ as a subgraph in $\mathbb{AG}(\mathcal{L})$, which is a contradiction. Therefore, $|U_{23}| = 1$. In this case, the vertices in $U_{13} \cup U_{12}$ are all end vertices, and, therefore, it does not affect the crosscap. Thus, the resulting graph is $K_{6,3} \cup \{(I_2, I_3)\}$, which is a subgraph of a graph given in Figure 2a, and, therefore, $\tilde{\gamma}(\mathbb{AG}(\mathcal{L})) = 2$.

Suppose $|U_1| \in \{5,4\}$. Then, according to Theorem 1a, we have $\tilde{\gamma}(\mathbb{AG}(\mathcal{L})) \geq 2$. If $U_{23} \neq \emptyset$, then the sets $X = U_1$ and $Y = U_2 \cup U_3 \cup U_{23}$ form $K_{5,4}$ as a subgraph of $\mathbb{AG}(\mathcal{L})$, and so $\tilde{\gamma}(\mathbb{AG}(\mathcal{L})) \geq 3$. Therefore, $U_{23} = \emptyset$. Let $|U_2| = 2$, $|U_{12}| \geq 0$, and $|U_{13}| \geq 0$. For the embedding of $\mathbb{AG}(\mathcal{L})$ in N_2, in the case of $|U_1| = 5$, we can obtain help from Figure 4a because the number of vertices and edges of $\mathbb{AG}(\mathcal{L})$ is less than that of in Figure 4a. Further, Figure 4b provides an N_2-embedding of $\mathbb{AG}(\mathcal{L})$ in the case of $|U_1| = 4$. Here, notice that the open neighborhood of each vertex in U_{13} is $\{I_2, I_2'\}$, and, in Figure 4a,b, there is a face in an N_2-embedding of $\mathbb{AG}(\mathcal{L})$ that contains both I_2 and I_2' so that every vertex of U_{13} can be embedded in N_2 no matter what its cardinality may be. Let $|U_2| = 3$. This implies that $|U_1| = 4$. If $U_{13} = \emptyset$ (recall that $U_{23} = \emptyset$), then $\mathbb{AG}(\mathcal{L})$ is a subgraph of the graph H_1 in Figure 1, and, therefore, according to Lemma 2, $\tilde{\gamma}(\mathbb{AG}(\mathcal{L})) = 2$. If not, consider that the subgraph $\mathbb{AG}(\mathcal{L}) - \{(I_3, I_1), (I_3, I_1'), (I_3, I_1''), (I_3, I_1''')\}$ contains $K_{3,6}$. By Euler's formula, any embedding of $K_{3,6}$ in N_2 has nine faces. Further, by solving the equations

$2|E| = 4f_4 + 6f_6$ and $|F| = f_4 + f_6$, we have all the faces as rectangular faces in any N_2-embedding of $K_{3,6}$. Now we try to recover the embedding of $\mathbb{AG}(\mathcal{L})$ by inserting all edges (I_3, I_1), (I_3, I'_1), (I_3, I''_1), (I_3, I'''_1) into the embedding of $K_{3,6}$. Since $deg_{K_{3,6}}(I_3) = 3$, the vertex I_3 is in the boundary of three rectangular faces of any N_2-embedding of $K_{3,6}$. In addition, note that, at the maximum, each rectangular face can adopt one edge incident with I_3. So, we cannot insert all four edges of I_3 into N_2 without crossing, which is a contradiction. Thus, $\tilde{\gamma}(\mathbb{AG}(\mathcal{L})) \geq 3$.

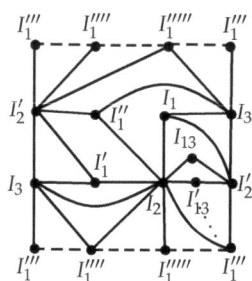 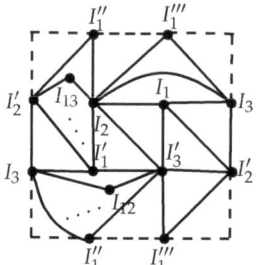

(a). $|\bigcup_{n=1}^3 U_n| = 9, |U_1| = 6$ and $U_{23} = \emptyset$ (b). $|\bigcup_{n=1}^3 U_n| = 8, |U_1| = 4, |U_2| = 2$ and $U_{23} = \emptyset$

Figure 4. N_2-embedding of $\mathbb{AG}(\mathcal{L})$.

Suppose $|U_1| = 3$. If $U_{ij} = \emptyset$ for all $1 \leq i < j \leq 3$, then, by Proposition 1c, we have $\tilde{\gamma}(\mathbb{AG}(\mathcal{L})) = 2$. Next, our claim is that $U_{ij} = \emptyset$ for all $1 \leq i < j \leq 3$.

Assume that $U_{12} \neq \emptyset$. Then the minor subgraph is

$$\mathbb{AG}(\mathcal{L}) - \{(I_1, I'_3), (I'_1, I'_3), (I''_1, I'_3), (I_2, [I_3, I_{12}]), (I'_2, [I_3, I_{12}]), (I''_2, [I_3, I_{12}])\} \cong K_{4,4}$$

with the partite sets $X = U_2 \cup \{[I_3, I_{12}]\}$ and $Y = U_1 \cup \{I'_3\}$. By Euler's formula, any N_2-embedding of $K_{4,4}$ has eight rectangular faces. Next, we attempt to obtain an N_2-embedding of $\mathbb{AG}(\mathcal{L})$ from any N_2-embedding of $K_{4,4}$. For this, we try to embed the six omitted edges of $\mathbb{AG}(\mathcal{L})$ into an arbitrary N_2-embedding of $K_{4,4}$. First, to embed the three edges $(I_1, I'_3), (I'_1, I'_3)$, and (I''_1, I'_3), three rectangular faces are required, denoted as F_1, F_2, and F_3, all of which contains I'_3 (refer to Figure 5a). Since $deg_{K_{4,4}}(I'_3) = 4$, exactly one more face should have I'_3; it is denoted as F_4. Intentionally, we label the diagonals of F_4 as the vertices I_2 and $[I_3, I_{12}]$ because F_4 can adopt one diagonal edge that can be used to embed the fourth edge $(I_2, [I_3, I_{12}])$. Finally, to embed the rest of the two edges $(I'_2, [I_3, I_{12}])$ and $(I''_2, [I_3, I_{12}])$, two distinct faces are required, denoted by F_5 and F_6, which should have the vertex $[I_3, I_{12}]$. Note that, in any N_k-embedding, every edge of a graph is in exactly two faces. Since the edge $(I_1, [I_3, I_{12}])$ is in F_2 and the edge $(I'_1, [I_3, I_{12}])$ is in F_4, the common edge between F_5 and F_6 must be $(I''_1, [I_3, I_{12}])$. Now, the choice for the unlabelled vertex of F_5 and F_6 is either I_1 or I'_1. Without a loss of generality, we label I_1 for F_5 and I'_1 for F_6 (refer to Figure 5b). Since any N_2-embedding of $K_{4,4}$ has eight faces, there are two more faces, lets say F_7 and F_8, that have to be formed using all of the remaining vertices and edges of $K_{4,4}$. Notice that, in any N_2-embedding of $K_{4,4}$, each vertex is present in exactly four faces, and each edge is present in exactly two faces. Since the vertices $I_2 \in X$ and $I'_1 \in Y$ are used twice in the faces $F_1, \ldots, F_6$, the faces F_7 and F_8 must share the edge (I_2, I'_1) (refer to Figure 5c). Now, the choices for the third and fourth vertices of F_7 and F_8 are $I'_2, I''_2 \in X$ and $I_1, I''_1 \in Y$, respectively. Clearly, we have to select distinct vertices for F_7 and F_8, in which one is from $\{I'_2, I''_2\}$ and the other is from $\{I_1, I''_1\}$. A contradiction to this fact is that the edges (I'_2, I_1) and (I''_2, I''_1) are used twice in the faces $F_1, \ldots, F_6$.

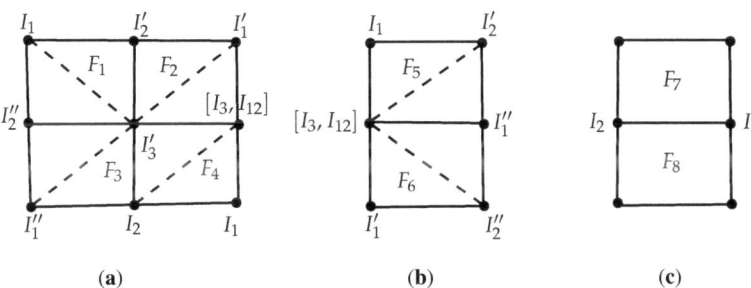

Figure 5. Representation of faces of N_2-embedding of $K_{4,4}$.

Assume that $U_{i3} \neq \emptyset$ for some $i \in \{1,2\}$. Then, the subgraph $\mathbb{AG}(\mathcal{L}) - \{I_{i3}, (I_i, I_3), (I'_i, I_3), (I''_i, I_3)\}$ contains $K_{4,4} - e$ with the partite sets $X = U_i \cup \{I_3\}$ and $Y = U_{i'} \cup \{I'_3\}$ where $i' \in \{1,2\} \setminus \{i\}$ and $e = (I_3, I'_3)$. By Proposition 2, any N_2-embedding of $K_{4,4} - e$ has one hexagonal and six rectangular faces. Note that the hexagonal face should have either I_3 or I'_3, and the vertex I_{i3} is adjacent to $\{I_{i'}, I'_{i'}, I''_{i'}\} \subset Y$. So, I_{i3} with its edges must be inserted into the hexagonal face, which implies that I_3 is in the hexagonal face. Since $\deg_{K_{4,4}-e}(I_3) = 3$, exactly two rectangular faces contain I_3 in which it is not possible to embed all of the three edges $(I_i, I_3), (I'_i, I_3)$, and (I''_i, I_3), which is a contradiction. Thus, $U_{ij} = \emptyset$ for all $i, j \in \{1, 2, 3\}$.

Case 3 Let $|\bigcup_{n=1}^{3} U_n| = 7$.

Suppose $|U_1| \in \{5, 4\}$. Clearly, $\mathbb{AG}(\mathcal{L})$ is either planar or projective when $U_{23} = \emptyset$ (refer to [19,20]), and $K_{5,4}$ is a subgraph of the contraction of $\mathbb{AG}(\mathcal{L})$ when $|U_{23}| \geq 2$. Therefore, $|U_{23}|$ will be one. Then, $\mathbb{AG}(\mathcal{L})$ is a subgraph of the graph given in Figure 4a when $|U_1| = 5$, and $\mathbb{AG}(\mathcal{L})$ is a subgraph of the graph given in Figure 4b when $|U_1| = 4$ so that $\tilde{\gamma}(\mathbb{AG}(\mathcal{L})) = 2$.

Assume that $|U_1| = |U_2| = 3$. Then, $\mathbb{AG}(\mathcal{L})$ is projective when $U_{i3} = \emptyset$ for all $i = 1, 2$, and the graph $\mathbb{AG}(\mathcal{L})$ contains $K_{3,7}$ as a subgraph when $|U_{i3}| \geq 3$ for some $i = 1, 2$. Suppose $U_{13} \neq \emptyset$ and $U_{23} \neq \emptyset$. Now, the graph $\mathbb{AG}(\mathcal{L}) - \{I_3\}$ is isomorphic to $K_{4,4} - \{e\}$ with the bipartite sets $\{I_1, I'_1, I''_1, I_{13}\}$ and $\{I_2, I'_2, I''_2, I_{23}\}$ where $e = (I_{13}, I_{23})$. Note that $\tilde{\gamma}(K_{4,4} - \{e\}) = 2$, and there are seven faces in any N_2-embedding of $K_{4,4} - \{e\}$, of which six are rectangular, and one is hexagonal. Since $\tilde{\gamma}(K_{4,4}) = 2$ and every face in any N_2-embedding of $K_{4,4}$ is rectangular, the hexagonal face of any N_2-embedding of $K_{4,4} - \{e\}$ must have the vertices I_{13} and I_{23}. Now, we try to recover an N_2-embedding of $\mathbb{AG}(\mathcal{L})$ from an N_2-embedding of $K_{4,4} - \{e\}$ by inserting I_3 with its edges. Here, I_3 is adjacent to the six vertices $I_1, I'_1, I''_1, I_2, I'_2$, and I''_2. However, the hexagonal face of $K_{4,4} - \{e\}$ does not contain two of them so that $\tilde{\gamma}(\mathbb{AG}(\mathcal{L})) \geq 3$. Therefore, either $U_{13} = \emptyset$ or $U_{23} = \emptyset$. Now, with the help of Figure 6, we have $\tilde{\gamma}(\mathbb{AG}(\mathcal{L})) = 2$ when $1 \leq |U_{i3}| \leq 2$ for a unique $i \in \{1, 2\}$.

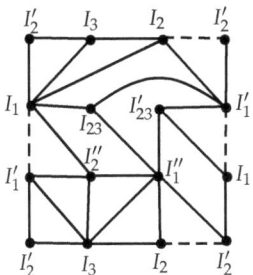

Figure 6. $|\bigcup_{n=1}^{3} U_n| = 7$ with $|U_1| = |U_2| = 3, U_{13} = \emptyset$ and $|U_{23}| = 2$.

Assume that $|U_1| = 3$ and $|U_2| = 2$. If $|U_{23}| \geq 3$, then $\mathbb{AG}(\mathcal{L})$ contains $K_{3,7}$ as a subgraph, and, if $U_{23} = \emptyset$, then, by Theorem 2.4iii [20], $\mathbb{AG}(\mathcal{L})$ is projective. Suppose $|U_{23}| = 2$. If $U_{1j} \neq \emptyset$ for $j = 2$ or 3, then consider a subgraph $G_1 = \mathbb{AG}(\mathcal{L}) - \{I_{1j}, I'_{23}, e_1, e_2, e_3, e_4\}$ where $e_1 = (I_2, I_3), e_2 = (I_2, I'_3), e_3 = (I'_2, I_3)$, and $e_4 = (I'_2, I'_3)$. Clearly, G_1 contains $K_{3,5}$ with the partite sets $X = \{I_1, I'_1, I''_1\}$ and $Y = \{I_2, I'_2, I_3, I'_3, I_{23}\}$. Note that any N_2-embedding of $K_{3,5}$ has one hexagonal and six rectangular faces. Now, we try to recover an N_2-embedding of $\mathbb{AG}(\mathcal{L})$ from any N_2-embedding of $K_{3,5}$. Since I'_{23} is adjacent to all three vertices of X, the embedding of I'_{23} requires the hexagonal face of $K_{3,5}$ to have I_1, I'_1, and I''_1. Notice that each rectangular face may adopt at most one edge into it. So, to insert e_fs, for $1 \leq f \leq 4$, into any N_2-embedding of $K_{3,5}$, four rectangular faces with diagonals as the end vertices of each e_f are required. At last, to insert I_{1j}, a rectangular face with the diagonals $I_{j'}$ and $I''_{j'}$ for $j' \in \{2,3\} \setminus \{j\}$ is required. Therefore, it requires one hexagonal face with five rectangular faces containing the vertices I_2, I'_2, I_3, and I'_3 in at least three different faces. Since the degree of I_2, I'_2, I_3, and I'_3 in $K_{3,5}$ is three, all four vertices are placed in exactly three faces of any N_2-embedding of $K_{3,5}$. So, the sixth rectangular face of $K_{3,5}$ could not be formed using the only left-out vertex in X (namely I_{23}), which is a contradiction. Thus, $U_{12} = U_{13} = \emptyset$, and an N_2-embedding of $\mathbb{AG}(\mathcal{L})$ for this case is provided in Figure 7a.

Suppose $|U_{23}| = 1$. If $U_{1j} \neq \emptyset$ for $j = 2$ and 3, then the minor subgraph is

$$G_2 = \mathbb{AG}(\mathcal{L}) - \{I_{13}, e_1, e_2, e_3, e_4, e_5\} \cong K_{4,4} - \{e\}, \tag{1}$$

with the bipartite sets $\{I_1, I'_1, I''_1, I_3\}$ and $\{I_2, I'_2, [I'_3, I_{12}], I_{23}\}$ where $e_1 = (I_1, I_3), e_2 = (I'_1, I_3)$, $e_3 = (I''_1, I_3), e_4 = (I_2, [I'_3, I_{12}]), e_5 = (I'_2, [I'_3, I_{12}])$, and $e = (I_3, I_{23})$. Note that any N_2-embedding of $K_{4,4} - \{e\}$ has six rectangular faces and a hexagonal face, and the hexagonal face must have the vertices I_3 and I_{23}. Let us denote the six rectangular faces by $F_1, \ldots, F_6$ and the hexagonal face by F_7. Now, let us try to recover an N_2-embedding of $\mathbb{AG}(\mathcal{L})$ by inserting the vertex I_{13} and the edges e_i for all $i = 1, \ldots, 5$. If we embed the edge e_4, the edge e_5, or the vertex I_{13} together with its edges into F_7, then we cannot insert the edges e_1, e_2, or e_3 into F_7. Since $deg_{G_2}(I_3) = 3$, the vertex I_3 is in exactly three faces of an N_2-embedding of G_2. So, in such cases, the edges e_1, e_2 and e_3 cannot be embedded in two rectangular faces which contains I_3. Therefore we have to add at least one of the edges e_1, e_2 or e_3 into F_7. For the best possibility, say e_1 and e_2 are embedded in F_7. Then, e_3 has to be embedded into one of the two rectangular faces that contains I_3, for example, F_1. Notice that there are two rectangular faces, say F_2 and F_3, that contain I_{23}, in which one should not embed any of e_4, e_5, or I_{13} with its edges. So, the edges e_4 and e_5 have to be embedded into different rectangular faces, say F_4 and F_5, respectively. Therefore, after embedding the edges from e_1 to e_5 nicely, we are left with the single rectangular face F_6 that could not be formed using the diagonal vertices I_2 and I'_2. Thus, $\tilde{\gamma}(\mathbb{AG}(\mathcal{L})) \geq 3$. Hence, either $U_{12} = \emptyset$ or $U_{13} = \emptyset$. In this case, with the help of Figure 7b, we obtain $\tilde{\gamma}(\mathbb{AG}(\mathcal{L})) = 2$.

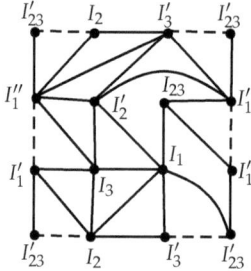 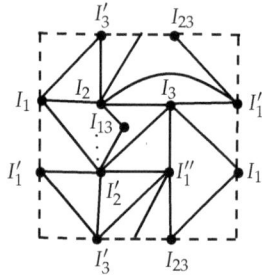

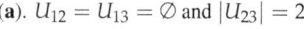

(**a**). $U_{12} = U_{13} = \emptyset$ and $|U_{23}| = 2$ (**b**). $U_{12} = \emptyset, |U_{13}| \geq 0$ and $|U_{23}| = 1$

Figure 7. $|\bigcup_{n=1}^{3} U_n| = 7$ with $|U_1| = 3$ and $|U_2| = 2$.

Case 4 Let $|\bigcup_{n=1}^{3} U_n| = 6$. Suppose $|U_1| = 4$. If $|U_{23}| \geq 3$, then $K_{4,5}$ is contained in $\mathbb{AG}(\mathcal{L})$, and if $|U_{23}| = 1$, then $\mathbb{AG}(\mathcal{L})$ is projective. Therefore $|U_{23}| = 2$. Clearly, $\mathbb{AG}(\mathcal{L})$(except for the end vertices) is a subgraph of the graph H_1 given in Figure 1a, and so Lemma 2 implies $\tilde{\gamma}(\mathbb{AG}(\mathcal{L})) = 2$.

Suppose $|U_1| = 3$. Then $\mathbb{AG}(\mathcal{L})$ contains $K_{3,7}$ when $|U_{23}| \geq 4$, and $\mathbb{AG}(\mathcal{L})$ is projective when $|U_{23}| \leq 1$. Thus, $2 \leq |U_{23}| \leq 3$. Then, $\mathbb{AG}(\mathcal{L}) - \{U_{13}\}$ is a subgraph of the graph H_2 (see Figure 2a), so that $\tilde{\gamma}(\mathbb{AG}(\mathcal{L}) - \{U_{13}\}) = 2$. Note that every vertex in U_{13} is adjacent to exactly two vertices of U_2 in $\mathbb{AG}(\mathcal{L})$. Therefore, replace the labels u_4 and u_5 with I_2 and I'_2, respectively, in the N_2-embedding of H_2 provided in Figure 2b, and then label all of the other vertices accordingly. Now, we can insert any number of vertices of U_{13} into a face that contains both I_2 and I'_2 so that $\tilde{\gamma}(\mathbb{AG}(\mathcal{L})) = 2$.

Moreover, if $|U_1| = 2$, then $\mathbb{AG}(\mathcal{L})$ is either planar or projective (refer to [19,20]).

Case 5 Let $|\bigcup_{n=1}^{3} U_n| = 5$. Then $\mathbb{AG}(\mathcal{L})$ is planar or projective when $|U_1| = 2$. This implies that $|U_1| = 3$. If $|U_{23}| \geq 5$, then $\mathbb{AG}(\mathcal{L})$ contains $K_{3,7}$ and, if $|U_{23}| \leq 2$, then $\mathbb{AG}(\mathcal{L})$ is projective. Thus, $|U_{23}| = 3$ or 4. Then, clearly, $\mathbb{AG}(\mathcal{L})$ is a subgraph of the graph H_1, as in Figure 2a, so that $\tilde{\gamma}(\mathbb{AG}(\mathcal{L})) = 2$. □

All of the results proved in this paper have a similar structure to that of those given in the statement of Theorem 3. To familiarize readers with the connection between the multipartite graph and the statement of Theorem 3, we illustrate two four-partite graphs, G and H, with $\tilde{\gamma}(G) = 2$ and $\tilde{\gamma}(H) \neq 2$, respectively, in the following example.

Example 1. Consider Case (iii)[c] in Theorem 3. Let $|U_1| = 3, |U_2| = 2, |U_3| = 2$, and $|U_{23}| = 1$. If $|U_{12}| = k \in \mathbb{Z}^+$ and $U_{13} = \emptyset$, then the corresponding four-partite graph G is a crosscap two, which is given in Figure 8a. Additionally, if $|U_{12}| = 1$ and $|U_{13}| = 1$, then the crosscap of the corresponding four-partite graph H, given in Figure 8b, is not equal to two. It is worth mentioning that the four-partite graph H in Figure 8b is minimal with respect to $\tilde{\gamma}(H) \neq 2$; that is, there exists an edge e in H such that $\tilde{\gamma}(H - e) = 2$. Further, the graph H may be realized as one of the forbidden subgraphs for a crosscap two surface.

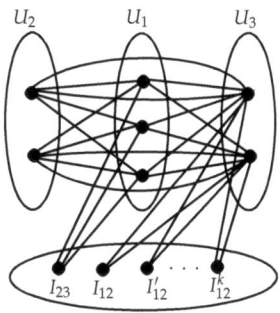 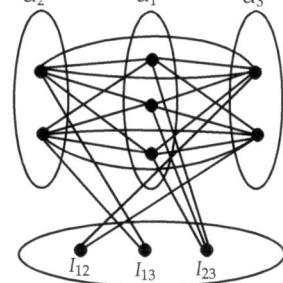

(**a**) A crosscap two 4-partite graph G (**b**) A minimal 4-partite graph H with crosscap $\neq 2$

Figure 8. Four-partite graphs.

By using the proof of Theorem 3, we establish the following points, which will be used in the subsequent results.

Remark 1. If a graph G is isomorphic to $K_{6,3} \cup (K_4 - e)$ or $K_{4,5} - e$ where e is an edge, then $\tilde{\gamma}(G) \geq 3$.

5. The Case When $|A(\mathcal{L})| = 4$

Next, we fix the number of atoms as four. As mentioned in the introduction, for $1 \leq i \neq j \leq 4$, we denote $U_{(ij)^c} = U_{k\ell}$ where $k, \ell \in \{1, 2, 3, 4\} \setminus \{i, j\}$, and the notation

$U_{(ij)^c}$ exists only when $U_{ij} \neq \emptyset$. Before going into the characterization of the crosscap two $\mathbb{AG}(\mathcal{L})$ with $|A(\mathcal{L})| = 4$, we provide modifications for Theorem 2.6 [20]. To be precise, the missing cases and the corresponding conditions for the projectiveness of $\mathbb{AG}(\mathcal{L})$ are given below.

(i) First of all, consider the missing case $|\bigcup_{n=1}^{4} U_n| = 4$. Then, $|U_i| = 1$ for all $1 \leq i \leq 4$. Clearly, $\mathbb{AG}(\mathcal{L})$ is planar whenever $\bigcup_{U_{ij} \neq \emptyset} U_{(ij)^c} = \emptyset$. Therefore, $\bigcup_{U_{ij} \neq \emptyset} U_{(ij)^c} \neq \emptyset$. If $|U_{ij} \cup U_{(ij)^c}| \geq 4$ with $U_{ij}, U_{(ij)^c} \neq \emptyset$, then the subgraph induced by the sets $X = U_i \cup U_j \cup U_{ij}$ and $Y = \bigcup_{k \neq i,j} U_k \cup U_{(ij)^c}$ contains $K_{4,4}$ or $K_{3,5}$ as a subgraph. This implies $\tilde{\gamma}(\mathbb{AG}(\mathcal{L})) \geq 2$. Therefore, $2 \leq |U_{ij} \cup U_{(ij)^c}| \leq 3$ if $U_{ij}, U_{(ij)^c} \neq \emptyset$ for $1 \leq i \neq j \leq 4$.

Suppose $|U_{ij} \cup U_{(ij)^c}| = 3$ for some $U_{ij}, U_{(ij)^c} \neq \emptyset$ with $1 \leq i \neq j \leq 4$. If $U_{k\ell}, U_{(k\ell)^c} \neq \emptyset$ for $k\ell \neq ij$, then the subgraph $\mathbb{AG}(\mathcal{L}) - \{U_{ij} \cup U_{(ij)^c}\}$ contains $K_{3,3}$ with the partite sets $X = U_k \cup U_\ell \cup U_{k\ell}$ and $Y = \bigcup_{m \neq k,\ell} U_m \cup U_{(k\ell)^c}$. Note that $\tilde{\gamma}(K_{3,3}) = 1$. Now, we try to embed all of the vertices of $U_{ij} \cup U_{(ij)^c}$ with their edges in any N_1-embedding of $K_{3,3}$. Since $|U_{ij} \cup U_{(ij)^c}| = 3$, either $|U_{ij}| = 2$ or $|U_{(ij)^c}| = 2$. Without a loss of generality, let $|U_{ij}| = 2$. Since the vertex $I_{(ij)^c} \in U_{(ij)^c}$ is adjacent to $I_{ij}, I'_{ij} \in U_{ij}$, all of the three vertices I_{ij}, I'_{ij}, and $I_{(ij)^c}$ must be embedded into a single face of the N_1-embedding of $K_{3,3}$, denoted as F_1. Now, draw the path $I_{ij} - I_{(ij)^c} - I'_{ij}$ into F_1 and then draw the edges $(I_{ij}, I_m), (I_{ij}, I_n), (I'_{ij}, I_m)$, and (I'_{ij}, I_n) where $m, n \notin \{i, j\}$. Now, the edges $(I_{(ij)^c}, I_i)$ and $(I_{(ij)^c}, I_j)$ cannot be embedded into F_1. Therefore, $\tilde{\gamma}(\mathbb{AG}(\mathcal{L})) \geq 2$. Thus, $\bigcup_{k\ell \neq ij, (ij)^c; U_{k\ell} \neq \emptyset} U_{(k\ell)^c} = \emptyset$.

Suppose $|U_{ij} \cup U_{(ij)^c}| = 2$ for all $U_{ij}, U_{(ij)^c} \neq \emptyset$ with $1 \leq i \neq j \leq 4$. Then, Figure 9 guarantees that $\tilde{\gamma}(\mathbb{AG}(\mathcal{L})) = 1$.

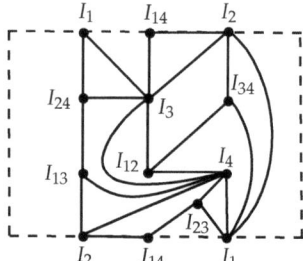

Figure 9. $|\bigcup_{n=1}^{4} U_n| = 4$ with $|U_{ij} \cup U_{(ij)^c}| \leq 2$ for all $U_{ij}, U_{(ij)^c} \neq \emptyset$.

(ii) Let $|\bigcup_{n=1}^{4} U_n| = 5$. Then, $|U_i| = 2$ for some $1 \leq i \leq 4$, and the condition for the projectiveness of $\mathbb{AG}(\mathcal{L})$ given in Theorem 2.6i [20] is that $|U_{jk}| = 1$ or 2, in which at most one of the U_{jk}s has exactly two elements for $1 \leq i \neq j \neq k \leq 4$. However, if $|U_{jk}| = 2$ with $U_{(jk)^c} \neq \emptyset$, then the sets $X = U_i \cup U_\ell \cup U_{(jk)^c}$ and $Y = U_j \cup U_k \cup U_{jk}$, where $\ell \notin \{i, j, k\}$, contain $K_{4,4}$ in $\mathbb{AG}(\mathcal{L})$ so that we obtain $\tilde{\gamma}(\mathbb{AG}(\mathcal{L})) \geq 2$. In fact, if $|U_{jk}| = 2$ for some $j, k \neq i$, then $\bigcup_{p,q \neq i; U_{pq} \neq \emptyset} U_{(pq)^c} = \emptyset$. Otherwise, the sets $X = U_j \cup U_k \cup U_{jk} \cup [I_{pq}, I_{(pq)^c}]$ and $Y = U_i \cup U_\ell$, where $\ell \notin \{i, j, k\}$, form $K_{5,3}$, so we can conclude that $\tilde{\gamma}(\mathbb{AG}(\mathcal{L})) \geq 2$. Further, if $|U_{jk}| \leq 1$ for all $j, k \neq i$, then $|\bigcup_{p,q \neq i; U_{pq} \neq \emptyset} U_{(pq)^c}| \leq 1$. For if $|U_{(pq)^c}| \geq 2$, then the sets $X = U_p \cup U_q \cup U_{pq}$ and $Y = U_i \cup U_r \cup U_{(pq)^c}$, where $r \notin \{i, p, q\}$, form $K_{3,5}$, and, if $|U_{(pq)^c}|, |U_{(p_1 q_1)^c}| = 1$ for some $1 \leq p_1 \neq q_1 \leq 4$ with $p_1 q_1 \neq pq$, then the sets $X = U_p \cup U_q \cup U_{pq} \cup \{[I_{p_1 q_1}, I_{(p_1 q_1)^c}]\}$ and $Y = U_i \cup U_r \cup U_{(pq)^c}$ form $K_{4,4} - \{e\}$ in $\mathbb{AG}(\mathcal{L})$ where $r \notin \{i, p, q\}$.

(iii) Let $|\bigcup_{n=1}^{4} U_n| = 6$. If there exists $|U_i| = 3$ for some $1 \leq i \leq 4$, then the statement of ([20] Theorem 2.6(ii)(a)) says that if $U_{jk\ell} = \emptyset$ for $1 \leq i \neq j \neq k \neq \ell \leq 4$, $|U_{jk}| \leq 1$, and at most one of the U_{jk}s has exactly one element, then $\mathbb{AG}(\mathcal{L})$ is projective. However, for instance, if $|U_{jk}| = 1$ with $U_{(jk)^c} = U_{i\ell} \neq \emptyset$, then the partite sets $X = U_i \cup U_\ell \cup U_{i\ell}$ and $Y = U_j \cup U_k \cup U_{jk}$ contain $K_{5,3}$ as a subgraph of $\mathbb{AG}(\mathcal{L})$ so that $\tilde{\gamma}(\mathbb{AG}(\mathcal{L})) \geq 2$. Therefore, the condition $U_{(jk)^c} = \emptyset$ has to be added to the statement of ([20] Theorem 2.6iia).

As a result of the above remarks (i), (ii), and (iii), we modify the statement of ([20] Theorem 2.6) as follows.

Theorem 4. *Let $\mathcal{L}$ be a lattice with $|A(\mathcal{L})| = 4$. Let $1 \leq i \neq j \neq k \neq \ell \leq 4$ and $1 \leq p \neq q \leq 4$. Then $\tilde{\gamma}(\mathbb{AG}(\mathcal{L})) = 1$ if and only if one of the following conditions hold:*

(i). *$|\bigcup_{n=1}^4 U_n| = 4$; there exist two non-empty sets U_{ij} and $U_{(ij)^c}$ such that $2 \leq |U_{ij} \cup U_{(ij)^c}| \leq 3$. Moreover, if $|U_{ij} \cup U_{(ij)^c}| = 3$, then $\bigcup_{pq \neq ij,(ij)^c; U_{pq} \neq \emptyset} U_{(pq)^c} = \emptyset$.*

(ii). *$|\bigcup_{n=1}^4 U_n| = 5$; there is U_i with $|U_i| = 2$, $|\bigcup_{p,q \neq i} U_{pq}| \leq 4$ in which at most one of the U_{pq}s has a maximum of two elements, and $|\bigcup_{U_{pq} \neq \emptyset} U_{(pq)^c}| \leq 1$. Moreover, if $|U_{pq}| = 2$, then $\bigcup_{U_{pq} \neq \emptyset} U_{(pq)^c} = \emptyset$, and, if $\bigcup_{p,q \neq i} U_{pq} = \emptyset$, then $U_{jk\ell} \neq \emptyset$.*

(iii). *$|\bigcup_{n=1}^4 U_n| = 6$, and one of the following is satisfied:*

  [a] *There is U_i with $|U_i| = 3$. If $|U_{jk\ell}| = 1$, then $U_{jk} = U_{j\ell} = U_{k\ell} = \emptyset$ and if $U_{jk\ell} = \emptyset$, then $|U_{jk} \cup U_{j\ell} \cup U_{k\ell}| \leq 1$. Moreover, $U_{(pq)^c} = \emptyset$ whenever $U_{pq} \neq \emptyset$.*

  [b] *There exist U_i and U_j such that $|U_i| = |U_j| = 2$ with $|U_{k\ell}| \leq 1$. Additionally, $U_{(pq)^c} = \emptyset$ whenever $U_{pq} \neq \emptyset$. Moreover, if $|U_{ik}|, |U_{i\ell}| \leq 1$ or $|U_{jk}|, |U_{j\ell}| \leq 1$, then $|U_{k\ell}| \leq 1$. Furthermore, if $|U_{ik}| = |U_{jk}| = 1$ or $|U_{i\ell}| = |U_{j\ell}| = 1$, then $U_{k\ell} = \emptyset$.*

(iv). *$|\bigcup_{n=1}^4 U_n| = 7$ and one of the following is satisfied:*

  [a] *There is U_i with $|U_i| = 4$ and $U_{jk\ell} = U_{jk} = \emptyset$.*

  [b] *There exist U_i and U_j such that $|U_i| = 3$ and $|U_j| = 2$. Additionally, $U_{k\ell} = \emptyset$, and $U_{jk\ell} = \emptyset$ whenever $U_{ik} = U_{i\ell} = U_{jk} = U_{j\ell} = \emptyset$.*

We are now in the position to state and prove the second result which classifies all lattices $\mathcal{L}$ with four atoms whose $\mathbb{AG}(\mathcal{L})$ has a crosscap two.

Theorem 5. *Let $\mathcal{L}$ be a lattice with $|A(\mathcal{L})| = 4$. Let $1 \leq i \neq j \neq k \neq \ell \leq 4$ and $1 \leq p, q, r, s, t \leq 4$. Then $\tilde{\gamma}(\mathbb{AG}(\mathcal{L})) = 2$ if and only if one of the following conditions hold:*

(i). *$|\bigcup_{n=1}^4 U_n| = 9$; there is U_i with $|U_i| = 6$ and $U_{jk} = U_{j\ell} = U_{k\ell} = U_{jk\ell} = \emptyset$.*

(ii). *$|\bigcup_{n=1}^4 U_n| = 8$, and one of the following cases is satisfied:*

  [a] *There is U_i with $|U_i| = 5$ and $U_{jk} = U_{j\ell} = U_{k\ell} = U_{jk\ell} = \emptyset$.*

  [b] *There exist U_i and U_j such that $|U_i| = 4$, $|U_j| = 2$ and $\bigcup_{pq \neq ij} U_{pq} = U_{jkl} = \emptyset$.*

  [c] *There exist U_i and U_j such that $|U_i| = |U_j| = 3$ and $\bigcup_{pq \neq ij} U_{pq} = U_{ik\ell} = U_{jk\ell} = \emptyset$.*

  [d] *There exist U_i, U_j, and U_k such that $|U_i| = 3, |U_j| = |U_k| = 2$, and $\bigcup U_{pq} = \bigcup_{pqr \neq ijk} U_{pqr} = \emptyset$ for $1 \leq p \neq q \neq r \leq 4$.*

(iii). *$|\bigcup_{n=1}^4 U_n| = 7$, and one of the following cases is satisfied:*

  [a] *There is U_i with $|U_i| = 4$ and $|\bigcup_{p,q \neq i} U_{pq} \cup U_{jk\ell}| = 1$. Moreover, $U_{(pq)^c} = \emptyset$ whenever $|U_{pq}| = 1$ for $p, q \neq i$.*

  [b] *There exist U_i and U_j such that $|U_i| = 3, |U_j| = 2$ and $|\bigcup_{p,q \neq i} U_{pq} \cup U_{jk\ell}| \leq 1$. Moreover, if $|\bigcup_{p,q \neq i} U_{pq} \cup U_{jk\ell}| = 1$, then $U_{(pq)^c} = \emptyset$ and $U_{ik} = U_{i\ell} = U_{ik\ell} = \emptyset$, and if $\bigcup_{p,q \neq i} U_{pq} \cup U_{jk\ell} = \emptyset$, then $|U_{ik} \cup U_{i\ell}| \in \{1, 2\}$.*

  [c] *There exist U_i, U_j, and U_k such that $|U_i| = |U_j| = |U_k| = 2$ with $|\bigcup U_{pq}| \leq 2$, in which at most one of the $U_{p\ell}$s has exactly one element, and, also, at most two distinct sets'*

U_{rst}s are non-empty for all $rst \neq ijk$. Moreover, if $|U_{pq}| = 2$ or $|U_{p\ell}| = 1$ for $p, q \neq \ell$, then at most one of the U_{rst}s is non-empty.

(iv). $|\bigcup_{n=1}^{4} U_n| = 6$, and one of the following cases is satisfied:

[a] There is U_i with $|U_i| = 3$, $|\bigcup_{p,q \neq i} U_{pq} \cup U_{jk\ell}| \in \{2,3\}$ in which $|U_{pq}| \leq 2$, and $|\bigcup_{U_{pq} \neq \emptyset} U_{(pq)^c}| \leq 1$. Moreover, if $|U_{pq}| \in \{1,2\}$ with $|U_{jk\ell}| = 2$, then $\bigcup_{U_{pq} \neq \emptyset} U_{(pq)^c} = \emptyset$.

[b] There exist U_i and U_j such that $|U_i| = |U_j| = 2$ and $|U_{ij} \cup U_{k\ell}| \leq 3$ with $|U_{ij}|, |U_{k\ell}| \leq 2$. Additionally, if $|U_{ij}| = 2$, then $|U_{k\ell}| \leq 1$ and $\bigcup_{pq \neq ij, k\ell} U_{pq} = U_{ik\ell} = U_{jk\ell} = \emptyset$, and, if $|U_{ij}| = 1$, then $|U_{k\ell}| \leq 1$ and $|\bigcup_{pq \neq ij, k\ell} U_{pq}| \leq 1$. Moreover, in the case of $U_{ij} = \emptyset$, one of the following hold:

[b1] If $|U_{k\ell}| = 2$, then $|\bigcup_{pq \neq ij, k\ell} U_{pq}| \leq 2$ in which $|U_{pq}| \leq 1$ and $\bigcup_{U_{pq} \neq \emptyset} U_{(pq)^c} = \emptyset$.

[b2] If $|U_{k\ell}| = 1$, then $|U_{rs}| \leq 3$ with $U_{(rs)^c} = \emptyset$ where $|U_{rs}| = \max_{pq \neq ij, k\ell} |U_{pq}|$ and $|\bigcup_{mn \neq ij, k\ell, rs, (rs)^c} U_{mn}| \leq 1$.

[b3] If $U_{k\ell} = \emptyset$, then $|\bigcup_{pq \neq ij, k\ell} U_{pq}| \leq 4$ in which at most three U_{pq}s are non-empty.

Furthermore, if $|U_{pq}| \in \{2,3\}$, then $U_{(pq)^c} = \emptyset$.

(v). $|\bigcup_{n=1}^{4} U_n| = 5$; there exists U_i such that $|U_i| = 2$ and $1 \leq |\bigcup_{p,q \neq i} U_{pq}| \leq 6$ in which $|U_{pq}| \leq 4$. Moreover,

[a] If $|U_{pq}| = 4$, then $U_{(pq)^c} = \emptyset$, $|\bigcup_{r,s \neq i; rs \neq pq} U_{rs}| \leq 1$, and $\bigcup_{U_{rs} \neq \emptyset} U_{(rs)^c} = \emptyset$.

[b] If $|U_{pq}| = 3$, then $U_{(pq)^c} = \emptyset$, $|\bigcup_{r,s \neq i; rs \neq pq} U_{rs}| \leq 2$ and $U_{(rs)^c} = \emptyset$ whenever $|U_{rs}| = 2$.

[c] In the case of $|U_{pq}| = 2$, one of the following holds

[c1] If $|\bigcup_{r,s \neq i; rs \neq pq} U_{rs}| = 4$, then $\bigcup_{U_{rs} \neq \emptyset} U_{(rs)^c} = \emptyset$.

[c2] If $|\bigcup_{r,s \neq i; rs \neq pq} U_{rs}| \in \{2,3\}$, then $|\bigcup_{U_{rs} \neq \emptyset} U_{(rs)^c}| \leq 1$. In addition, $|\bigcup_{U_{rs} \neq \emptyset} U_{(rs)^c}| = 1$ whenever $|\bigcup_{r,s \neq i; rs \neq pq} U_{rs}| = 2$ in which exactly two U_{rs}s are non-empty.

[c3] If $|\bigcup_{r,s \neq i; rs \neq pq} U_{rs}| \leq 1$, then either $U_{(pq)^c} = \emptyset$ with $1 \leq |\bigcup_{U_{rs} \neq \emptyset} U_{(rs)^c}| \leq 2$ or $U_{(rs)^c} = \emptyset$ with $|U_{(pq)^c}| \leq 1$.

[d] If $|U_{pq}| \leq 1$ for all $1 \leq p \neq q \neq i \leq 4$, then $2 \leq |\bigcup_{U_{pq} \neq \emptyset} U_{(pq)^c}| \leq 3$ in which at most two distinct $U_{(pq)^c}$s are non-empty.

(vi). $|\bigcup_{n=1}^{4} U_n| = 4$; there exist two non-empty sets U_{ij} and $U_{(ij)^c}$ such that $2 \leq |U_{ij} \cup U_{(ij)^c}| \leq 5$, and one of the following cases is satisfied:

[a] If $|U_{ij} \cup U_{(ij)^c}| = 5$, then either $|U_{ij}| = 4$ or $|U_{(ij)^c}| = 4$. Further, $\bigcup_{pq \neq ij, (ij)^c; U_{pq} \neq \emptyset} U_{(pq)^c} = \emptyset$.

[b] If $|U_{ij} \cup U_{(ij)^c}| = 4$, then $|U_{pq} \cup U_{(pq)^c}| = 2$ whenever $U_{pq}, U_{(pq)^c} \neq \emptyset$ for $pq \neq ij$. Further, if $|U_{ij}| = |U_{(ij)^c}| = 2$, then at most one pair of $U_{pq}, U_{(pq)^c}$ is nonempty for all $pq \neq ij$.

[c] If $|U_{ij} \cup U_{(ij)^c}| = 3$, then $|U_{pq} \cup U_{(pq)^c}| \in \{2,3\}$ whenever $U_{pq}, U_{(pq)^c} \neq \emptyset$ for $pq \neq ij$. Further, if $U_{(rs)^c} \neq \emptyset$ for $1 \leq r \neq s \leq 4$ and $rs \neq pq, ij$, then $|U_{rs} \cup U_{(rs)^c}| \in \{2,3\}$ with $|(U_{pq} \cup U_{(pq)^c}) \cup (U_{rs} \cup U_{(rs)^c})| \in \{4,5\}$.

Proof. Assume that $\tilde{\gamma}(\mathbb{AG}(\mathcal{L})) = 2$. Then, by Theorem 1b, we have $|\bigcup_{n=1}^4 U_n| \leq 9$. So, $4 \leq |\bigcup_{n=1}^4 U_n| \leq 9$.

Case 1 Let $|\bigcup_{n=1}^4 U_n| = 9$. Then, by Theorem 1b, $\tilde{\gamma}(\mathbb{AG}(\mathcal{L})) = 2$ implies $|U_1| = 6$. If $U_{ij} \neq \emptyset$ or $U_{ijk} \neq \emptyset$ for some $i \neq 1$, then the sets $X = U_1$ and $Y = V(\mathbb{AG}(\mathcal{L})) \setminus U_1$ contain $K_{6,4}$, which has a crosscap four. So, $U_{ij}, U_{ijk} = \emptyset$ for all $i \neq 1$. Here, remember that every vertex in U_{1jk} is an end vertex, and every vertex in U_{1j} is of degree two. Let G_{12} be the induced subgraph of $\mathbb{AG}(\mathcal{L})$ induced by the vertex subset $\bigcup_{n=1}^4 U_n$. It is clear that $G_{12} \cong K_{6,1,1,1}$, and G_{12} is a subgraph of the graph H_2 given in Figure 2a with the labels $u_\ell \in U_1$ (for $\ell = 1, \ldots, 6$), $I_2 = v_1$, $I_3 = v_2$, and $I_4 = v_3$. By Figure 2b, the N_2-embedding of G_{12} contains three different faces with vertices I_2, I_3; I_3, I_4; and I_2, I_4, respectively. So, any number of vertices in U_{1j} can be embedded into the N_2-embedding of G_{12} without edge-crossing. Thus, $\tilde{\gamma}(\mathbb{AG}(\mathcal{L})) = 2$.

Case 2 Let $|\bigcup_{n=1}^4 U_n| = 8$.

Case 2.1 Suppose $|U_1| \in \{5, 4\}$. If $U_{ij} \neq \emptyset$ or $U_{ijk} \neq \emptyset$ for some $i \neq 1$, then $\mathbb{AG}(\mathcal{L})$ contains $K_{5,4}$ as a subgraph, which is a contradiction. Therefore, $U_{ij} = \emptyset$ and $U_{ijk} = \emptyset$ for all $i \neq 1$. Now, if $|U_1| = 5$, then $\mathbb{AG}(\mathcal{L})$ is a subgraph of the annihilating-ideal graph in Case 1 with $|U_1| = 6$ so that $\tilde{\gamma}(\mathbb{AG}(\mathcal{L})) = 2$. Suppose $|U_1| = 4$. Here, $|U_2| = 2$. If $I \in \bigcup_{i \neq 1} U_{ij} \cup U_{234}$, then $\mathbb{AG}(\mathcal{L})$ contains a copy of $K_{4,5}$ where the partite sets are U_1 and $U_2 \cup U_3 \cup U_4 \cup \{I\}$ so that $\tilde{\gamma}(\mathbb{AG}(\mathcal{L})) \geq 3$. If $U_{1j} \neq \emptyset$ for some $j \in \{3, 4\}$, then $\mathbb{AG}(\mathcal{L})$ contains $K_{5,4} - e$ as a subgraph with the partition sets $U_1 \cup U_{1j}$ and $U_2 \cup U_3 \cup U_4$ so that, by Remark 1, we have $\tilde{\gamma}(\mathbb{AG}(\mathcal{L})) \geq 3$. Therefore, $\bigcup_{ij \neq 12} U_{ij} = \emptyset$ and $U_{234} = \emptyset$. In this case, one can retrieve an N_2-embedding of $\mathbb{AG}(\mathcal{L})$ from Figure 4b by changing the label I_3' to I_4 and its related edges such that $\tilde{\gamma}(\mathbb{AG}(\mathcal{L})) = 2$.

Case 2.2 Suppose $|U_1| = 3$. Let $|U_2| = 3$. If $U_{ij} \neq \emptyset$ or $U_{ijk} \neq \emptyset$ for $ij \neq 12$, then $\mathbb{AG}(\mathcal{L})$ contains $K_{4,5} - e$, which is a contradiction. Therefore, $U_{ij} = \emptyset$ and $U_{ijk} = \emptyset$ for all $ij \neq 12$. In this case, the crosscap of $\mathbb{AG}(\mathcal{L})$ is same as the crosscap of $K_{3,3,1,1}$ so that $\tilde{\gamma}(\mathbb{AG}(\mathcal{L})) = 2$. Let $|U_2| = 2$ and $I \in \bigcup_{ijk \neq 123} U_{ij} \cup U_{ijk}$.

- In the case that $I \in U_{ij}$ for $ij \in \{12, 13\}$, the contraction of $\mathbb{AG}(\mathcal{L})$ induced by the partite sets $X = U_i \cup U_4$ and $Y = U_j \cup \{I_k, [I_k', I_{ij}]\}$, where $k \notin \{i, j, 4\}$, forms a copy of H_4.
- In the case that $I \in U_{ij}$ for $ij \in \{14, 23, 24, 34\}$, the graph $\mathbb{AG}(\mathcal{L})$ contains $K_{5,4}$ with the partite sets $U_i \cup U_j \cup U_{ij}$ and $U_k \cup U_\ell$ where $k, \ell \notin \{i, j\}$.
- In the case that $I \in \bigcup_{ijk \neq 123} U_{ijk}$, the contraction of $\mathbb{AG}(\mathcal{L})$ induced by $(\bigcup_{n=1}^4 U_n \setminus \{I_\ell\}) \cup \{[I_\ell, I]\}$ forms H_4 where ℓ is the least integer in $\{1, 2, 3, 4\} \setminus \{i, j, k\}$.

Thus, $\bigcup_{ijk \neq 123} U_{ij} \cup U_{ijk} = \emptyset$, and, so, the crosscap of $\mathbb{AG}(\mathcal{L})$ is the crosscap of $K_{3,2,2,1}$, which is two.

Case 2.3 Suppose $|U_1| = 2$. Then, $K_{2,2,2,2}$ is a subgraph of $\mathbb{AG}(\mathcal{L})$. Suppose $\tilde{\gamma}(K_{2,2,2,2}) = 2$. Then, by Euler's formula, the number of faces in an N_2 embedding of $K_{2,2,2,2}$ is 16 so that all the faces are triangular, which contradicts the fact that $K_{2,2,2,2}$ has no triangular embedding (see [27]). Thus, $\tilde{\gamma}(\mathbb{AG}(\mathcal{L})) \geq 3$.

Case 3 Let $|\bigcup_{n=1}^4 U_n| = 7$.

Case 3.1 Suppose $|U_1| = 4$. If $|\bigcup_{i \neq 1} U_{ij} \cup U_{ijk}| \geq 2$, then $\mathbb{AG}(\mathcal{L})$ contains $K_{4,5}$ with one partite set $X = U_1$, and, so, $\tilde{\gamma}(\mathbb{AG}(\mathcal{L})) \geq 3$. Further, by Theorem 4iv, $\mathbb{AG}(\mathcal{L})$ is projective whenever $U_{ij} = U_{ijk} = \emptyset$ for all $i \neq 1$. Therefore, $|\bigcup_{i \neq 1} U_{ij} \cup U_{ijk}| = 1$, and let $I \in \bigcup_{i \neq 1} U_{ij} \cup U_{ijk}$. Now, if $U_{1j} = \emptyset$ for all $2 \leq j \leq 4$, then it is easy to verify that $\mathbb{AG}(\mathcal{L})$ is isomorphic to a subgraph of the graph H_1 (see Figure 1a). Therefore, by Lemma 2, we have $\tilde{\gamma}(\mathbb{AG}(\mathcal{L})) = 2$. So, let $U_{1j} \neq \emptyset$ for some $2 \leq j \leq 4$. Suppose $U_{k\ell} = \emptyset$ for $2 \leq j \neq k \neq \ell \leq 4$. Here, the open neighbor of each vertex in U_{1j} is I_k and I_ℓ in $\mathbb{AG}(\mathcal{L})$. Let G_{13} be the induced subgraph of $\mathbb{AG}(\mathcal{L})$ induced by the vertex subset $\bigcup_{n=1}^{4} U_n \cup \{I\}$. Clearly, G_{13} is a subgraph of the graph H_1 given in Figure 1a with the labels $u_\ell \in U_1$ (for $\ell = 1, \ldots, 4$), $v_1 = I_2, v_2 = I_3, v_3 = I_4$, and $v_4 = I$. Since $(I_3, I_4), (I_2, I_4), (I_2, I_3) \in E(\mathbb{AG}(\mathcal{L}))$, any number of vertices in U_{1j} (for $2 \leq j \leq 4$) can be embedded in the N_2-embedding of G_{13} without edge-crossing, and, therefore, $\tilde{\gamma}(\mathbb{AG}(\mathcal{L})) = 2$. Now, take $U_{k\ell} \neq \emptyset$ for $2 \leq j \neq k \neq \ell \leq 4$. Note that the set $U_{k\ell}$ is nothing but the singleton set $\{I\}$. Now, consider the subgraph $G_{14} = \mathbb{AG}(\mathcal{L}) - \{I_{1j}, (I_j, I_k), (I_k, I_\ell), (I_j, I_\ell), (I, I_j)\}$, which is isomorphic to $K_{4,4}$ with the partition sets $X = U_1$ and $Y = \{I_j, I_k, I_\ell, I\}$. Note that any N_2-embedding of G_{14} has eight rectangular faces so that each face shares exactly two vertices from X and Y. In $\mathbb{AG}(\mathcal{L})$, the vertex I_{1j} is adjacent to three vertices of Y, namely I_k, I_ℓ, and I. Therefore, one cannot insert I_{1j} with its edges into N_2 without crossing, which is a contradiction.

Case 3.2 Suppose $|U_1| = 3$. Then, $|U_2| = 2$. If $|\bigcup_{i \neq 1} U_{ij} \cup U_{ijk}| \geq 2$, then it is easy to check that the contraction of $\mathbb{AG}(\mathcal{L})$ contains either $K_{4,5} - e$ or $K_{3,6} \cup (K_4 - e)$ as a subgraph, and, so, by Remark 1, we have $\tilde{\gamma}(\mathbb{AG}(\mathcal{L})) \geq 3$. Therefore, $|\bigcup_{i \neq 1} U_{ij} \cup U_{ijk}| \leq 1$.

Assume $|\bigcup_{i \neq 1} U_{ij} \cup U_{ijk}| = 1$. If $U_{ij} \neq \emptyset$, then $U_{(ij)^c} = \emptyset$; otherwise, the graph induced by the partition sets $X = U_1 \cup U_3$ and $Y = U_2 \cup U_4 \cup [I_{ij}, I_{(ij)^c}]$ form H_4 in $\mathbb{AG}(\mathcal{L})$ so that $\tilde{\gamma}(\mathbb{AG}(\mathcal{L})) \geq 3$. Further, if $I \in U_{13} \cup U_{14} \cup U_{134}$, then consider the graph $\mathbb{AG}(\mathcal{L}) - \{I, e_1, e_2, e_3, e_4, e_5\} \cong K_{4,4} - e$ with the bipartite sets $\{I_1, I'_1, I''_1, I_j\}$ and $\{I_i, I'_i, I_k, I_{ijk}\}$ where $e_1 = (I_1, I_j), e_2 = (I'_1, I_j), e_3 = (I''_1, I_j), e_4 = (I_i, I_k), e_5 = (I'_i, I_k)\}$, and $e = (I_j, I_{ijk})$. Now, a similar argument given for G_2 (refer to Equation 1) leads to $\tilde{\gamma}(\mathbb{AG}(\mathcal{L})) \geq 3$. Therefore, $|\bigcup_{i \neq 1} U_{ij} \cup U_{ijk}| = 1$ with $U_{13} = U_{14} = U_{134} = \emptyset$. In this case, with the help of Figure 10a, we obtain $\tilde{\gamma}(\mathbb{AG}(\mathcal{L})) = 2$. Notice that in Figure 10a, we take $|U_{34}| = 1$.

Assume $\bigcup_{i \neq 1} U_{ij} \cup U_{ijk} = \emptyset$. If $|U_{1j}| \geq 3$ for some $j \in \{3, 4\}$, then the sets $X = U_2 \cup U_{j'}$ and $Y = U_1 \cup U_j \cup U_{1j}$, where $j' \in \{3, 4\} \setminus \{j\}$, form $K_{3,7}$. So, $|U_{1j}| \leq 2$ for $j = 3, 4$. Suppose $|U_{13} \cup U_{14}| \geq 3$. Let $|U_{1j}| \geq 2$ and $|U_{1k}| \geq 1$ for $j, k \in \{3, 4\}$. Then, the subgraph $\mathbb{AG}(\mathcal{L}) - \{I_{1k}, (I_1, I_j), (I'_1, I_j), (I''_1, I_j)\}$ contains $K_{3,6}$ with the partite sets $X = U_2 \cup U_k$ and $Y = U_1 \cup U_j \cup U_{1j}$. Since $deg_{K_{3,6}}(I_j) = 3$, I_j is contained in exactly three rectangular faces in any N_2-embedding of $K_{3,6}$. Since $\{I_1, I'_1, I''_1, I_j\} \subset Y$, to embed the edges $(I_1, I_j), (I'_1, I_j)$, and (I''_1, I_j), the vertices I_1, I'_1, and I''_1 on the diagonals of the three rectangular faces that contain I_j, respectively, are required. Now, after embedding the three edges, I_j is in exactly six triangular faces, all of which were formed by using two vertices from Y and one vertex from X. Therefore, the vertex I_{1k} cannot be embedded because it is adjacent to I_j as well as two vertices from X. So, $|U_{13} \cup U_{14}| \leq 2$. However, $\mathbb{AG}(\mathcal{L})$ is projective if $U_{13} \cup U_{14} = \emptyset$. Thus, $1 \leq |U_{13} \cup U_{14}| \leq 2$. Now, one can obtain help from Figure 10b to say that $\tilde{\gamma}(\mathbb{AG}(\mathcal{L})) = 2$.

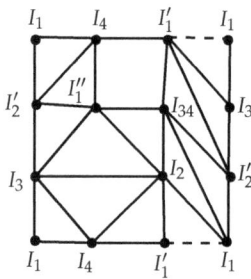 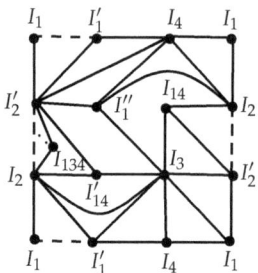

(**a**). $|\bigcup_{i \neq 1} U_{ij} \cup U_{ijk}| = 1$ and $U_{13} = U_{14} = U_{134} = \emptyset$ (**b**). $\bigcup_{i \neq 1} U_{ij} \cup U_{ijk} = \emptyset$ and $1 \leq |U_{13} \cup U_{14}| \leq 2$

Figure 10. $|\bigcup_{n=1}^{4} U_n| = 7$ with $|U_1| = 3$.

Case 3.3 Suppose $|U_1| = 2$.

Claim A: At most two distinct U_{ij}s are non-empty in which at most one U_{i4} is non-empty for $1 \leq i \neq j \leq 4$. Additionally, at most two distinct $U_{\ell mn}$s are non-empty for $\ell mn \neq 123$.

Assume on the contrary that at least three U_{ij}s are non-empty for $1 \leq i, j \leq 4$; say, $U_{i_1 i_2}, U_{i_3 i_4}$ and $U_{i_5 i_6}$ are non-empty. Let $p \in \{1, 2, 3\} \setminus \{i_1, i_2\}, q \in \{1, 2, 3\} \setminus \{p, i_3, i_4\}$ and $r \in \{1, 2, 3\} \setminus \{p, q, i_5, i_6\}$. If r exists, then the minor subgraph induced by the vertices $[I_p, I_{i_1 i_2}], I'_p, [I_q, I_{i_3 i_4}], I'_q, [I_r, I_{i_5 i_6}], I'_r$, and I_4 forms K_7 in $\mathbb{AG}(\mathcal{L})$, which is a contradiction. If r does not exist, then take r as $\{1, 2, 3\} \setminus \{p, q\}$ and form a minor of $\mathbb{AG}(\mathcal{L})$ with the partite sets $X = \{I_r, I'_r, I_4, I_{r4}\}$ and $Y = \{[I_p, I_{i_1 i_2}], I'_p, [I_q, I_{i_3 i_4}], I'_q\}$, which is isomorphic to either H_3 or H_4, as in Figure 3. So, by Lemma 3, we have $\tilde{\gamma}(\mathbb{AG}(\mathcal{L})) \geq 3$. Therefore, only at most two distinct U_{ij}s can be non-empty for $1 \leq i \neq j \leq 4$. Further, if $U_{m4}, U_{n4} \neq \emptyset$ for some $1 \leq m \neq n \leq 4$, then the subgraph induced by the sets $X = U_m \cup U_{m4} \cup \{I_k\}$ and $Y = U_n \cup U_4 \cup \{[I'_k, I_{n4}]\}$, where $k \neq m$ or n, form H_4 which has a crosscap of at least three.

Note that all the vertices in U_{123} are end vertices in $\mathbb{AG}(\mathcal{L})$. If $U_{ijk}, U_{\ell mn}$, and U_{pqr} are non-empty for $ijk, \ell mn, pqr \neq 123$, then the minor subgraph induced by $\{[I_{(ijk)^c}, I_{ijk}], I'_{(ijk)^c}, [I_{(\ell mn)^c}, I_{\ell mn}], I'_{(\ell mn)^c}, [I_{(prq)^c}, I_{pqr}], I'_{(pqr)^c}, I_4\}$ is K_7, which is a contradiction. Therefore, at most two distinct $U_{\ell mn}$s are non-empty for $\ell mn \neq 123$.

Claim B: $|U_{ij}| \leq 2$ and $|U_{i4}| \leq 1$ for all $1 \leq i < j \leq 3$.

If $|U_{ij}| \geq 3$ for some $1 \leq i, j \leq 3$, then $\mathbb{AG}(\mathcal{L})$ contains $K_{7,3}$ as a subgraph with the partite sets $X = U_i \cup U_j \cup U_{ij}$ and $Y = U_k \cup U_4$ where $k \in \{1, 2, 3\} \setminus \{i, j\}$. Additionally, if $|U_{i4}| \geq 2$ for some $1 \leq i \leq 3$, then $\mathbb{AG}(\mathcal{L})$ contains $K_{5,4}$ as a subgraph with the partite sets $X = U_i \cup U_4 \cup U_{i4}$ and $Y = U_j \cup U_k$ where $j, k \in \{1, 2, 3\} \setminus \{i\}$. Thus, $|U_{ij}| \leq 2$ and $|U_{i4}| \leq 1$ for all $1 \leq i < j \leq 3$.

Assume $|U_{ij}| = 2$ for some $1 \leq i, j \leq 3$. Suppose $U_{k\ell} \neq \emptyset$ for some $1 \leq k < \ell \leq 4$ and $k\ell \neq ij$. Let us take $j \notin \{k, \ell\} \cap \{i, j\}$. Then, $\mathbb{AG}(\mathcal{L})$ contains $K_{6,3} \cup (K_4 - e)$ with the partite sets $X = \{I_i, I'_i, I_j, [I'_j, I_{k\ell}], I_{ij}, I'_{ij}\}$ and $Y = U_m \cup U_4$ where $m \in \{1, 2, 3\} \setminus \{i, j\}$. So, by Remark 1, $\tilde{\gamma}(\mathbb{AG}(\mathcal{L})) \geq 3$. Therefore, $U_{k\ell} = \emptyset$. In this case, the number of U_{ijk} cannot be more than one because here $\mathbb{AG}(\mathcal{L})$ contains $K_{6,3} \cup (K_4 - e)$. For the remaining cases, by Figure 11a, we obtain $\tilde{\gamma}(\mathbb{AG}(\mathcal{L})) = 2$.

Assume $|U_{ij}| \leq 1$ for all $1 \leq i, j \leq 3$. Suppose $|U_{k4}| = 1$ for some $1 \leq k \leq 3$. If there are two $U_{\ell mn}$s that are non-empty for $\ell mn \neq 123$, then it is not hard to verify that $\mathbb{AG}(\mathcal{L})$ contains a subgraph similar to the structure of H_3, which has a crosscap of at least three. For all the remaining cases, that is $|U_{ij}| = |U_{k4}| = 1$ with unique $U_{\ell mn} \neq \emptyset$ or $|U_{ij}| \leq 1$ and $|U_{pq}| \leq 1$ with at most two $U_{\ell mn}$s that are non-empty for $1 \leq i, j, k, p, q \leq 3$ and $\ell mn \neq 123$, one can use Figure 11b to obtain $\tilde{\gamma}(\mathbb{AG}(\mathcal{L})) = 2$.

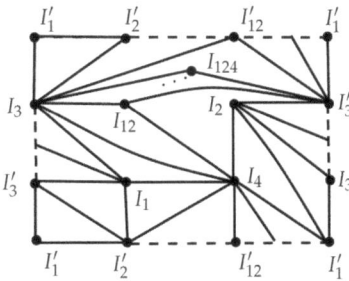
(a). $|U_{ij}| = 2$, $U_{k\ell} = \emptyset \ \forall \ k\ell \neq ij$ and at most one $U_{ijk} \neq \emptyset$ for $ijk \neq 123$

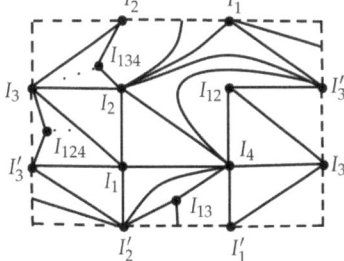
(b). $|U_{ii}|, |U_{pq}| \leq 1$ and at most two $U_{ijk} \neq \emptyset$ for $ijk \neq 123$ if $U_{i4} = \emptyset$

Figure 11. $|\bigcup_{n=1}^{4} U_n| = 7$ with $|U_1| = 2$.

Case 4 Let $|\bigcup_{n=1}^{4} U_n| = 6$.

Case 4.1 Suppose $|U_1| = 3$. Note that each vertex of U_{ij} for $i = 1$ is adjacent to exactly two vertices $I_{i'}$ and $I_{j'}$ for $i', j' \notin \{i, j\}$ and $(I_{i'}, I_{j'}) \in E(\mathbb{AG}(\mathcal{L}))$, so we do not want to bother about U_{1j} and U_{1jk} for all $2 \le j < k \le 4$. If $|U_{ij}| \ge 3$ for some $i \ne 1$, then $\mathbb{AG}(\mathcal{L})$ contains $K_{4,5}$ as a subgraph with the partite sets $X = U_1 \cup U_k$ and $Y = U_i \cup U_j \cup U_{ij}$ where $k \in \{2,3,4\} \setminus \{i,j\}$, which is a contradiction. So, $|U_{ij}| \le 2$ for all $i \ne 1$.

(i). Assume $|U_{ij}| = 2$ for some $i \ne 1$. If $U_{(ij)^c} \ne \emptyset$, then the sets $X = U_i \cup U_j \cup U_{ij}$ and $Y = U_1 \cup U_k \cup U_{(ij)^c}$ form $K_{4,5}$ in $\mathbb{AG}(\mathcal{L})$, and, if $U_{k\ell} \ne \emptyset$ for some $k \ne 1$ with $k\ell \ne ij$ or $U_{234} \ne \emptyset$, then $\mathbb{AG}(\mathcal{L})$ contains $K_{4,5} - e$ so that $\tilde{\gamma}(\mathbb{AG}(\mathcal{L})) \ge 3$. If not, that is $U_{(ij)^c}, U_{k\ell}, U_{234} = \emptyset$ for all $k \ne 1$ with $k\ell \ne ij$, then by Figure 12a, we have $\tilde{\gamma}(\mathbb{AG}(\mathcal{L})) = 2$.

(ii). Assume $|U_{ij}| \le 1$ for all $i \ne 1$. If $U_{(i_1 j_1)^c} \ne \emptyset$ and $U_{(i_2 j_2)^c} \ne \emptyset$ for some $U_{i_1 j_1} \ne \emptyset$ and $U_{i_2 j_2} \ne \emptyset$, then the sets $X = U_{i_1} \cup U_{j_1} \cup U_{i_1 j_1} \cup \{[I_{i_2 j_2}, I_{(i_2 j_2)^c}]\}$ and $Y = U_1 \cup U_m \cup U_{(i_1 j_1)^c}$, where $m \ne i_1, j_1$, contains $K_{4,5} - e$ in $\mathbb{AG}(\mathcal{L})$. Additionally, if $|U_{(ij)^c}| \ge 3$, then the sets $X = U_i \cup U_j \cup U_{ij}$ and $Y = U_1 \cup U_m \cup U_{(ij)^c}$, where $m \ne i, j$, form $K_{3,7}$ in $\mathbb{AG}(\mathcal{L})$, which is a contradiction. So, at most one of the sets $U_{(ij)^c}$ is non-empty with $|U_{(ij)^c}| \le 2$.

Let $|U_{(ij)^c}| = 2$. If $I \in \bigcup_{k\ell \ne ij} U_{k\ell} \cup U_{234}$, then the sets $X = \{I_i, I_j, I_{ij}\}$ and $Y = \{I_1, I_1', [I_1'', I], I_m, I_{(ij)^c}, I'_{(ij)^c}\}$, where $m \ne i, j$, form $K_{3,6} \cup (K_4 - e)$ so that, by Remark 1, $\tilde{\gamma}(\mathbb{AG}(\mathcal{L})) \ge 3$. Therefore, $\bigcup_{k \ne 1; k\ell \ne ij} U_{k\ell} \cup U_{234} = \emptyset$. For this case, readers can verify the N_2-embedding of $\mathbb{AG}(\mathcal{L})$.

Let $|U_{(ij)^c}| = 1$. If $I, J \in \bigcup_{k \ne 1; k\ell \ne ij} U_{k\ell} \cup U_{234}$ with $|U_{k\ell}| \le 1$, then the sets $\{I_i, I_j, I_m, I_1, [I_1', I], [I_1'', J], [I_{ij}, I_{(ij)^c}]\}$ form K_7. Therefore, $|\bigcup_{k \ne 1; k\ell \ne ij} U_{k\ell} \cup U_{234}| = 1$.

Let $\bigcup_{i \ne 1} U_{(ij)^c} = \emptyset$. Then, by Theorem 4iii[a], $\mathbb{AG}(\mathcal{L})$ is projective if $|\bigcup_{i \ne 1} U_{ij} \cup U_{ijk}| \le 1$. If $|\bigcup_{i \ne 1} U_{ij} \cup U_{ijk}| \ge 4$, then $K_{3,7}$ is a subgraph of $\mathbb{AG}(\mathcal{L})$ with the partite sets $X = U_1$ and $Y = V(\mathbb{AG}(\mathcal{L})) \setminus U_1$. So, in the case of $\bigcup_{i \ne 1} U_{(ij)^c} = \emptyset$, $\tilde{\gamma}(\mathbb{AG}(\mathcal{L})) = 2$ whenever $2 \le |\bigcup_{i \ne 1} U_{ij} \cup U_{ijk}| \le 3$ with $|U_{ij}| \le 1$ (refer to Figure 12b).

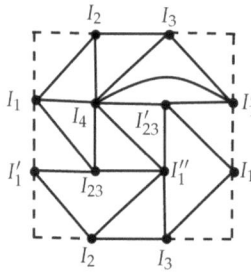

(a). Unique $|U_{ij}| = 2$ for $i \ne 1$ and $U_{k\ell}, U_{234} = \emptyset \ \forall \ k \ne 1$ and $k\ell \ne ij$

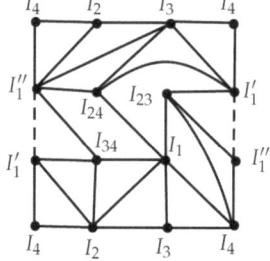

(b). $|U_{ij}| = 1$ for all $i \ne 1$

Figure 12. $|\bigcup_{n=1}^{4} U_n| = 6$ with $|U_1| = 3$.

Case 4.2 Suppose $|U_1| = 2$. Then, $|U_2| = 2$ and $|U_3| = |U_4| = 1$. If $|U_{34}| \ge 3$, then the partite sets $X = U_1 \cup U_2$ and $Y = U_3 \cup U_4 \cup U_{34}$ form $K_{4,5}$ as a subgraph in $\mathbb{AG}(\mathcal{L})$, which is a contradiction.

Case 4.2.1 Assume $|U_{34}| = 2$. Then, $U_{(pq)^c} = \emptyset$ for all $U_{pq} \ne \emptyset$; otherwise, the sets $X = U_1 \cup U_2$ and $Y = U_3 \cup U_4 \cup U_{34} \cup \{[I_{pq}, I_{(pq)^c}]\}$ form $K_{4,5}$ in $\mathbb{AG}(\mathcal{L})$. In particular, $U_{12} = \emptyset$.

If $|U_{ij}| \ge 2$ for some $ij \ne 12, 34$ and $i < j$, then the subgraph $\mathbb{AG}(\mathcal{L}) - \{I_{34}, I'_{34}, (I_i, I_j), (I'_i, I_j)\}$ contains $K_{3,5}$ with the partite sets $X = U_i \cup U_j \cup U_{ij}$ and $Y = U_{i'} \cup U_{j'}$ where $i' \in$

$\{1,2\} \setminus \{i\}$ and $j' \in \{3,4\} \setminus \{j\}$. Note that any N_2-embedding of $K_{3,5}$ has one hexagonal and six rectangular faces, and the vertices I_{34} and I'_{34} are adjacent to $I_i, I'_i, I_{i'}$ and $I'_{i'}$. So, to insert I_{34} and I'_{34} into an N_2-embedding of $K_{3,5}$, we require two faces, say F_1 and F_2, which contains $I_i, I'_i, I_{i'}$, and $I'_{i'}$. If either F_1 or F_2 is hexagonal, then the corresponding face may adopt one of the edges (I_i, I_j) or (I'_i, I_j). Let us take that the edge (I_i, I_j) is embedded. Now, to insert an edge (I'_i, I_j), a rectangular face containing I'_i and I_j as diagonals is required. However, no such rectangular face exists because the edges $(I'_i, I_{i'})$ and $(I'_i, I'_{i'})$ have been used twice in F_1 and F_2, which is a contradiction.

For all of the remaining cases, that is $|\bigcup_{ij \neq 12,34} U_{ij}| \leq 2$ with $|U_{ij}| \leq 1$ and $U_{(pq)^c} = \emptyset$ when $U_{pq} \neq \emptyset$ for $1 \leq p \neq q \leq 4$, we have $\tilde{\gamma}(\mathbb{AG}(\mathcal{L})) = 2$ (refer to Figure 13a).

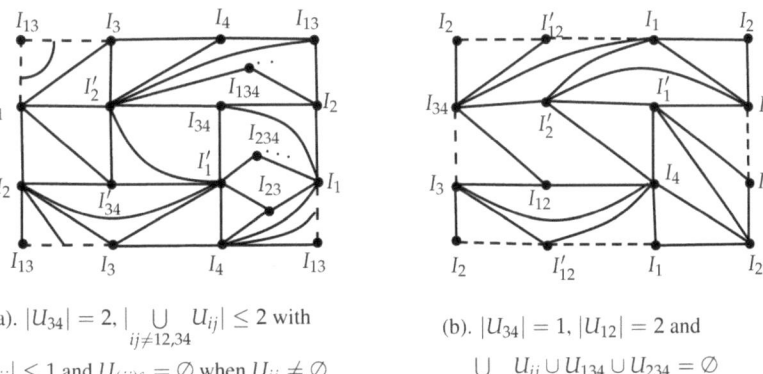

(a). $|U_{34}| = 2$, $|\bigcup_{ij \neq 12,34} U_{ij}| \leq 2$ with $|U_{ij}| \leq 1$ and $U_{(ij)^c} = \emptyset$ when $U_{ij} \neq \emptyset$

(b). $|U_{34}| = 1, |U_{12}| = 2$ and $\bigcup_{ij \neq 12,34} U_{ij} \cup U_{134} \cup U_{234} = \emptyset$

Figure 13. $|\bigcup_{n=1}^{4} U_n| = 6$ with $|U_1| = 2$.

Case 4.2.2 Assume that $|U_{34}| = 1$. Let us take $ij \neq 12, 34$.

Let $|U_{12}| \geq 3$, then the subgraph of $\mathbb{AG}(\mathcal{L})$ induced by the sets $X = U_3 \cup U_4 \cup U_{34}$ and $Y = U_1 \cup U_2 \cup U_{12}$ contains $K_{3,7}$ so that $\tilde{\gamma}(\mathbb{AG}(\mathcal{L})) \geq 3$. Thus, $|U_{12}| \leq 2$.

Let $|U_{12}| = 2$. If $I \in \bigcup_{ij \neq 12,34} U_{ij} \cup U_{134} \cup U_{234}$, then $\mathbb{AG}(\mathcal{L})$ contains $K_{3,6} \cup (K_4 - e)$, so that, by Remark 1, $\tilde{\gamma}(\mathbb{AG}(\mathcal{L})) \geq 3$. Therefore, $\bigcup_{ij \neq 34,12} U_{ij} \cup U_{134} \cup U_{234} = \emptyset$, and in this case, by Figure 13b, we obtain $\tilde{\gamma}(\mathbb{AG}(\mathcal{L})) = 2$.

Let $|U_{12}| = 1$. If $|U_{ij}| \geq 2$, then the partite sets $X = U_{i'} \cup U_{j'}$ and $Y = \{I_i, I'_i, I_j, I_{ij}, I'_{ij}, [I_{34}, I_{12}]\}$ where $i' \in \{1,2\} \setminus \{i\}$ and $j' \in \{3,4\} \setminus \{j\}$ form a minor subgraph $K_{3,6} \cup (K_4 - e)$ in $\mathbb{AG}(\mathcal{L})$ so that, by Remark 1, $\tilde{\gamma}(\mathbb{AG}(\mathcal{L})) \geq 3$. If $U_{ij}, U_{k\ell} \neq \emptyset$ for $ij, k\ell \neq 12,34$ where $\{i,j\} \cap \{k,\ell\} = j = \ell$, then the partite sets $X = \{I_i, [I'_i, I_{k\ell}], I_\ell, I_{ij}\}$ and $Y = \{I_k, I'_k, I_m, [I_{34}, I_{12}]\}$ where $m \notin \{i,j,k\}$ form $(H_4 \cup (u_2, u_3)) - (u_1, u_4)$. A slight modification of the proof for H_4 in Lemma 3 yields $\tilde{\gamma}(\mathbb{AG}(\mathcal{L})) \geq 3$. Further, minor changes to the labels in Figure 13a give $\tilde{\gamma}(\mathbb{AG}(\mathcal{L})) = 2$ whenever $|\bigcup_{ij \neq 12,34} U_{ij}| \leq 1$.

Let $U_{12} = \emptyset$. Then $U_{(pq)^c} = \emptyset$ for all $U_{pq} \neq \emptyset$; otherwise, $\mathbb{AG}(\mathcal{L})$ contains $K_8 - 4e$, which is isomorphic to $(H_4 \cup (u_1, u_3)) - (v_1, v_2)$, so Lemma 3 gives us $\tilde{\gamma}(\mathbb{AG}(\mathcal{L})) \geq 3$. If $|U_{ij}| \geq 4$, then the partite sets $X = U_i \cup U_j \cup U_{ij}$ and $Y = U_{i'} \cup U_{j'}$ where $i' \in \{1,2\} \setminus \{i\}$ and $j' \in \{3,4\} \setminus \{j\}$ contain $K_{7,3}$ in $\mathbb{AG}(\mathcal{L})$, which is a contradiction. Suppose $|U_{ij}| \in \{2,3\}$. If $|U_{k\ell}| \geq 2$ for some $k\ell \neq ij$ where $\{k,\ell\} \cap \{i,j\} = k = i$, then the subgraph $G_{15} = \mathbb{AG}(\mathcal{L}) - \{I_{34}, I_{k\ell}, I'_{k\ell}, (I_i, I_j), (I'_i, I_j)\}$ contains $K_{5,3}$ with the partite sets $X = U_i \cup U_j \cup U_{ij}$ and $Y = U_{i'} \cup U_{j'}$ where $i', j' \notin \{i,j\}$. Note that any N_2-embedding of $K_{5,3}$ has one hexagonal and six rectangular faces. Further, in $\mathbb{AG}(\mathcal{L})$, I_{34} is adjacent to $I_i, I'_i, I_{i'}, I'_{i'}$, and, also, $I_{k\ell}, I'_{k\ell}$ are adjacent to $I_{i'}, I'_{i'}, I_j$. So, to embed the vertices $I_{34}, I_{k\ell}$, and $I'_{k\ell}$, one hexagonal and two rectangular faces containing both $I_{i'}$ and $I'_{i'}$ are required. In such a case, one cannot find two rectangular faces with the diagonal vertices I_i, I_j and I'_i, I_j. So, either the edge (I_i, I_j) or (I'_i, I_j) cannot be drawn without crossing, which is a contradiction. Thus, we obtain the result as in the statement-(iv)[b2].

Case 4.2.3 Suppose $U_{34} = \emptyset$.

If $|U_{ij} \cup U_{(ij)^c}| \geq 4$ for some $ij \notin \{12, 34\}$, then the sets $X = U_i \cup U_j \cup U_{ij}$ and $Y = U_{i'} \cup U_{j'} \cup U_{(ij)^c}$ where $i', j' \notin \{i, j\}$ form a complete bipartite graph whose crosscap is more than two.

Let $|U_{ij}| \in \{2, 3\}$ for some $ij \notin \{12, 34\}$. Then, clearly, $U_{(ij)^c}$ must be empty. Let $k\ell \notin \{12, 34, ij, (ij)^c\}$. If $|U_{ij} \cup U_{k\ell} \cup U_{(k\ell)^c}| \geq 5$, then the sets $X = U_i \cup U_j \cup U_{ij} \cup \{[I_{k\ell}, I_{k\ell^c}]\}$ and $Y = U_{i'} \cup U_{j'}$ where $i' \in \{1,2\} \setminus \{i\}$ and $j' \in \{3,4\} \setminus \{j\}$ form $K_{6,3} \cup (K_4 - e)$ and, by Remark 1, $\tilde{\gamma}(\mathbb{AG}(\mathcal{L})) \geq 3$. Therefore, $2 \leq |U_{ij} \cup U_{k\ell} \cup U_{(k\ell)^c}| \leq 4$. Now, there are at most three possibilities:

(i). $|U_{ij}| = 3$ and $|U_{k\ell}| = 1$; this case is pictured in Figure 14.

(ii). $|U_{ij}| = 2$ and $|U_{k\ell}| = |U_{(k\ell)^c}| = 1$; this case is pictured in Figure 15a.

(iii). $|U_{ij}| = |U_{k\ell}| = 2$; this case is pictured in Figure 15b.

Thus, in all these cases, we have $\tilde{\gamma}(\mathbb{AG}(\mathcal{L})) = 2$.

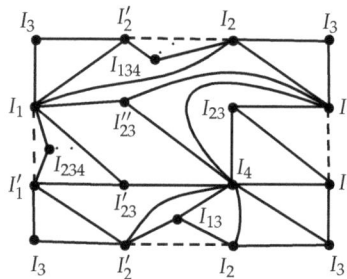

$U_{34} = \emptyset$ with $|U_{ij}| = 3$ and $|U_{k\ell}| = 1$ for some $ij, k\ell \neq 12, 34$

Figure 14. $|\bigcup_{n=1}^{4} U_n| = 6$ with $|U_1| = |U_2| = 2$.

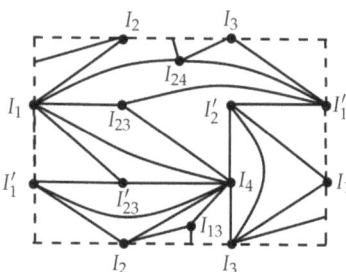
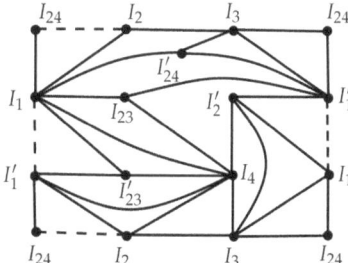

(**a**). $U_{34} = \emptyset$ with $|U_{ij}| = 2$ and $|U_{k\ell}| = |U_{(k\ell)^c}| = 1$ for some $ij, k\ell \neq 12, 34$

(**b**). $U_{34} = \emptyset$ with $|U_{ij}| = |U_{k\ell}| = 2$ for some $ij, k\ell \neq 12, 34$

Figure 15. $|\bigcup_{n=1}^{4} U_n| = 6$ with $|U_1| = |U_2| = 2$.

Let $|U_{ij}| \leq 1$ for all $ij \notin \{12, 34\}$. Then, at least one $U_{ij} = \emptyset$ for $ij \notin \{12, 34\}$. Otherwise, the graph induced by $\{I_1, I'_1, I_2, I'_2, I_3, I_4, [I_{13}, I_{24}], [I_{14}, I_{23}]\}$ forms $K_8 - 3e$ in $\mathbb{AG}(\mathcal{L})$. Clearly, $\tilde{\gamma}(K_8 - 3e) \geq 3$ because the number of faces in the N_2-embedding of $K_8 - 3e$ is 17, which contradicts the well-known fact that $\frac{2|E|}{|F|}$ must be greater than the girth value (refer to Observation 1). Therefore, $|\bigcup_{ij \neq 12, 34} U_{ij}| \leq 3$. Thus, by [20, Theorem 2.6iib)], we have $\tilde{\gamma}(\mathbb{AG}(\mathcal{L})) = 2$ whenever $|\bigcup_{ij \neq 12, 34} U_{ij}| = 3$.

Case 5 Let $|\bigcup_{n=1}^{4} U_n| = 5$. Then, $|U_1| = 2$. If $U_{ij} = \emptyset$ for all $1 \leq i < j \leq 4$, then $\tilde{\gamma}(\mathbb{AG}(\mathcal{L})) \leq 1$. Observe that we do not want to consider the sets U_{ij} for $i \neq 1$ whenever $U_{(ij)^c} = \emptyset$ because every vertex in U_{ij} is adjacent to I_i, I_j and $(I_i, I_j) \in E(\mathbb{AG}(\mathcal{L}))$. If $|U_{ij}| \geq 5$ for some $i \neq 1$, then the sets $X = U_i \cup U_j \cup U_{ij}$ and $Y = U_{i'} \cup U_{j'}$ where $i', j' \notin \{i, j\}$ form $K_{3,7}$ in $\mathbb{AG}(\mathcal{L})$, which is a contradiction.

Case 5.1 Assume $|U_{ij}| = 4$ for some $i \neq 1$. Then, $U_{(mn)^c} = \emptyset$ whenever $U_{mn} \neq \emptyset$; otherwise, the sets $X = U_i \cup U_j \cup U_{ij} \cup \{[I_{mn}, I_{(mn)^c}]\}$ and $Y = U_{i'} \cup U_{j'}$ where $i', j' \notin \{i, j\}$ form $K_{7,3}$ as a minor of $\mathbb{AG}(\mathcal{L})$. Similarly, $U_{(ij)^c} = \emptyset$; otherwise $K_{6,4}$ is a minor of $\mathbb{AG}(\mathcal{L})$. If $|U_{k\ell}| \geq 2$ for some $k \neq 1$ and $k\ell \neq ij$, then the subgraph $G_{16} = \mathbb{AG}(\mathcal{L}) - \{I_{k\ell}, I'_{k\ell}, (I_i, I_j)\}$ contains $K_{6,3}$ with the partition sets $X = U_i \cup U_j \cup U_{ij}$ and $Y = U_1 \cup U_{i'}$ where $i' \notin \{1, i, j\}$. Since $\{i, j\} \cap \{k, \ell\} \neq \emptyset$, let $\{i, j\} \cap \{k, \ell\} = i = k$. Clearly, $j \in \{2, 3, 4\} \setminus \{k, \ell\}$. Note that each face in any N_2-embedding of $K_{6,3}$ is rectangular, and the vertices $I_{k\ell}, I'_{k\ell}$ are adjacent to I_1, I'_1 and I_j. Therefore, to insert $I_{k\ell}$ and $I'_{k\ell}$, two rectangular faces that contain I_1, I'_1 and I_j are required. Next, to insert the edge (I_i, I_j), a rectangular face with the diagonals I_i and I_j is required. However, the edges (I_1, I_j) and (I'_1, I_j) have been used twice to form the first two rectangular faces. So, one cannot construct another rectangular face that contains I_i and I_j with a single left-out vertex of Y, which is a contradiction.

Therefore, for the remaining case, that is, $|U_{k\ell}| \leq 1$ for all $k \neq 1$ and $k\ell \neq ij$ with $U_{(mn)^c} = \emptyset$ whenever $U_{mn} \neq \emptyset$, by using Figure 16a, one can have $\tilde{\gamma}(\mathbb{AG}(\mathcal{L})) = 2$.

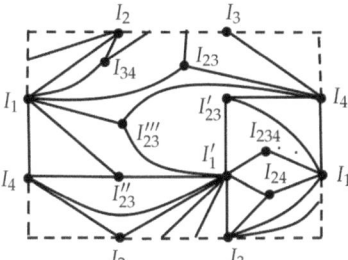
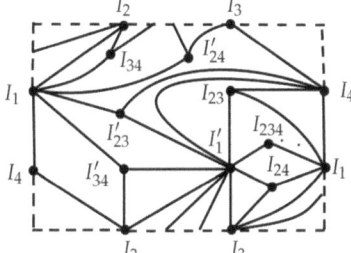
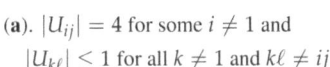

(a). $|U_{ij}| = 4$ for some $i \neq 1$ and $|U_{k\ell}| \leq 1$ for all $k \neq 1$ and $k\ell \neq ij$

(b). $|U_{ij}| = 2$ and $U_{(ij)^c} = \emptyset$ for all $i \neq 1$

Figure 16. $|\bigcup_{n=1}^{4} U_n| = 5$ with $|U_1| = 2$.

Case 5.2 Assume $|U_{ij}| = 3$ for some $i \neq 1$. Let $p \notin \{1, i, j\}$. Clearly, $U_{(ij)^c} = \emptyset$; otherwise, the sets $X = U_i \cup U_j \cup U_{ij}$ and $Y = U_1 \cup U_p \cup U_{(ij)^c}$ form $K_{5,4}$.

If $|U_{k\ell}| = 3$ for some $k \neq 1$ and $k\ell \neq ij$, then the subgraph $G'_{15} = \mathbb{AG}(\mathcal{L}) - \{I_{k\ell}, I'_{k\ell}, I''_{k\ell}, (I_i, I_j), (I_1, I_p), (I'_1, I_p)\}$ has a similar structure of G_{15} with the partite sets $X = U_i \cup U_j \cup U_{ij}$ and $Y = U_1 \cup U_p$, and so $\tilde{\gamma}(\mathbb{AG}(\mathcal{L})) \geq 3$. Suppose $|U_{k\ell}|, |U_{mn}| = 2$ for $k, m \neq 1$ and $k\ell, mn \neq ij$. Let $\{i, j\} \cap \{k, \ell\} = i = k$. Then, $G_{17} = \mathbb{AG}(\mathcal{L}) - \{I_{k\ell}, I'_{k\ell}, I_{mn}, I'_{mn}, (I_i, I_j)\}$ has $K_{5,3}$ with the partite sets $X = U_i \cup U_j \cup U_{ij}$ and $Y = U_1 \cup U_\ell$. Any N_2-embedding of $K_{5,3}$ has one hexagonal and six rectangular faces. Notice that $I_{k\ell}, I'_{k\ell}$ are adjacent to I_1, I'_1, I_j, and I_{mn}, I'_{mn} are adjacent to I_1, I'_1, I_i. So, to embed $I_{k\ell}, I'_{k\ell}, I_{mn}$, and I'_{mn}, one hexagonal and two rectangular faces containing both I_1 and I'_1 are required. However, the edge (I_i, I_j) cannot be drawn without crossing, which is a contradiction. Therefore, $|\bigcup_{k \neq 1; k\ell \neq ij} U_{k\ell}| \leq 3$ and $|U_{k\ell}| \neq 3$.

Suppose $|\bigcup_{k \neq 1; k\ell \neq ij} U_{k\ell}| = 3$. Since $|U_{k\ell}| \neq 3$ for all $k \neq 1$ and $k\ell \neq ij$, we have $|U_{k\ell}| = 2$ and $|U_{mn}| = 1$ for some $m \neq 1$ and $mn \neq ij, k\ell$. Next, we claim that $U_{(k\ell)^c} = U_{(mn)^c} = \emptyset$. If $U_{(k\ell)^c} \neq \emptyset$, then by letting $\{i, j\} \cap \{k, \ell\} = i = k$, $K_{7,3}$ can be formed by the sets $X = U_i \cup U_j \cup U_{ij} \cup U_{k\ell}$ and $Y = U_1 \cup \{[I_\ell, I_{(k\ell)^c}]\}$. If $U_{(mn)^c} \neq \emptyset$, then $\mathbb{AG}(\mathcal{L})$ has a similar structure to G_{15}, so that $\tilde{\gamma}(\mathbb{AG}(\mathcal{L})) \geq 3$.

Suppose $|\bigcup_{k \neq 1; k\ell \neq ij} U_{k\ell}| \leq 2$. As mentioned, $U_{(k\ell)^c} = \emptyset$ when $|U_{k\ell}| = 2$ for $k \neq 1$ and $k\ell \neq ij$. Suppose $|U_{k\ell}| = 1$ and $|U_{(k\ell)^c}| \geq 2$. Then, $\mathbb{AG}(\mathcal{L}) - \{I_{k\ell}, I_{(k\ell)^c}, I'_{(k\ell)^c}, (I_i, I_j), (I_1, I_\ell),$ and $(I'_1, I_\ell)\}$ has $K_{5,3}$ with the partite sets $X = U_i \cup U_j \cup U_{ij}$ and $Y = U_1 \cup U_\ell$. Note that any N_2-embedding of $K_{5,3}$ has one hexagonal and six rectangular faces, $I_{k\ell}$ is adjacent to $I_1, I'_1, I_j, I_{(k\ell)^c}, I'_{(k\ell)^c}$, and $I_{(k\ell)^c}, I'_{(k\ell)^c}$ are adjacent to $I_k, I_\ell, I_{k\ell}$. So, the three vertices $I_{k\ell}, I_{(k\ell)^c}, I'_{(k\ell)^c}$ together with the edges $(I_i, I_j), (I_1, I_\ell), (I'_1, I_\ell)$ cannot be embedded, and, also

, $\tilde{\gamma}(\mathbb{AG}(\mathcal{L})) \geq 3$. Therefore, $|U_{k\ell} \cup U_{(k\ell)^c}| \leq 2$. Further, if $|U_{k\ell} \cup U_{(k\ell)^c}| = |U_{\ell m} \cup U_{(\ell m)^c}| = 2$ for $k\ell \neq ij$ and $\ell m \neq ij, k\ell$, then $\mathbb{AG}(\mathcal{L})$ contains $K_{3,7}$, which is a contradiction.

Thus, an N_2-embedding of $\mathbb{AG}(\mathcal{L})$ can be retrieved from Figure 16a for $|\bigcup_{pq \neq ij} U_{pq}| \leq 3$ with $U_{(pq)^c} = \emptyset$ if $|U_{pq}| = 2$.

Case 5.3 Assume $|U_{ij}| = 2$ for some $i \neq 1$. Clearly, $|U_{(ij)^c}| \leq 1$; otherwise, the sets $X = U_i \cup U_j \cup U_{ij}$ and $Y = U_1 \cup U_p \cup U_{(ij)^c}$ where $p \notin \{1, i, j\}$ form $K_{5,4}$.

If $|U_{k\ell}|, |U_{mn}| = 2$ for $k, m \neq 1$ and $k\ell, mn \neq ij$, then $U_{(ij)^c}, U_{(k\ell)^c}, U_{(mn)^c} = \emptyset$. Further, an N_2-embedding of $\mathbb{AG}(\mathcal{L})$ in the case of $|U_{ij}| = |U_{k\ell}| = |U_{mn}| = 2$ is given in Figure 16b so that $\tilde{\gamma}(\mathbb{AG}(\mathcal{L})) = 2$.

Suppose $|U_{k\ell}| = 2, |U_{mn}| \leq 1$ for $k, m \neq 1$ and $k\ell, mn \neq ij$. If $U_{(ij)^c}, U_{(k\ell)^c} \neq \emptyset$, then the sets $X = U_1 \cup U_p \cup U_{(ij)^c}$ and $Y = U_i \cup U_j \cup U_{ij} \cup \{[I_{(k\ell)}, I_{(k\ell)^c}]\}$ where $p \notin \{1, i, j\}$ form $K_{5,4} - e$ in $\mathbb{AG}(\mathcal{L})$ so that, by Remark 1, we have $\tilde{\gamma}(\mathbb{AG}(\mathcal{L})) \geq 3$. Further, since $|U_{k\ell}| = 2$, we have $|U_{(k\ell)^c}| \leq 1$. Therefore, $|U_{(ij)^c} \cup U_{(k\ell)^c}| \leq 1$. Suppose $|U_{(ij)^c} \cup U_{(k\ell)^c}| = 1$, say $U_{(ij)^c} \neq \emptyset$. Then, $U_{(mn)^c} = \emptyset$; otherwise, $X = U_1 \cup U_p \cup U_{(ij)^c}$ and $Y = U_i \cup U_j \cup U_{ij} \cup \{[I_{(mn)}, I_{(mn)^c}]\}$ where $p \notin \{1, i, j\}$ form $K_{4,5} - e$ in $\mathbb{AG}(\mathcal{L})$. So, $|U_{mn} \cup U_{(mn)^c}| \leq 1$. Suppose not, that is, $U_{(ij)^c}, U_{(k\ell)^c} = \emptyset$, then $|U_{(mn)^c}| \leq 1$; otherwise, $\mathbb{AG}(\mathcal{L}) - \{I_{ij}, I'_{ij}, I_{k\ell}, I'_{k\ell}, (I_m, I_n), (I_1, I_{m'}), (I'_1, I_{m'})\} \cong K_{5,3}$ with the partite sets $X = U_1 \cup U_{m'} \cup U_{(mn)^c}$ and $Y = U_m \cup U_n \cup U_{mn}$ where $m' \notin \{1, m, n\}$ is a similar structure to G_{17} which has a crosscap of at least three. So, $|U_{mn} \cup U_{(mn)^c}| \leq 2$.

Suppose $|U_{k\ell}|, |U_{mn}| \leq 1$ for $k, m \neq 1$ and $k\ell, mn \neq ij$. Then, by Theorem 4(ii), $\tilde{\gamma}(\mathbb{AG}(\mathcal{L})) = 2$ provided $|\bigcup_{k \neq 1; k\ell \neq ij} U_{k\ell}| = 2$ with $|\bigcup_{p \neq 1} U_{(pq)^c}| = 1$ or $|\bigcup_{k \neq 1; k\ell \neq ij} U_{k\ell}| = 1$ with $|U_{(ij)^c}| = 1$, $U_{(k\ell)^c} = \emptyset$ or $U_{(ij)^c} = \emptyset$, $|U_{(k\ell)^c}| \leq 2$ or $\bigcup_{k \neq 1; k\ell \neq ij} U_{k\ell} = \emptyset$ with $|U_{(ij)^c}| = 1$.

Hence, $\tilde{\gamma}(\mathbb{AG}(\mathcal{L})) = 2$ whenever $4 \leq |\bigcup_{i \neq 1} U_{ij} \cup U_{(ij)^c}| \leq 6$ with $|\bigcup_{i \neq 1} U_{(ij)^c}| \leq 1$ or $|\bigcup_{i \neq 1} U_{ij}| = 3$ with $|U_{ij} \cup U_{(ij)^c}| \leq 3$ and a unique $U_{(ij)^c} \neq \emptyset$ or $\bigcup_{i \neq 1} U_{ij} = 2$ with $|U_{(ij)^c}| = 1$.

Case 5.4 Assume $|U_{ij}| = 1$ for all $i \neq 1$. Then, $|U_{(ij)^c}| \leq 3$; otherwise, the sets $X = U_i \cup U_j \cup U_{ij}$ and $Y = U_1 \cup U_{i'} \cup U_{(ij)^c}$ where $i' \notin \{1, i, j\}$ form $K_{3,7}$.

Suppose $|U_{k\ell}| = |U_{mn}| = 1$ for $k, m \neq 1$ and $k\ell, mn \neq ij$. If $U_{(ij)^c}, U_{(k\ell)^c}, U_{(mn)^c} \neq \emptyset$, then the sets $X = U_1 \cup U_2 \cup U_3$ and $Y = \{I_4, [I_{ij}, I_{(ij)^c}], [I_{k\ell}, I_{(k\ell)^c}], [I_{mn}, I_{(mn)^c}]\}$ form H_4 as a minor of $\mathbb{AG}(\mathcal{L})$, which is a contradiction. Assume that $|U_{(ij)^c}| = 3$. If $I \in U_{(k\ell)^c} \cup U_{(mn)^c}$, then $G_{18} = \mathbb{AG}(\mathcal{L}) - \{I, I_{k\ell}, I_{mn}, (I_i, I_j), (I_1, I_{i'}), (I'_1, I_{i'})\}$ contains $K_{6,3}$ with the partite sets $X = U_1 \cup U_{i'} \cup U_{(ij)^c}$ and $Y = U_i \cup U_j \cup U_{ij}$ and any N_2-embedding of $K_{3,6}$ has nine rectangular faces. Here, it is not hard to verify that all the left-out vertices and edges cannot be embedded into the nine rectangular faces so that $\tilde{\gamma}(\mathbb{AG}(\mathcal{L})) \geq 3$. Therefore, $U_{(k\ell)^c} \cup U_{(mn)^c} = \emptyset$. Here, the graph $\mathbb{AG}(\mathcal{L}) - \{I_{k\ell}, I_{mn}\}$ is a subgraph of the graph in Figure 2a, and the suitable labels in Figure 2b give two different faces in the N_2-embedding of $\mathbb{AG}(\mathcal{L}) - \{I_{k\ell}, I_{mn}\}$ that contains the vertices $N(I_{k\ell})$ and $N(I_{mn})$ so that $\tilde{\gamma}(\mathbb{AG}(\mathcal{L})) = 2$. Assume $|U_{(ij)^c}| \leq 2$. If $|U_{(ij)^c} \cup U_{(k\ell)^c}| \geq 4$, then the subgraph $\mathbb{AG}(\mathcal{L}) - \{I_{(k\ell)^c}, I'_{(k\ell)^c}, I_{mn}, (I_i, I_j), (I_1, I_{i'}), (I'_1, I_{i'})\}$ has a similar structure to G_{15} so that we have $\tilde{\gamma}(\mathbb{AG}(\mathcal{L})) \geq 3$. Additionally, by Theorem 4ii, $\mathbb{AG}(\mathcal{L})$ is projective when $|\bigcup_{i \neq 1} U_{(ij)^c}| \leq 1$. For all of the remaining cases, $\tilde{\gamma}(\mathbb{AG}(\mathcal{L})) = 2$ can be verified by drawing the N_2-

embedding.

Thus, $\tilde{\gamma}(\mathbb{AG}(\mathcal{L})) = 2$ when $2 \leq |\bigcup_{i \neq 1} U_{(ij)^c}| \leq 3$ with at least one of the sets' $U_{(ij)^c} = \emptyset$.

Suppose $|U_{k\ell}| = 1$ and $U_{mn} = \emptyset$ for $k, m \neq 1$ and $k\ell, mn \neq ij$. If $|U_{(ij)^c}| = 3$ and $U_{(k\ell)^c} \neq \emptyset$, then the subgraph $\mathbb{AG}(\mathcal{L}) - \{I_{(k\ell)^c}, I_{k\ell}, (I_i, I_j), (I_1, I_{i'}), (I'_1, I_{i'})\}$ has a similar structure to G_{18}, and, if $|U_{(ij)^c}| = |U_{(k\ell)^c}| = 2$, then the subgraph $\mathbb{AG}(\mathcal{L}) - \{I_{(k\ell)^c}, I'_{(k\ell)^c}, I_{k\ell}, (I_i, I_j), (I_1, I_{i'}), (I'_1, I_{i'})\}$ has a similar structure to G_{15} so that $\tilde{\gamma}(\mathbb{AG}(\mathcal{L})) \geq 3$. Further, $\mathbb{AG}(\mathcal{L})$ is projective if $|U_{(ij)^c} \cup U_{(k\ell)^c}| \leq 1$. Thus, $\tilde{\gamma}(\mathbb{AG}(\mathcal{L})) = 2$ whenever $|U_{(ij)^c} \cup U_{(k\ell)^c}| \in \{2, 3\}$.

Suppose $U_{k\ell}, U_{mn} = \emptyset$ for $k, m \neq 1$ and $k\ell, mn \neq ij$. Then, $\tilde{\gamma}(\mathbb{AG}(\mathcal{L})) = 2$ whenever $2 \leq |U_{(ij)^c}| \leq 3$.

Case 6 Let $|\bigcup_{n=1}^{4} U_n| = 4$. Then, by Theorem 4(i), $|U_{ij} \cup U_{(ij)^c}| \geq 3$ for some $U_{ij}, U_{(ij)^c} \neq \emptyset$. Further, if $|U_{ij} \cup U_{(ij)^c}| \geq 6$ with $U_{ij}, U_{(ij)^c} \neq \emptyset$, then the subgraph induced by the sets $X = U_i \cup U_j \cup U_{ij}$ and $Y = \bigcup_{k \neq i,j} U_k \cup U_{(ij)^c}$ contains one of the graph's $K_{3,7}$, $K_{4,6}$, or $K_{5,5}$ as a subgraph so that $\tilde{\gamma}(\mathbb{AG}(\mathcal{L})) \geq 3$. Therefore, $3 \leq |U_{ij} \cup U_{(ij)^c}| \leq 5$ for some $U_{ij}, U_{(ij)^c} \neq \emptyset$.

(i) Suppose $|U_{ij} \cup U_{(ij)^c}| = 5$ for $U_{ij}, U_{(ij)^c} \neq \emptyset$. If either $|U_{ij}| = 3$ or $|U_{(ij)^c}| = 3$, then the sets $X = U_i \cup U_j \cup U_{ij}$ and $Y = \bigcup_{k \neq i,j} U_k \cup U_{(ij)^c}$ form $K_{4,5}$, which is a contradiction. So, either $|U_{ij}| = 4$ or $|U_{(ij)^c}| = 4$. With no loss of generality, assume that $|U_{ij}| = 4$. If $U_{k\ell}, U_{(k\ell)^c} \neq \emptyset$ for $k\ell \neq ij, (ij)^c$, then clearly $|\{i,j\} \cap \{k,\ell\}| = 1$ and $|\{m,n\} \cap \{k,\ell\}| = 1$ where $m, n \in \{1, 2, 3, 4\} \setminus \{i, j\}$. So, let us take $\{i, j\} \cap \{k, \ell\} = \{j\}$ and $\{m, n\} \cap \{k, \ell\} = \{m\}$. This implies that $(I_{k\ell}, I_i), (I_{(k\ell)^c}, I_m) \in E(\mathbb{AG}(\mathcal{L}))$. Then, the subgraph $\mathbb{AG}(\mathcal{L}) - \{I_i, I_{k\ell}, I_{(k\ell)^c}\}$ contains $K_{5,3}$ with the partite sets $X = U_j \cup U_{ij}$ and $Y = U_m \cup U_n \cup U_{(ij)^c}$. Now, the path $I_i - I_{k\ell} - I_{(k\ell)^c}$ has to be embedded into a single face of any N_2-embedding of $K_{5,3}$. Further, the vertices I_i and $I_{(k\ell)^c}$ are adjacent to I_j and I_m. So, after embedding these four edges, the edge $(I_{k\ell}, I_n)$ cannot be embedded, which means $\tilde{\gamma}(\mathbb{AG}(\mathcal{L})) \geq 3$. Therefore, $U_{(k\ell)^c} = \emptyset$ when $U_{k\ell} \neq \emptyset$ for all $k\ell \neq ij, (ij)^c$, and, in such cases, $\tilde{\gamma}(\mathbb{AG}(\mathcal{L})) = 2$.

(ii) Suppose $|U_{ij} \cup U_{(ij)^c}| = 4$ for $U_{ij}, U_{(ij)^c} \neq \emptyset$. If $|U_{k\ell} \cup U_{(k\ell)^c}| \geq 3$ for $k\ell \neq ij$, then the subgraph $\mathbb{AG}(\mathcal{L}) - \{U_{k\ell} \cup U_{(k\ell)^c}\}$ contains a crosscap two graph $K_{5,3}$ or $K_{4,4}$ with the partite sets $X = U_i \cup U_j \cup U_{ij}$ and $Y = \bigcup_{m \neq i,j} U_m \cup U_{(ij)^c}$. Since $|U_{k\ell} \cup U_{(k\ell)^c}| \geq 3$, we can take $|U_{k\ell}| \geq 2$. Notice that the path $I_{k\ell} - I_{(k\ell)^c} - I'_{k\ell}$ together with the edges $(I_{k\ell}, I_m), (I_{k\ell}, I_i), (I'_{k\ell}, I_m)$, and $(I'_{k\ell}, I_i)$ should be embedded into a single face of an N_2-embedding of $K_{5,3}$. Thereafter, the face cannot adopt the edges $(I_{(k\ell)^c}, I_j)$ and $(I_{(k\ell)^c}, I_n)$ where $n \notin \{i, j, m\}$, which implies that $\tilde{\gamma}(\mathbb{AG}(\mathcal{L})) \geq 3$. Therefore, $|U_{k\ell} \cup U_{(k\ell)^c}| = 2$ for all $U_{k\ell}, U_{(k\ell)^c} \neq \emptyset$ with $k\ell \neq ij$ and $1 \leq i, j \leq 4$.

If $|U_{ij}| = 3$, then, by Figure 17a, we obtain $\tilde{\gamma}(\mathbb{AG}(\mathcal{L})) = 2$. If not, then $|U_{ij}| = 2$. Suppose $|U_{k\ell} \cup U_{(k\ell)^c}| = |U_{mn} \cup U_{(mn)^c}| = 2$ for $U_{k\ell}, U_{(k\ell)^c}, U_{mn}, U_{(mn)^c} \neq \emptyset$ with $k\ell, mn \neq ij$. Then, the subgraph $\mathbb{AG}(\mathcal{L}) - \{[I_{k\ell}, I_{(k\ell)^c}], [I_{mn}, I_{(mn)^c}]\}$ contains $K_{4,4}$ with the partite sets $X = U_i \cup U_j \cup U_{ij}$ and $Y = U_{i'} \cup U_{j'} \cup U_{(ij)^c}$, where $i', j' \notin \{i, j\}$. Note that every face of any N_2-embedding of $K_{4,4}$ is rectangular, and the vertices $[I_{k\ell}, I_{(k\ell)^c}]$ and $[I_{mn}, I_{(mn)^c}]$ are adjacent to the four vertices $I_i, I_j, I_{i'}$, and $I_{j'}$. So, to embed the vertices $[I_{k\ell}, I_{(k\ell)^c}]$ and $[I_{mn}, I_{(mn)^c}]$, two distinct rectangular faces with boundaries $I_i, I_j, I_{i'}$, and $I_{j'}$ are required, which is a contradiction. Therefore, at least one $U_{(k\ell)^c} = \emptyset$ when $U_{k\ell} \neq \emptyset$ for $k\ell \neq ij$ and $1 \leq i \neq j \leq 4$. In this case, an N_2-embedding of $\mathbb{AG}(\mathcal{L})$ is given in Figure 17b.

(iii) Suppose $2 \leq |U_{ij} \cup U_{(ij)^c}| \leq 3$ for all $U_{ij}, U_{(ij)^c} \neq \emptyset$ with $1 \leq i \neq j \leq 4$. Then, by Theorem 4i, there exists $U_{k\ell}$ such that $U_{k\ell}, U_{(k\ell)^c} \neq \emptyset$ with $|U_{k\ell} \cup U_{(k\ell)^c}| = 3$ and $\bigcup_{mn \neq k\ell, (k\ell)^c; U_{mn} \neq \emptyset} U_{(mn)^c} \neq \emptyset$.

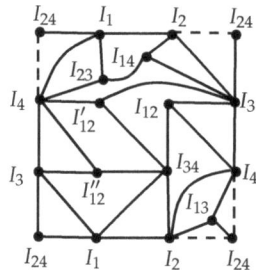
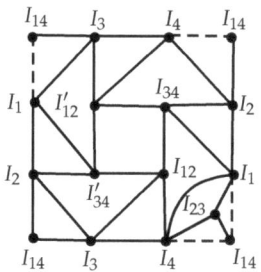

(**a**). $|U_{12}| = 3$ and $|U_{13} \cup U_{24}| = |U_{14} \cup U_{23}| = 2$ (**b**). $|U_{12}| = |U_{34}| = 2$ and $|U_{14} \cup U_{23}| = 2$

Figure 17. $|\bigcup_{n=1}^{4} U_n| = 4$ with $|U_{12} \cup U_{34}| = 4$.

Suppose $|U_{ij} \cup U_{(ij)^c}| = 3$ for all $1 \leq i \neq j \leq 4$. That is, $|U_{12} \cup U_{34}| = |U_{13} \cup U_{24}| = |U_{14} \cup U_{23}| = 3$. Without a loss of generality, we let $|U_{12}| = |U_{13}| = |U_{14}| = 2$. Now, consider the bipartite graph $G_{19} = \mathbb{AG}(\mathcal{L}) - \{(I_2, I_3), (I_2, I_4), (I_3, I_4), (I_2, I_{34}), (I_3, I_{24}), (I_4, I_{23})\}$ with the partite sets $X = U_1 \cup U_{12} \cup U_{13} \cup U_{14}$ and $Y = U_2 \cup U_3 \cup U_4 \cup U_{34} \cup U_{24} \cup U_{23}$. Note that $\tilde{\gamma}(G_{19}) = 2$ and the faces of any N_2-embedding of G_{19} have one of the following possibilities:

- Nine rectangular and two hexagonal faces;
- Ten rectangular faces and one octagonal face.

Since, in G_{19}, the only common neighbor for I_2 and I_{34} in X is I_1, no rectangular face has both I_2 and I_{34}. Therefore, the edge (I_2, I_{34}) should be embedded in a face of a length of more than four; so the edges are (I_3, I_{24}) and (I_4, I_{23}). Thus, we have to embed the three mutually disjoint edges of $\langle Y \rangle$ in either two hexagonal faces or one octagonal face. However, in any case, the faces may adopt at most two mutually disjoint edges of $\langle Y \rangle$, and, so, $\tilde{\gamma}(\mathbb{AG}(\mathcal{L})) \geq 3$. For the remaining cases, we have $\tilde{\gamma}(\mathbb{AG}(\mathcal{L})) = 2$. □

Remark 2. As an illustration, we consider the case (v)[a] in Theorem 5. Let $|U_1| = |U_2| = |U_3| = |U_4| = 1$ and $|U_{23}| = 4$. If $|U_{24}| = |U_{34}| = 1$, then the corresponding five-partite graph, as in Figure 18a, has a crosscap two. Additionally, if $|U_{24}| = 2$, then the crosscap of the corresponding five-partite graph, given in Figure 18b, is not equal to two. Moreover, the five-partite graph G in Figure 18b is minimal with respect to $\tilde{\gamma}(G) \neq 2$.

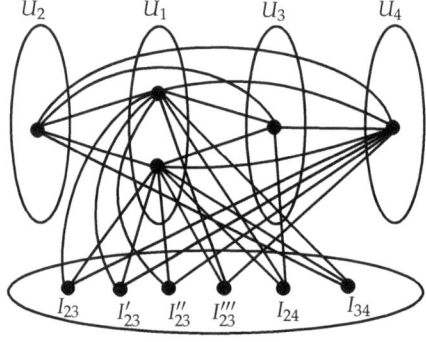
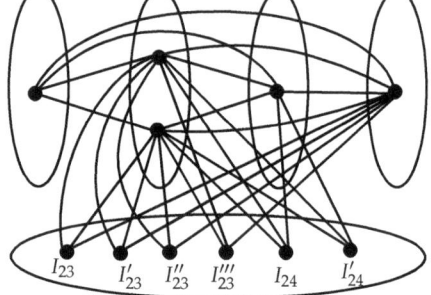

(**a**) A crosscap two 5-partite graph   (**b**) A minimal 5-partite graph with crosscap $\neq 2$

Figure 18. Five-partite graphs.

6. Conclusions

The forbidden subgraphs for a crosscap two surface (a Klein bottle) are not known yet. In this regard, an open problem will be to determine a family of graphs that has a crosscap number two. This paper provides a class of r-partite graphs, where $2 \leq r \leq 5$, that can be both embedded and not embedded in a crosscap two surface. This was completed by using the classification of all lattices with at most four atoms whose annihilating-ideal graph has a crosscap two.

Author Contributions: Conceptualization, T.A.; methodology, T.A.; investigation, K.M.; writing—original draft preparation, T.A. and K.M.; writing—review and editing, J.A.A.-B. and W.M.F.; project administration, J.A.A.-B.; funding acquisition, W.M.F. All authors have read and agreed to the published version of the manuscript.

Funding: This research project was funded by the Deanship of Scientific Research (DSR) at King Abdulaziz University, under grant no. KEP-44-130-42. The first, third, and fourth authors, therefore, acknowledge the DSR for its technical and financial support.

Institutional Review Board Statement: Not applicable.

Informed Consent Statement: Not applicable.

Acknowledgments: The The authors gratefully thank to the referees for the constructive comments and recommendations which definitely help to improve the readability of the paper.

Conflicts of Interest: The authors declare no conflict of interest.

References

1. Robertson, N.; Seymour, P. Graph minors. XX. Wagners conjecture. *J. Comb. Theory Ser. B* **2004**, *92*, 325–357. [CrossRef]
2. Kawarabayashi, K.; Mohar, B. Some recent progress and applications in graph minor theory. *Graphs Combin.* **2007**, *23*, 1–46. [CrossRef]
3. Thomassen, C. A simpler proof of the excluded minor theorem for higher surfaces. *J. Comb. Theory Ser. B* **1997**, *70*, 306–311. [CrossRef]
4. Archdeacon, D. A Kuratowski Theorem for the Projective Plane. Ph.D. Thesis, The Ohio State University, Columbus, OH, USA, 1980.
5. Glover, H.; Huneke, J.P.; Wang, C.S. 103 graphs that are irreducible for the projective plane. *J. Comb. Theory Ser. B* **1979**, *27*, 332–370. [CrossRef]
6. Beck, I. Coloring of commutative rings. *J. Algebra* **1988**, *116*, 208–226. [CrossRef]
7. Halaš, R.; Jukl, M. On Beck's coloring of posets. *Discrete Math.* **2009**, *309*, 4584–4589. [CrossRef]
8. Estaji, E.; Khashyarmanesh, K. The zero-divisor graph of a lattice. *Results Math.* **2012**, *61*, 1–11. [CrossRef]
9. Anderson, D.F.; Asir, T.; Tamizh Chelvam, T.; Badawi, A. *Graphs from Rings*, 1st ed.; Springer International Publishing: New York, NY, USA, 2021.
10. Behboodi, M.; Rakeei, Z. The annihilating-ideal graph of commutative rings I. *J. Algebra Appl.* **2011**, *10*, 727–739. [CrossRef]
11. Afkhami, M.; Bahrami, S.; Khashyarmanesh, K.; Shahsavar, F. The annihilating-ideal graph of a lattice. *Georgian Math. J.* **2016**, *23*, 1–7. [CrossRef]
12. Asir, T.; Mano, K. Classification of rings with crosscap two class of graphs. *Discrete Appl. Math.* **2019**, *256*, 13–21. [CrossRef]
13. Asir, T. The genus two class of graphs arising from rings. *J. Algebra Appl.* **2018**, *17*, 1850193. [CrossRef]
14. Asir, T.; Mano, K. Classification of non-local rings with genus two zero-divisor graphs. *Soft Comput.* **2020**, *24*, 237–245. [CrossRef]
15. Chiang-Hsieh, H.-J. Classification of rings with projective zero-divisor graphs. *J. Algebra.* **2008**, *319*, 2789–2802. [CrossRef]
16. Chiang-Hsieh, H.-J.; Smith, N.O.; Wang, H.-J. Commutative rings with toroidal zero-divisor graphs. *Houston J. Math.* **2010**, *36*, 1–31.
17. Pucanović, Z.S.; Petrović, Z.Z. Toroidality of intersection graphs of ideals of commutative rings. *Graphs Combin.* **2014**, *30*, 707–716. [CrossRef]
18. Smith, N.O. Planar zero-divisor graphs. *Int. J. Commut. Rings* **2003**, *2*, 177–188.
19. Shahsavar, F. On the planar and outer planar annihilating-ideal graphs of a lattice. *Algebras Groups Geom.* **2015**, *32*, 479–494.
20. Parsapour, A.; Ahmad Javaheri, K. The embedding of annihilating-ideal graphs associated to lattices in the projective plane. *Bull. Malays. Math. Sci. Soc.* **2019**, *42*, 1625–1638. [CrossRef]
21. Parsapour, A.; Ahmad Javaheri, K. When a line graph associated to annihilating-ideal graph of a lattice is planar or projective. *Czech. Math. J.* **2018**, *68*, 19–34. [CrossRef]
22. Parsapour, A.; Ahmad Javaheri, K. Line graphs associated to annihilating-ideal graph attached to lattices of genus one. *Trans. Comb.* **2023**, *12*, 175–190.

23. Nation, J.B. *Notes on Lattice Theory*; University of Hawaii: Honolulu, HI, USA, 1998; pp. 1–143.
24. Davey, B.A.; Priestley, H.A. *Introduction to Lattices and Order*; Cambridge University Press: Cambridge, MA, USA, 2002.
25. White, A.T. *Graphs, Groups and Surfaces*; Elsevier: Amsterdam, The Netherlands, 1973.
26. Ellingham, M.N.; Stephens, C.; Zhab, X. The nonorientable genus of complete tripartite graphs. *J. Comb. Theory Ser. B* **2006**, *96*, 529–559. [CrossRef]
27. Jungerman, M. The non-orientable genus of the symmetric quadripartite graph. *J. Comb. Theory Ser. B* **1979**, *26*, 154–158. [CrossRef]

Disclaimer/Publisher's Note: The statements, opinions and data contained in all publications are solely those of the individual author(s) and contributor(s) and not of MDPI and/or the editor(s). MDPI and/or the editor(s) disclaim responsibility for any injury to people or property resulting from any ideas, methods, instructions or products referred to in the content.

Article

On the Planarity of Graphs Associated with Symmetric and Pseudo Symmetric Numerical Semigroups

Yongsheng Rao [1], Muhammad Ahsan Binyamin [2,*], Adnan Aslam [3], Maria Mehtab [2] and Shazia Fazal [2]

[1] Institute of Computing Science and Technology, Guangzhou University, Guangzhou 510006, China
[2] Department of Mathematics, GC University, Faisalabad 38000, Pakistan
[3] Department of Natural Sciences and Humanities, University of Engineering and Technology, Lahore 54000, Pakistan
* Correspondence: ahsanbanyamin@gmail.com

Abstract: Let $S(m,e)$ be a class of numerical semigroups with multiplicity m and embedding dimension e. We call a graph G_S an $S(m,e)$-graph if there exists a numerical semigroup $S \in S(m,e)$ with $V(G_S) = \{x : x \in g(S)\}$ and $E(G_S) = \{xy \Leftrightarrow x + y \in S\}$, where $g(S)$ denotes the gap set of S. The aim of this article is to discuss the planarity of $S(m,e)$-graphs for some cases where S is an irreducible numerical semigroup.

Keywords: numerical semigroup; Frobenius number; genus; clique number; planarity

MSC: 05C25; 16U60

1. Introduction and Preliminaries

In the last couple of decades, researchers have been assigning graphs to various kinds of algebraic structures, which opens new horizons to study algebraic structures with the help of graphs' theoretic properties and vice versa. The first paper in this direction was the work by Beck [1], where he assigned a graph with the zero divisor elements of a commutative ring and called it a zero divisor graph. After that, many generalizations of this concept were provided by different researchers. Presently, assigning a graph to an algebraic object and studying the interplay between the properties of algebraic objects and with properties of the graph is an active area of research. The most studied concepts among these are the zero divisor graph [2], extended zero divisor graph [3], Cayley graph [4], nilpotent graphs [5], etc. Recently, Binyamin et al. [6] assigned a graph to the numerical semigroup and studied some properties of this graph. In a similar way, a graph is assigned to the ideal of a numerical semigroup by Binyamin et al. [7] who studied its metric dimension [8] and planarity [9].

Let $\mathbb{N}$ be the set of non-negative integers. A subset $S \subset \mathbb{N}$ is said to be numerical semigroup if $0 \in S$, $x + y \in S$ for all $x, y \in S$, and $\mathbb{N} \setminus S$ is finite. The least positive integer $x \in S$ is called the multiplicity of S and the set $\mathbb{N} \setminus S$ is called the gap set of S. We use the notations $m(S)$ and $g(S)$ to denote the multiplicity and gap set of S, respectively. The number of elements of $g(S)$ is called the genus of S. The largest integer that belongs to the set $g(S)$ is called the Frobenius number and is denoted by $F(S)$ or simply F. A numerical semigroup is said to be symmetric if for any $x \in \mathbb{N} \setminus S$, then $F - x \in S$. Similarly, a numerical semigroup is said to be pseudo symmetric if for any $x \in \mathbb{N} \setminus S$, either $F - x \in S$ or $x = \frac{F}{2}$. An important property of numerical semigroup is that it is always finitely generated and there exists a minimal system of generators of S. Let $x_1, x_2, \ldots, x_n$ be a minimal system of generators of S, then we write $S = \langle x_1, x_2, \ldots, x_n \rangle$. The number of elements in the minimal system of generators of S is called the embedding dimension of S and is denoted by $e(S)$. A numerical semigroup is called irreducible if it cannot be written as an intersection of two numerical semigroups containing it properly. It is well-known that an irreducible numerical semigroup is either symmetric or pseudo-symmetric [10]. To read more about the theory of numerical semigroups, the readers can see the book by [11].

Let G be a simple graph with the vertex set and edge set denoted by V and E, respectively. The degree of a vertex $x \in V$ is the number of edges incident to it. A graph is called complete if every pair of vertices has an edge between them. A complete graph on n vertices is denoted by K_n. A complete subgraph of a graph G is called clique and the clique of largest possible size in G is called a maximum clique of G. The number of vertices in the maximum clique of G is called clique number and is denoted by $cl(G)$. A graph G is called bipartite if its vertex set V can be partitioned into two sets, V_1 and V_2, and the edges are from elements of V_1 to the elements of V_2. If all the vertices of V_1 are adjacent to all vertices of V_2, then G is called a complete bipartite graph. If $\mid V_1 \mid = m$ and $\mid V_1 \mid = n$, $K_{m,n}$ denotes the complete bipartite graph. A graph is called planar if it can be embedded in a plane. In other words, a graph is planar if it can be drawn in a plane such that its edges intersect at end points (or no edges cross each other). A graph H is called minor of G if H can be formed by deleting edges and vertices and by contracting edges. The planarity of a graph can be checked using the famous Wagner's Theorem which states that a graph G is planar if and only if it contains neither K_5 nor $K_{3,3}$ as a graph minor [12].

We use the notation $S(m, e)$ to denote the class of numerical semigroups with multiplicity m and embedding dimension e. Following the idea of Binyamin et al. [6], a graph G can be assigned to any numerical semigroup S by considering the vertex set of G as the gap set $g(S)$ and any two vertices are adjacent if their sum belongs to S. In this work, we introduced the notion of $S(m, e)$ graph. We call a graph G_S an $S(m, e)$-graph if there exist a numerical semigroup $S \in S(m, e)$ with $V(G_S) = \{x : x \in g(S)\}$ and $E(G_S) = \{xy \Leftrightarrow x + y \in S\}$, where $g(S)$ denotes the gap set of S. Now, finding a closed subset of $g(S)$ is equivalent to finding a clique of graph G_S (which is very difficult to compute in general). In this article, we computed a clique of graph G_S of order 5 and as a consequence, we deduced that the graph G_S is non-planar. The aim of this article is to discuss the planarity of $S(m, e)$-graphs for some cases when S is an irreducible numerical semigroup.

2. Planarity of Graphs Associated with Numerical Semigroups of Embedding Dimension 2

In this section, we discuss the planarity of the graph G_S associated with the numerical semigroup $S \in S(m, 2)$. It is well-known that every numerical semigroup of embedding dimension 2 is symmetrical and for any $S \in S(m, 2)$, we have $\mid g(S) \mid = \frac{F+1}{2}$. We prove that if $\mid G_S \mid > 4$, then G_S is always non-planar. The following results can be immediately obtained from Theorem 1 [6].

Proposition 1 ([6]). *Every $S(m, e)$-graph for $m > 3$, is not a complete graph.*

Proposition 2 ([6]). *If $S(3,2)$-graph is complete then $G_S \cong K_3$ or K_4.*

Proposition 3 ([6]). *If $S(3,3)$-graph is complete then $G_S \cong K_2$ or K_3.*

Proposition 4 ([6]). *Every $S(2,2)$-graph is complete.*

Lemma 1. *Let G_S be a graph associated with $S = \langle m, b \rangle$. If $|G_S| > 4$, then one of the following conditions hold:*

1. *If $m = 3$ then $\{F, F-3, F-6, F-9, F-b\} \subseteq g(\langle m,b \rangle)$.*
2. *If $m \geq 4$ then $\{F, F-m, F-2m, F-b, F-(m+b)\} \subseteq g(\langle m,b \rangle)$.*

Proof. If $m = 3$ then clearly $0, 3, 6, 9, b \in S$, and therefore $F, F-3, F-6, F-9, F-b \notin S$. Furthermore, $|G_S| > 4$ gives $F \geq 11$ and $b \geq 7$. Please note that

$$F - b = b - 3.$$

This implies
$$F-3, F-6, F-9, F-b > 0,$$
and therefore
$$F, F-3, F-6, F-9, F-b \in g(\langle m, b \rangle).$$

Since $0, m, 2m, b, b+m \in S$, therefore, $F, F-m, F-2m, F-b, F-(m+b) \notin S$. Also
$$F - m = mb - b - 2m = (m-1)b - 2m,$$
$$F - 2m = mb - b - 3m = (m-1)b - 3m,$$
$$F - b = mb - m - 2b = (m-2)b - m,$$
and
$$F - (m+b) = mb - 2m - 2b = (m-2)b - 2m.$$

If $m \geq 4$, then clearly
$$F - m, F - 2m, F - b, F - (m+b) > 0.$$

This implies
$$F, F-m, F-2m, F-b, F-(m+b) \in g(\langle m, b \rangle).$$

□

Theorem 1. *Let G_S be an $S(m, 2)$-graph, where $m \geq 2$. If $|G_S| > 4$ then $cl(G_S) \geq 5$.*

Proof. We may assume that $S = <m, b>$. If $m = 2$ then from Proposition 4, we have $G_S \cong K_n$ with $n \geq 5$, as $|G_S| > 4$. This gives $cl(G_S) \geq 5$ in this case.
Now if $m = 3$ then from Lemma 1, we have
$$\{F, F-3, F-6, F-9, F-b\} \subseteq g(\langle m, b \rangle).$$

Clearly $2F - 3, 2F - 6, 2F - 9, 2F - b \in S$. Now we need to show
$$2F - 12, 2F - 15, 2F - (3+b), 2F - (6+b), 2F - (9+b) \in S.$$

Since $|G_S| > 4$ therefore $F \geq 11$ and $b \geq 7$. Please note that
$$F - (2F - 12) = 12 - F \notin S,$$
$$F - (2F - 15) = 15 - F \notin S,$$
$$F - (2F - (3+b)) = (3+b) - F = 3 - (F - b) \notin S,$$
$$F - (2F - (6+b)) = (6+b) - F = 9 - b \notin S,$$
$$F - (2F - (9+b)) = (6+b) - F = 12 - b \notin S.$$

This gives
$$2F - 12, 2F - 15, 2F - (3+b), 2F - (6+b), 2F - (9+b) \in S,$$
and therefore $cl(G_S) \geq 5$ (see Figure 1).

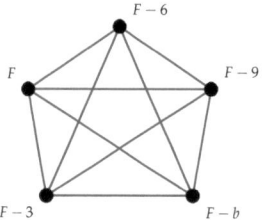

Figure 1. Minimum possible clique for the case $m = 3$.

If $m \geq 4$ then again from Lemma 1, we have

$$\{F, F - m, F - 2m, F - b, F - (m + b)\} \subseteq g(\langle m, b \rangle).$$

Clearly, $2F - m, 2F - 2m, 2F - b, 2F - (m + b) \in S$. Please note that

$$F - (2F - 3m) = 3m - F = m - (F - 2m) \notin S,$$

$$F - (2F - (2m + b)) = 2m + b - F = m - (F - (m + b)) \notin S,$$

$$F - (2F - (3m + b)) = 3m + b - F.$$

This implies $3m + b - F = 4m + (2 - m)b$ or $3m + b - F = (4 - b)m + 2b$. Since $4 \leq m < b$, therefore, both possibilities give $3m + b - F \notin S$. Furthermore,

$$F - (2F - (m + 2b)) = m + 2b - F.$$

We have either $m + 2b - F = 2m + (3 - m)b$ or $3m + b - F = (2 - b)m + 3b$. Again $4 \leq m < b$, give $m + 2b - F \notin S$. This implies

$$2F - 3m, 2F - (2m + b), 2F - (3m + b), 2F - (m + 2b) \in S.$$

Consequently, we obtain $cl(G_S) \geq 5$ (see Figure 2). □

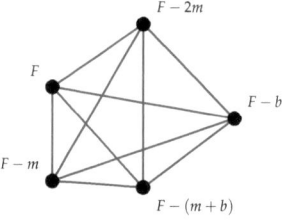

Figure 2. Minimum possible clique for the case $m \geq 4$.

Corollary 1. *For $m \geq 2$, every $S(m, 2)$-graph, whose order is greater than 4 is non-planar.*

3. Planarity of Graphs Associated with Irreducible Numerical Semigroups of Maximal Embedding Dimension

A numerical semigroup S is said to have a maximal embedding dimension if its multiplicity and embedding dimension are the same. It is proved in [10] that a numerical semigroup of maximal embedding dimension is irreducible if its embedding dimension is either 2 or 3. In this section, we discuss the planarity of the graph G_S in the case $S \in S(3,3)$.

Lemma 2. *Let $S = \langle 3, 3 + x, 3 + 2x \rangle$, where x is not a multiple of 3. If $|g(S)| > 6$, then*

$$\{F, F - 3, F - 6, F - 9, \frac{F}{2}\} \subseteq g(S).$$

Proof. Please note that $x > 5$ and $F > 10$, as $|g(S)| > 6$. This implies $F - 3, F - 6, F - 9 > 0$. Since S is pseudo symmetric and $3, 6, 9 \in S$, therefore,

$$\{F, F - 3, F - 6, F - 9, \frac{F}{2}\} \subseteq g(S).$$

□

Theorem 2. *Let G_S be an $S(m, e)$-graph, where S is an irreducible numerical semigroup of maximal embedding dimension. If $|G_S| > 4$ then $cl(G_S) \geq 4$.*

Proof. Since S is an irreducible numerical semigroup of maximal embedding dimension, then from Proposition 6 of [10], it follows that either $m = 2 = e$ or $m = 3 = e$. If $m = 2 = e$, then from Proposition 4, it follows that $cl(G_S) \geq 5$. Now if $m = 3 = e$, then from Proposition 7 of [10], we have $S = \langle 3, 3 + x, 3 + 2x \rangle$, where x is not a multiple of 3.

If $|G_S| = 5$ then $x = 4$. This implies $S = \langle 3, 7, 11 \rangle$ and $g(S) = \{1, 2, 4, 5, 8\}$ such that $1 + 4 \notin S$ and

$$2 + 4, 2 + 5, 2 + 8, 4 + 5, 4 + 8, 5 + 8 \in S.$$

This gives $cl(G_S) = 4$. Similarly, If $|G_S| = 6$ then $x = 5$, therefore, $S = \langle 3, 8, 13 \rangle$ and $g(S) = \{1, 2, 4, 5, 7, 10\}$. Clearly $cl(G_S) = 4$.
Now if $|G_S| > 6$ then from Lemma 2, we have

$$\{F, F - 3, F - 6, F - 9, \frac{F}{2}\} \subseteq g(S).$$

Clearly, $2F - 3, 2F - 6, 2F - 9, \frac{3F}{2} \in S$. Now we show that $2F - 9, 2F - 12, \frac{3F}{2} - 3, 2F - 15, \frac{3F}{2} - 6, \frac{3F}{2} - 9 \in S$. This is easy to see that none of $2F - 9, 2F - 12, \frac{3F}{2} - 3, 2F - 15, \frac{3F}{2} - 6$ and $\frac{3F}{2} - 9$ is equal to $\frac{F}{2}$. Please note that

$$F - (2F - 9) = 9 - F = 3 - (F - 6),$$

$$F - (2F - 12) = 12 - F = 3 - (F - 9),$$

$$F - (2F - 15) = 15 - F,$$

$$F - (\frac{3F}{2} - 3) = 3 - \frac{F}{2},$$

$$F - (\frac{3F}{2} - 6) = 6 - \frac{F}{2}$$

and

$$F - (\frac{3F}{2} - 9) = 9 - \frac{F}{2}.$$

Since $F - 6, F - 9, \frac{F}{2} \in g(S)$, therefore, $9 - F, 12 - F, 3 - \frac{F}{2} \notin S$. Furthermore, since $F \geq 14$, therefore, $15 - F, 6 - \frac{F}{2}, 9 - \frac{F}{2} \notin S$. This implies $cl(G_S) \geq 5$ (see Figure 3). □

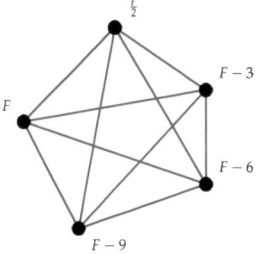

Figure 3. Minimum possible clique for the case $m = e = 3$ and $|G_S| > 6$.

Corollary 2. *Let G_S be an $S(m,e)$-graph, where S is an irreducible numerical semigroup of maximal embedding dimension. If $|G_S| > 5$ then G_S is non-planar.*

Proof. If $m = 2 = e$, then the result follows immediately from Theorem 1. If $m = 3 = e$, then $S = <3, x+3, 2x+3>$ and $F = 2x$. Now, if $|G_S| = 6$ then $x = 5$ and therefore $S = <3, 8, 13>$. This implies $cl(G_S) = 4$ (see Figure 4). By contraction of $e_4 e_5$ and by removing multiple edges, we obtain the minor of G_S isomorphic to K_5 (see Figure 5). Now if $|G_S| > 6$ then from Theorem 2 it follows that $cl(G_S) \geq 5$. Hence G_S is non-planar. □

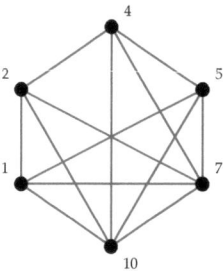

Figure 4. Graph G_S for $S = <3, 8, 13>$.

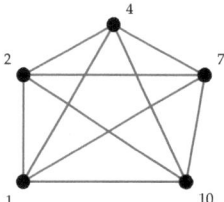

Figure 5. Minor of G_S for $S = <3, 8, 13>$.

4. Planarity of Graphs Associated with Irreducible Numerical Semigroups of Arbitrary Embedding Dimension

In this section, we discuss the planarity of different classes of irreducible numerical semigroups of arbitrary embedding dimensions.

Lemma 3. *Let G_S be an $S(m,e)$-graph, where $S = \langle m, m+1, qm+2q+2, \ldots, qm+(m-1) \rangle$ with $m \geq 2q+3$, $e = m-2q$ and $q \geq 1$. Then,*

$$\{F, F - m, F - (m+1), F - (2m+1), F - (qm+2q+2)\} \subseteq g(S).$$

Proof. Since $0, m, m+1, 2m+1, qm+2q+2 \in S$, therefore, $F, F-m, F-(m+1), F-(2m+1), F-(qm+2q+2) \notin S$. From Lemma 1 of [13], it follows that S is symmetric and $F = 2qm+2q+1$. Please note that

$$F = 2qm + 2q + 1 = (m+1) + (2q-1)m + 2q.$$

Since $q \geq 1$, therefore, $F > m+1$. This implies $F-m, F-(m+1) > 0$ and therefore $F-m, F-(m+1) \in g(S)$. Now consider

$$F - (2m+1) = 2qm + 2q + 1 - 2m - 1 = (2q-2)m + 2q > 0,$$

$$F - (qm+2q+2) = 2qm + 2q + 1 - qm - 2q - 2 = qm - 1 > 0.$$

This gives $F - (2m+1), F - (qm+2q+2) \in g(S)$. Consequently, we obtain the required result. □

Theorem 3. Let G_S be an $S(m,e)$-graph, where $S = \langle m, m+1, qm+2q+2, \ldots, qm+(m-1) \rangle$ with $m \geq 2q+3$, $e = m-2q$ and $q \geq 1$. Then, G_S is nonplanar.

Proof. From Lemma 3, we have

$$\{F, F-m, F-(m+1), F-(2m+1), F-(qm+2q+2)\} \subseteq g(S).$$

Clearly $2F-m, 2F-(m+1), 2F-(2m+1), 2F-(qm+2q+2) \in S$. We need to show $2F-(3m+1), 2F-(3m+2), 2F-((q+1)m+2q+2), 2F-((q+1)m+2q+3), 2F-((q+2)m+2q+3) \in S$. For this, we consider

$$F-(2F-(3m+1)) = (3m+1) - F = m - (F-(2m+1)) \notin S,$$

$$F-(2F-(3m+2)) = (3m+2) - F = (3-2q)m - (2q-1).$$

For $q = 1$, we have $F-(2F-(3m+2)) = m-1$ and for $q > 1$, $F-(2F-(3m+2)) < 0$. Both cases give $F-(2F-(3m+2)) \notin S$.

$$F-(2F-((q+1)m+2q+2)) = ((q+1)m+2q+2) - F,$$

$$= m - (F-(qm+2q+2)) \notin S.$$

$$F-(2F-((q+1)m+2q+3)) = ((q+1)m+2q+3) - F,$$

$$= (1-q)m + 2 \notin S.$$

$$F-(2F-((q+2)m+2q+3)) = ((q+2)m+2q+3) - F = (2-q)m + 2.$$

For $q = 1$, we have $F-(2F-((q+2)m+2q+3)) = m+2$, for $q = 2$, we have $F-(2F-((q+2)m+2q+3)) = 2$ and for $q > 2$, $F-(2F-((q+2)m+2q+3)) < 0$. All three cases give $F-(2F-((q+2)m+2q+3)) \notin S$. This implies $cl(G_S) \geq 5$ and consequently G_S is non-planar (see Figure 6). □

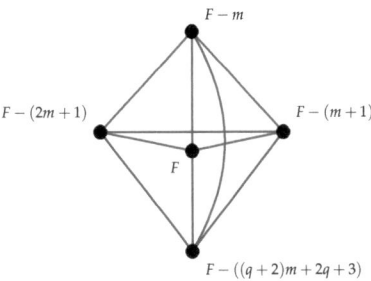

Figure 6. Minimum possible clique for the case $m \geq 2q+3$, $e = m-2q$ and $q \geq 1$.

Lemma 4. Let G_S be an $S(m,e)$-graph, where $S = \langle m, m+1, (q+1)m+q+2, \ldots, (q+1)m+m-q-2 \rangle$ with $m \geq 2q+4$, $e = m-2q-1$ and $q \geq 0$.
1. If $q = 0$ and $|G_S| > 6$, then $\{F, F-m, F-(m+1), F-(m+2), F-(m+3)\} \subseteq g(S)$.
2. If $q > 0$ then $\{F, F-m, F-2m, F-(m+1), F-(2m+1)\} \subseteq g(S)$.

Proof. Since $0, m, m+1, m+2, m+3, 2m, 2m+1 \in S$, therefore, $F, F-m, F-2m, F-(m+1), F-(m+2), F-(m+3), F-(2m+1) \notin S$. From Lemma 3 of [13], it follows that S is symmetric and $F = 2(q+1)m - 1$.

If $q = 0$ and $|G_S| > 6$ then $F = 2m-1$ with $m > 6$. Please note that $F - m = m-1 > 0$, $F-(m+1) = m-2 > 0$, $F-(m+2) = m-3 > 0$ and $F-(m+3) = m-4 > 0$. This implies

$$\{F, F-m, F-(m+1), F-(m+2), F-(m+3)\} \subseteq g(S).$$

Now if $q > 0$, then $F \geq 4m - 1$ with $m \geq 6$. We have $F - m \geq 3m - 1 > 0$, $F - 2m \geq 2m - 1 > 0$, $F - (m+1) \geq 3m - 2 > 0$ and $F - (2m+1) \geq 2m - 2 > 0$. This gives

$$\{F, F - m, F - 2m, F - (m+1), F - (2m+1)\} \subseteq g(S).$$

□

Theorem 4. *Let G_S be an $S(m,e)$-graph, where $S = \langle m, m+1, (q+1)m + q + 2, \ldots, (q+1)m + m - q - 2 \rangle$ with $m \geq 2q + 4$, $e = m - 2q - 1$ and $q \geq 0$.*
1. *If $q = 0$ and $|G_S| > 6$, then G_S is non-planar.*
2. *If $q > 0$, then G_S is non-planar.*

Proof. If $q = 0$ and $|G_S| > 6$, then from Lemma 4, it follows that

$$\{F, F - m, F - (m+1), F - (m+2), F - (m+3)\} \subseteq g(S).$$

Clearly, $2F - m, 2F - (m+1), 2F - (m+2), 2F - (m+3) \in S$. Also

$$F - (2F - (2m+1)) = 2m + 1 - F = m - (F - (m+1)) \notin S.$$
$$F - (2F - (2m+2)) = 2m + 2 - F = m - (F - (m+2)) \notin S.$$
$$F - (2F - (2m+3)) = 2m + 3 - F = m - (F - (m+3)) \notin S.$$
$$F - (2F - (2m+4)) = 2m + 4 - F = 5 \notin S.$$
$$F - (2F - (2m+5)) = 2m + 5 - F = 6 \notin S.$$

Now if $q > 0$, then again from Lemma 4, we have

$$\{F, F - m, F - 2m, F - (m+1), F - (2m+1)\} \subseteq g(S).$$

Clearly, $2F - m, 2F - 2m, 2F - (m+1), 2F - (2m+1) \in S$. We have to show $2F - 3m, 2F - (3m+1), 2F - (4m+1), 2F - (3m+2) \in S$. For this, we consider

$$F - (2F - 3m) = 3m - F = m - (F - 2m) \notin S.$$
$$F - (2F - (3m+1)) = 3m + 1 - F = m - (F - (2m+1)) \notin S.$$
$$F - (2F - (4m+1)) = 4m + 1 - F = m - 2((1-q)m + 1) \notin S.$$
$$F - (2F - (3m+2)) = 3m + 2 - F = m - 2(1-q)m + 3 \notin S.$$

Both cases implies $cl(G_S) \geq 5$, therefore, G_S is non-planar (see Figures 7 and 8). □

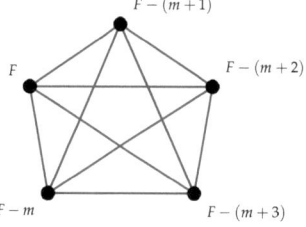

Figure 7. Minimum possible clique for the case $m \geq 2q + 4$, $e = m - 2q - 1$ and $q = 0$.

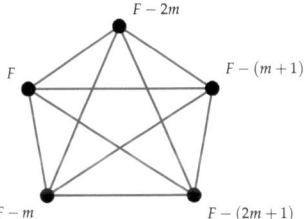

Figure 8. Minimum possible clique for the case $m \geq 2q+4$, $e = m-2q-1$ and $q > 0$.

Lemma 5. *Let G_S be an $S(m,e)$-graph, where $S = \langle m, m+1, (q+1)m+q+2, \ldots, (q+1)m+m-q-3, (q+1)m+(m-1) \rangle$ with $m \geq 2q+5$, $e = m-2q-1$ and $q \geq 0$. Then,*

$$\{F, \frac{F}{2}, F-m, F-(m+1), F-((q+1)m+q+2)\} \subseteq g(S).$$

Proof. Since $m, m+1, (q+1)m+q+2 \in S$, therefore, $F-m, F-(m+1), F-((q+1)m+q+2) \notin S$. From Lemma 2 of [14], it follows that S is pseudo-symmetric and $F = 2(q+1)m-2$. This implies

$$F - m = (2q+1)m - 2 > 0.$$
$$F - (m+1) = (2q+1)m - 3 > 0.$$
$$F - ((q+1)m+q+2) = (q+1)m - (q+4) > 0,$$

since $m \geq 2q+5$. This gives

$$\{F, \frac{F}{2}, F-m, F-(m+1), F-((q+1)m+q+2)\} \subseteq g(S).$$

□

Theorem 5. *Let G_S be an $S(m,e)$-graph, where $S = \langle m, m+1, (q+1)m+q+2, \ldots, (q+1)m+m-q-3, (q+1)m+(m-1) \rangle$ with $m \geq 2q+5$, $e = m-2q-1$ and $q \geq 0$. If $m \geq 6$ then G_S is non-planar.*

Proof. From Lemma 5, we have

$$\{F, \frac{F}{2}, F-m, F-(m+1), F-((q+1)m+q+2)\} \subseteq g(S).$$

Then $\frac{3F}{2}, 2F-m, 2F-(m+1), 2F-((q+1)m+q+2) \in S$. Now consider

$$F - (\frac{3F}{2} - m) = m - \frac{F}{2} \notin S.$$

$$F - (\frac{3F}{2} - (m+1)) = m+1 - \frac{F}{2} = 2 - qm \notin S.$$

$$F - (\frac{3F}{2} - ((q+1)m+q+2)) = (q+1)m+q+2 - \frac{F}{2} = q+3 \notin S,$$

since $q+3 < m$.

$$F - (2F - (m+1)) = 2m+1 - F = m - (F-(m+1)) \notin S.$$

$$F - (2F - ((q+2)m+q+2)) = (q+2)m+q+2 - F = (1-m)q + 4 \notin S.$$

$$F - (2F - ((q+2)m+q+3)) = (q+2)m+q+3 - F = (1-m)q + 5 \notin S.$$

This implies $cl(G_S) \geq 5$ and therefore G_S is non-planar (see Figure 9). □

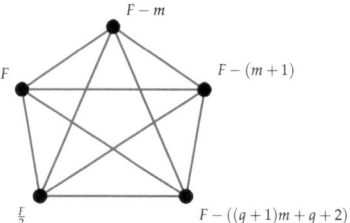

Figure 9. Minimum possible clique for the case $m \geq 2q + 5$, $e = m - 2q - 1$ and $q \geq 0$.

Lemma 6. *Let G_S be an $S(m,e)$-graph, where $S = \langle m, m+1, qm+2q+3, \ldots, qm+m-1, (q+1)m+q+2 \rangle$ with $m \geq 2q+4$, $e = m - 2q$ and $q \geq 1$. Then,*

$$\{F, \frac{F}{2}, F-m, F-(m+1), F-2m\} \subseteq g(S).$$

Proof. Since $m, m+1, 2m \in S$, therefore, $F-m, F-(m+1), F-2m \notin S$. From Lemma 4 of [14], it follows that S is pseudo-symmetric and $F = 2qm + 2q + 2$. This implies

$$F - m = (2q-1)m + q + 2 > 0.$$
$$F - (m+1) = (2q-1)m + q + 1 > 0.$$
$$F - 2m = (2q-2)m + q + 2 > 0.$$

This gives

$$\{F, \frac{F}{2}, F-m, F-(m+1), F-2m\} \subseteq g(S).$$

□

Theorem 6. *Let G_S be an $S(m,e)$-graph, where $S = \langle m, m+1, qm+2q+3, \ldots, qm+m-1, (q+1)m+q+2 \rangle$ with $m \geq 2q+4$, $e = m - 2q$ and $q \geq 1$. Then,*

$$\{F, \frac{F}{2}, F-m, F-(m+1), F-2m\} \subseteq g(S).$$

Proof. From Lemma 6, it follows that

$$\{F, \frac{F}{2}, F-m, F-(m+1), F-2m\} \subseteq g(S).$$

Note that $\frac{3F}{2}, 2F-m, 2F-2m, 2F-(m+1) \in S$. Now consider

$$F - (\frac{3F}{2} - m) = m - \frac{F}{2} \notin S.$$

$$F - (\frac{3F}{2} - 2m) = 2m - \frac{F}{2} = (2-q)m - (q+1) \notin S,$$

$$F - (\frac{3F}{2} - (m+1)) = m + 1 - \frac{F}{2} = (1-q)m - q \notin S,$$

since $m > q + 1$.

$$F - (2F - 3m) = 3m - F = m - (F - 2m) \notin S.$$
$$F - (2F - (2m+1)) = 2m + 1 - F = m - (F - (m+1)) \notin S.$$
$$F - (2F - (3m+1)) = 3m + 1 - F = (3-2q)m - (2q+1) \notin S,$$

since $m > 2q + 1$. This gives $cl(G_S) \geq 5$ and hence G_S is non-planar (see Figure 10). □

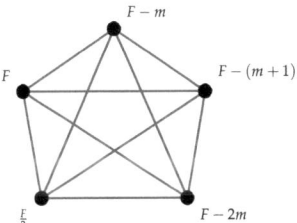

Figure 10. Minimum possible clique for the case $m \geq 2q+4$, $e = m - 2q$ and $q \geq 1$.

5. Conclusions

Numerical semigroups have applications in many fields. One of the important applications of a numerical semigroup is in finding the non-negative solutions of linear diophantine equations. Following the idea of Binyamin et al. [6], we introduced the concept of $S(m,e)$ graph. In this work, we discussed the planarity of $S(m,e)$-graphs in the case when the numerical semigroup is either symmetric or pseudo-symmetric. To answer the planarity of any general $S(m,e)$ graph is still an open problem.

Author Contributions: Conceptualization, M.A.B.; Methodology, Y.R., M.A.B., A.A. and S.F.; Validation, Y.R., M.A.B., A.A., M.M. and S.F.; Formal analysis, Y.R., M.A.B., M.M. and S.F.; Investigation, Y.R., A.A., M.M. and S.F.; Writing—original draft, M.A.B., M.M. and S.F.; Writing—review & editing, A.A. All authors have read and agreed to the published version of the manuscript.

Funding: This work was supported by the National Natural Science Foundation of China (No. 62172116) and the Natural Science Research Projects of Department of Education of Guizhou Province (No. QianJiaoHe KY[2021]250).

Data Availability Statement: Not applicable.

Conflicts of Interest: The authors declare no conflict of interest.

References

1. Beck, I. Coloring of commutative rings. *J. Algebra* **1988**, *116*, 208–226. [CrossRef]
2. Anderson, D.F.; Livingston, P.S. The Zero-Divisor Graph of a Commutative Ring. *J. Algebra* **1999**, *217*, 434–447. [CrossRef]
3. Bakhtyiari, M.; Nikmehr, M.J.; Nikandish, R. The extended zero-divisor graph of a commutative ring I. *Hokkaido Math. J.* **2017**, *46*, 381–393. [CrossRef]
4. Meier, J. *Groups Graphs and Trees: An Introduction to the Geometry of Infinite Groups*; Cambridge University Press: Cambridge, UK, 2008.
5. Kumar, B.D.; Ajay, S.; Rahul, D. Nilpotent Graph. *Theory Appl. Graphs* **2021**, *8*, 2.
6. Binyamin, M.A.; Siddiqui, H.M.A.; Khan, N.M.; Aslam, A.; Rao, Y. Characterization of graphs associated with numerical semigroups. *Mathematics* **2019**, *7*, 557. [CrossRef]
7. Xu, P.; Binyamin, M.A.; Aslam, A.; Ali, W.; Mahmood, H.; Zhou, H. Characterization of graphs associated with the ideal of numerical semigroups. *J. Math.* **2020**, *2020*, 60944372. [CrossRef]
8. Wang, Y.; Binyamin, M.A.; Ali, W.; Aslam, A.; Rao, Y. Graphs associated with the ideals of a Numerical Semigroup having metric dimension 2. *Math. Probl. Eng.* **2021**, *2021*, 6697980. [CrossRef]
9. Binyamin, M.A.; Ali, W.; Aslam, A.; Mahmood, H. A complete classification of planar graphs associated with the ideal of the numerical semigroup. *Iran. J. Sci. Technol. Transection Sci.* **2022**, *46*, 491–498. [CrossRef]
10. Rosales, J.C.; Branco, M.B. Irreducible numerical seimgroups. *Pac. J. Math.* **2003**, *209*, 131–143. [CrossRef]
11. Rosales, J.C.; Garcia-Sanchez, P.A. Numerical Semigroups. In *Developments in Mathematics*; Springer: New York, NY, USA, 2009; Volume 20. [CrossRef]
12. Bondy, A.; Murty, U.S.R. Graph Theory. In *Graduate Texts in Mathematics*, 1st ed.; Springer: London, UK, 2008; Volume XII, p. 663.
13. Rosales, J.C. Symmetric numerical semigroups with arbitrary multiplicity and embedding dimension. *Proc. Am. Math. Soc.* **2001**, *129*, 2197–2203. [CrossRef]
14. Rosales, J.C.; Branco, M.B. Irreducible numerical semigroups with arbitrary multiplicity and embedding dimension. *J. Algebra* **2003**, *264*, 305–315. [CrossRef]

Disclaimer/Publisher's Note: The statements, opinions and data contained in all publications are solely those of the individual author(s) and contributor(s) and not of MDPI and/or the editor(s). MDPI and/or the editor(s) disclaim responsibility for any injury to people or property resulting from any ideas, methods, instructions or products referred to in the content.

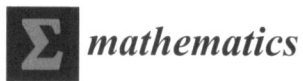

Article

On the Independence Number of Cayley Digraphs of Clifford Semigroups

Krittawit Limkul [1] and Sayan Panma [2,*]

[1] Doctoral Program in Mathematics, Graduate School, Chiang Mai University, Chiang Mai 50200, Thailand; krittawit_lim@cmu.ac.th
[2] Department of Mathematics, Faculty of Science, Chiang Mai University, Chiang Mai 50200, Thailand
* Correspondence: sayan.panma@cmu.ac.th

Abstract: Let S be a Clifford semigroup and A a subset of S. We write $Cay(S, A)$ for the Cayley digraph of a Clifford semigroup S relative to A. The (weak, path, weak path) independence number of a graph is the maximum cardinality of an (weakly, path, weakly path) independent set of vertices in the graph. In this paper, we characterize maximal connected subdigraphs of $Cay(S, A)$ and apply these results to determine the (weak, path, weak path) independence number of $Cay(S, A)$.

Keywords: Cayley digraph; Clifford semigroup; independent set; independence number

MSC: 05C69; 05C25

Citation: Limkul, K.; Panma, S. On the Independence Number of Cayley Digraphs of Clifford Semigroups. *Mathematics* **2023**, *11*, 3445. https://doi.org/10.3390/math11163445

Academic Editors: Irina Cristea and Alessandro Linzi

Received: 2 July 2023
Revised: 3 August 2023
Accepted: 6 August 2023
Published: 8 August 2023

Copyright: © 2023 by the authors. Licensee MDPI, Basel, Switzerland. This article is an open access article distributed under the terms and conditions of the Creative Commons Attribution (CC BY) license (https://creativecommons.org/licenses/by/4.0/).

1. Introduction

In algebraic graph theory, Cayley graphs are an important concept relating semigroup theory and graph theory. One of the appealing subjects in the study of Cayley graphs of semigroups is considering how to apply the results obtained from the Cayley graphs of groups to the case of semigroups.

Let S be a semigroup and A a subset of S. The *Cayley digraph* $Cay(S, A)$ of a semigroup S relative to A (which is simply called Cayley graph) is defined as the digraph with the vertex set S, and the arc set $E(Cay(S, A))$ consisting of those ordered pairs (x, y) such that $y = xa$ for some $a \in A$, i.e., $E(Cay(S, A)) = \{(x, xa) | x \in S, a \in A\}$.

The motivation for considering Clifford semigroups lies in their unique and intriguing algebraic properties; Clifford semigroups represent one of the important types of semigroups, which are a union of groups. These semigroups serve as a natural bridge between the worlds of semigroups and groups, providing an avenue to explore the interplay between these two fundamental algebraic structures. Consequently, it can be inferred that the Cayley digraphs of Clifford semigroups contain the Cayley digraphs of groups.

Investigating the Cayley digraph can yield valuable insights into network optimization and communication protocols. In [1] Heydemann has undertaken a comprehensive examination of diverse classes of Cayley graphs of groups, which have been subject to extensive scrutiny as models for interconnection networks. It subsequently presents a detailed analysis of outcomes and issues pertaining to network routings, with a particular focus on evaluating the loads of nodes and links during the routing processes. Xiao and Parhami [2] explored the Cayley digraphs of groups and their coset graphs concerning subgroups, deriving general results on homomorphisms and broadcasting. Additionally, practical applications were discussed in well-known interconnection networks such as butterfly network, de Bruijn network, cube-connected cycles network, and shuffle-exchange network. Consequently, these results can be effectively applied to the Cayley digraph of Clifford semigroups by specifying a certain collection of groups.

Numerous papers have undertaken the study of characterizations concerning the Cayley graphs of different types of semigroups (see [3–6] and their references). Notably, specific conditions delineating the characteristics of Cayley graphs of Clifford semigroups have been provided in reference [7]. Recently, Ilić-Georgijević [8] focused on presenting conditions that precisely characterize the Cayley graphs of a particular group known as homogeneous semigroups. It is important to highlight that this class encompasses, among others, the category of Clifford semigroups.

The independence number is a graph parameter that measures the size of the largest vertex set in a graph that induces no edge. There have been many research topics on the independence numbers of graphs and digraphs. The independence number of finite connected simple graphs was studied by Harant and Schiermeyer [9,10]. They gave lower bounds of the independence number in terms of the order, size and degrees. In [11], Löwenstein et al. proved several tight lower bounds of the order and average degree for the independence number of connected graphs. Some results on the upper and lower bounds of the independence number of graphs have been obtained by many authors (see for examples, refs. [12–17]). In their work [18], The authors presented the zero forcing number for specific classes of graphs and digraphs. It is worth noting that in certain classes of digraphs, such as cycles or trees, we observed that the zero forcing number is less than or equal to the independence number. As a result, the zero forcing set demonstrates a relationship with the independent set.

The independent sets are interesting topics in the study of Cayley digraphs. In [19], Panma and Nupo studied independent sets and some generalizations of independent sets such as weakly independent, path independent, and weakly path independent sets in Cayley digraphs of rectangular groups. They gave lower and upper bounds for the independence, weak independence, path independence, and weak path independence numbers by using some algebraic properties of groups.

It is natural to investigate the Cayley digraph of Clifford semigroups and consider how the results from the group case exist. The purpose of this work is to find the independence, weak independence, path independence, and weak path independence numbers of Cayley digraphs of Clifford semigroups by using the properties of groups.

In order to attain these results, our approach initiates with an exploration of the independent sets of small size within the Cayley digraph of the Clifford semigroup. It is noteworthy that the independence number of a graph can be expressed as the summation of the independence numbers of its maximal connected subdigraphs. Building upon this fundamental fact, we progress to the second step, which involves a dedicated focus on characterizing a maximal connected subdigraph of the Cayley digraph (Section 3).

Subsequently, we determine the independence number of the Cayley graphs (Section 4) and the weak independence number of the components (Section 5). In continuation, we define a partial order on the set of all left cosets in all subgroups of the Clifford semigroup, effectively representing a path within the component. This facilitates the determination of the path independence number for any given component (Section 6). Lastly, we delve into the investigation of the weak path independence number (Section 7).

2. Preliminaries

Some basic definitions and relevant notations are presented in this section. We refer to [20] for more information on graph theory and [21] for semigroup theory. All sets mentioned in this paper are assumed to be finite. Because, in this work, all mentioned graphs are directed graphs, we will refer to a directed path as a path for convenience.

Let D be a digraph with a vertex set $V(D)$ and an arc set $E(D)$. The vertices u and v in D are said to be:

- *independent* if $(u,v) \notin E(D)$ and $(v,u) \notin D$;
- *weakly independent* if $(u,v) \notin E(D)$ or $(v,u) \notin E(D)$;
- *path independent* if there is neither a path from u to v nor from v to u;
- *weakly path independent* if there are no paths from u to v or no paths from v to u.

The non-empty subset I of $V(D)$ is called an *independent* (respectively, *weakly independent, path independent, weakly path independent*) set if any two vertices in I are independent (respectively, weakly independent, path independent, weakly path independent).

The *independence* (respectively, *weak independence, path independence, weak path independence*) the number of D is the maximum cardinality among all independent (respectively, weakly independent, path independent, weakly path independent) sets of D.

Let $\alpha(D)$ (respectively, $\alpha_w(D)$, $\alpha_p(D)$, $\alpha_{wp}(D)$) denote the independence (respectively, weak independence, path independence, weak path independence) number of D.

The independent (respectively, weakly independent, path independent, weakly path independent) set of D is called an $\alpha-$set (respectively α_w-set, α_p-set, $\alpha_{wp}-$set) of D if the cardinality of I is equal to $\alpha(D)$ (respectively, $\alpha_w(D)$, $\alpha_p(D)$, $\alpha_{wp}(D)$).

The digraph D is said to be *connected* if the underlying graph, obtained by replacing all directed edges of D with undirected edges, is connected. It is said to be *strongly connected* if there exists a path from u to v and a path from v to u for all $u, v \in V(D)$. It is a well-known result that for any group G and a non-empty subset A of G, the Cayley digraph $Cay(\langle A \rangle, A)$ is strongly connected where $\langle A \rangle$ is a subgroup of G generated by A. Let $G_1 = (V_1, E_1)$, $G_2 = (V_2, E_2)$ be digraphs. The *union* $G_1 \cup G_2$ of G_1 and G_2 is the digraph with vertex set $V_1 \cup V_2$ and arc set $E_1 \cup E_2$. The *disjoint union* $G_1 \dot\cup G_2$ of G_1 and G_2 is the union of G_1 and G_2 with $V_1 \cap V_2 = \emptyset$. In view of [7], we obtain the following helpful lemma.

Lemma 1 ([7]). *Let G be a group and $\emptyset \neq A \subseteq G$. Then $Cay(G, A) \cong \bigcup_{i \in I} (V_i, E_i)$ where $I = \{1, 2, \ldots, \frac{|G|}{|\langle A \rangle|}\}$ and $(V_i, E_i) \cong Cay(\langle A \rangle, A)$ for all $i \in I$.*

Let $(Y, \leq)$ be a partially ordered set and X is a non-empty subset of Y, we say that an element c of Y is a *lower bound* of X if $c \leq y$ for every y in X. A lower bound element c of X is called the *greatest lower bound (meet)* of X if $b \leq c$ for every lower bound b in X. An *upper bound* and the *least upper bound (join)* are defined dually. The meet (join) of $\{a, b\}$ will be denoted by $a \wedge b$ ($a \vee b$).

A partially ordered set Y is called a *meet (join) semilattice* if $x \wedge y$ ($x \vee y$) $\in Y$ for all $x, y \in Y$. A partially ordered set Y is called a *semilattice* if it is a meet semilattice or a join semilattice. In this work, we suppose that all semilattices are meet semilattices. For join semilattices, the results are proved dually.

An element e of a semigroup S is *idempotent* if $e^2 = e$. An element a of a semigroup S is *completely regular* if there exists an element $x \in S$ such that $a = axa$ and $ax = xa$.

A semigroup S is *completely regular* if all its elements are completely regular. A semigroup S is a *Clifford semigroup* if it is completely regular and all its idempotents commute with all elements of S. It can be readily deduced that if S is a group, then the identity element e is the only idempotent element in S such that $ea = ae$ for all $a \in S$ and every element a is a completely regular because $a = aa^{-1}a$ and $aa^{-1} = a^{-1}a$ where a^{-1} is an inverse of a. This then implies that every group is a Clifford semigroup.

Let Y be a semilattice and $\{(G_\beta, \circ_\beta) | \beta \in Y\}$ be a family of groups indexed by Y where $G_\beta \cap G_\lambda = \emptyset$ for any $\beta \neq \lambda \in Y$. Suppose that, for all $\beta \geq \lambda$ in Y, there exists a group homomorphism $f_{\beta, \lambda} : G_\beta \to G_\lambda$ such that

(i) for all $\lambda \in Y$, $f_{\lambda, \lambda} = id_{G_\lambda}$ is the identity mapping on G_λ,
(ii) $f_{\beta, \lambda} f_{\gamma, \beta} = f_{\gamma, \lambda}$ for all $\lambda, \beta, \gamma \in Y$ with $\gamma \geq \beta \geq \lambda$,

and the multiplication on $S = \bigcup_{\beta \in Y} G_\beta$ is defined for $x \in G_\beta$ and $y \in G_\lambda$ by
$xy = f_{\beta, \beta \wedge \lambda}(x) \circ_{\beta \wedge \lambda} f_{\lambda, \beta \wedge \lambda}(y)$.

It is easy to check that $S = \bigcup_{\beta \in Y} G_\beta$ under that multiplication is a semigroup, and called a *strong semilattice of groups*. We write $S = [Y; G_\beta, f_{\beta, \lambda}]$. For convenience, we will refer to $f_{\beta, \beta \wedge \lambda}(x) \circ_{\beta \wedge \lambda} f_{\lambda, \beta \wedge \lambda}(y)$ as $f_{\beta, \beta \wedge \lambda}(x) f_{\lambda, \beta \wedge \lambda}(y)$.

In 1995, Howie [21] showed a necessary and sufficient condition for a Clifford semigroup that S is a Clifford semigroup if and only if S is a strong semilattice of groups. Thus, every Clifford semigroup can be written in the form $[Y; G_\beta, f_{\beta,\lambda}]$ for some semilattice Y, group G_β and structure homomorphism $f_{\beta,\lambda}$. Henceforth, whenever we state that $[Y; G_\beta, f_{\beta,\lambda}]$ is a Clifford semigroup, it is to be understood that G_β is a group for every $\beta \in Y$. Consequently, we will use the term strong semilattice of groups instead of Clifford semigroup.

3. Characterizations of Maximal Connected Subdigraphs in $Cay(S, A)$

Clearly, the independence number of a graph is a summation of the independence numbers of all its maximal connected subdigraphs. Thus we begin this work with the characterization of maximal connected subdigraphs of $Cay(S, A)$.

Hereafter, we let $S = [Y; G_\beta, f_{\beta,\lambda}]$ be a Clifford semigroup, $Y' = \{\gamma \in Y : G_\gamma \cap A \neq \emptyset\}$ and $A_\beta = \{f_{\gamma,\beta}(a_\gamma) : a_\gamma \in G_\gamma \cap A, \gamma \geq \beta\}$ where $\emptyset \neq A \subseteq S$. For $X \subseteq S$, let us denote by $[X]$ the subdigraph of $Cay(S, A)$ induced by X.

Since the minimum element of Y exists it follows that in each maximal connected subdigraph of $Cay(S, A)$, there exists $\beta \in Y$ such that $\beta \wedge \gamma = \beta$ for all $\gamma \in Y'$. Let $B = \{\beta \in Y : \beta \wedge (\bigwedge_{\gamma \in Y'} \gamma) = \beta\}$. Clearly, $(\lambda \wedge (\bigwedge_{\gamma \in Y'} \gamma)) \wedge (\bigwedge_{\gamma \in Y'} \gamma) = \lambda \wedge (\bigwedge_{\gamma \in Y'} \gamma)$ for all $\lambda \in Y$. Then we obtain the following lemma.

Lemma 2. $\lambda \wedge (\bigwedge_{\gamma \in Y'} \gamma) \in B$ for all $\lambda \in Y$.

By Lemma 2, we obtain for each $\lambda \in Y$ there exists $\beta \in B$ such that $\lambda \wedge (\bigwedge_{\gamma \in Y'} \gamma) = \beta$. We then define $Y_\beta = \{\lambda \in Y : \lambda \wedge (\bigwedge_{\gamma \in Y'} \gamma) = \beta\}$ for all $\beta \in B$.

Lemma 3. $\{Y_\beta : \beta \in B\}$ is a partition of Y.

Proof. Clearly, $\beta \in Y_\beta$ for every $\beta \in B$. Thus $Y_\beta \neq \emptyset$ for all $\beta \in B$. By Lemma 2, we obtain $\bigcup_{\beta \in B} Y_\beta = Y$. Now, assume that $\mu \in Y_\beta \cap Y_{\beta'}$. Then $\mu \wedge (\bigwedge_{\gamma \in Y'} \gamma) = \beta$ and $\mu \wedge (\bigwedge_{\gamma \in Y'} \gamma) = \beta'$ which implies $\beta = \beta'$. Therefore $\{Y_\beta : \beta \in B\}$ is a partition of Y. □

Example 1. Let $Y = \{\lambda_1, \lambda_2, \ldots, \lambda_6\}$ be a semilattice with a partial order that represented by the Hasse diagram in Figure 1. For $I = \{1, 2, \ldots, 6\}$, we let $\{G_{\lambda_i} : i \in I\}$ be a family of groups, indexed by the semilattice Y where $G_{\lambda_i} = \mathbb{Z}_4 = \{\bar{0}_{\lambda_i}, \bar{1}_{\lambda_i}, \bar{2}_{\lambda_i}, \bar{3}_{\lambda_i}\}$ is an additive group of integers modulo 4, for all $i \in I$. Let $f_{\lambda_i, \lambda_j}(\bar{x}_{\lambda_i}) = \bar{x}_{\lambda_j}$ for every $\bar{x}_{\lambda_i} \in G_{\lambda_i}$, $\bar{x}_{\lambda_j} \in G_{\lambda_j}$ and $i > j$. Then $S = [Y; G_{\lambda_i}, f_{\lambda_i, \lambda_j}]$ is a Clifford semigroup.

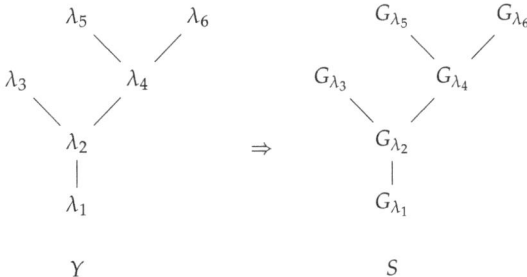

Figure 1. The Hasse diagram of the semilattice $Y = \{\lambda_1, \lambda_2, \ldots, \lambda_6\}$ and the family of groups $\{G_{\lambda_i} = \mathbb{Z}_4 : i = 1, 2, 3, 4, 5, 6\}$.

If we put $A = \{\bar{2}_{\lambda_6}\}$ where $\bar{2}_{\lambda_6} \in G_{\lambda_6}$, then we get

(i) $Y' = \{\lambda_6\}$ and $B = \{\lambda_1, \lambda_2, \lambda_4, \lambda_6\}$,
(ii) $Y_{\lambda_1} = \{\lambda_1\}$, $Y_{\lambda_2} = \{\lambda_2, \lambda_3\}$, $Y_{\lambda_4} = \{\lambda_4, \lambda_5\}$ and $Y_{\lambda_6} = \{\lambda_6\}$,
(iii) $\{Y_{\lambda_1}, Y_{\lambda_2}, Y_{\lambda_4}, Y_{\lambda_6}\}$ is a partition of Y.

Lemma 4. $f_{\lambda,\eta}(g\langle A_\lambda\rangle) \subseteq f_{\lambda,\eta}(g)\langle A_\eta\rangle$ for all $\eta, \lambda \in Y$, such that $\eta \leq \lambda$.

Proof. Let $h \in f_{\lambda,\eta}(g\langle A_\lambda\rangle)$. Then $h = f_{\lambda,\eta}(ga)$ for some $a = a_1^{t_1} a_2^{t_2} \ldots a_m^{t_m} \in \langle A_\lambda\rangle$ where $a_i \in A_\lambda$ and $t_i \in \mathbb{Z}$ for all $1 \leq i \leq m$. For each $a_i \in A_\lambda$, we obtain $a_i = f_{\gamma_i,\lambda}(b_{\gamma i})$ for some $b_{\gamma i} \in A \cap G_{\gamma_i}$ where $\lambda \leq \gamma_i$ and we then obtain $f_{\lambda,\eta}(f_{\gamma_i,\lambda}(b_{\gamma i})) = f_{\gamma_i,\eta}(b_{\gamma i}) \in A_\eta$ for all $1 \leq i \leq m$. Consider

$$\begin{aligned}
h = f_{\lambda,\eta}(ga) &= f_{\lambda,\eta}(ga_1^{t_1} a_2^{t_2} \ldots a_m^{t_m}) \\
&= f_{\lambda,\eta}(g) f_{\lambda,\eta}(f_{\gamma_1,\lambda}(b_{\gamma 1})^{t_1} f_{\gamma_2,\lambda}(b_{\gamma 2})^{t_2} \ldots f_{\gamma_m,\lambda}(b_{\gamma m})^{t_m}) \\
&= f_{\lambda,\eta}(g) f_{\lambda,\eta}(f_{\gamma_1,\lambda}(b_{\gamma 1}))^{t_1} f_{\lambda,\eta}(f_{\gamma_2,\lambda}(b_{\gamma 2}))^{t_2} \ldots f_{\lambda,\eta}(f_{\gamma_m,\lambda}(b_{\gamma m}))^{t_m} \\
&= f_{\lambda,\eta}(g) f_{\gamma_1,\eta}(b_{\gamma 1})^{t_1} f_{\gamma_2,\eta}(b_{\gamma 2})^{t_2} \ldots f_{\gamma_m,\eta}(b_{\gamma m})^{t_m}.
\end{aligned}$$

Hence $h = f_{\lambda,\eta}(g) f_{\gamma_1,\eta}(b_{\gamma 1})^{t_1} f_{\gamma_2,\eta}(b_{\gamma 2})^{t_2} \ldots f_{\gamma_m,\eta}(b_{\gamma m})^{t_m} \in f_{\lambda,\eta}(g)\langle A_\eta\rangle$. Therefore $f_{\lambda,\eta}(g\langle A_\lambda\rangle) \subseteq f_{\lambda,\eta}(g)\langle A_\eta\rangle$. □

Let D be a digraph and $v \in V(D)$. The set of in-neighbors and the set of out-neighbors of a vertex v are defined by $N^-(v) = \{u \in V(D) : (u,v) \in E(D)\}$ and $N^+(v) = \{u \in V(D) : (v,u) \in E(D)\}$, respectively. In addition, we use $N(v) = N^-(v) \cup N^+(v)$, the set of neighbors of the vertex v.

From Lemma 1, we observe that the Cayley digraph $Cay(G_\lambda, A_\lambda) \cong \bigcup_{i \in I}(V_i, E_i)$ for all $\lambda \in Y$ where $I = \{1, 2 \ldots, \frac{|G_\lambda|}{|\langle A_\lambda\rangle|}\}$ and $(V_i, E_i) = [g_i\langle A_\lambda\rangle] \cong Cay(\langle A_\lambda\rangle, A_\lambda)$ for all $i \in I$ where $g_i\langle A_\lambda\rangle \in G_\lambda / \langle A_\lambda\rangle$ and $[g_i\langle A_\lambda\rangle]$ is an induced subdigraph of $Cay(S, A)$.

Lemma 5. Let x be a vertex in $Cay(S, A)$ and let $\beta \in B$. Then $N(x) \subseteq \bigcup_{\substack{g \in g_\beta\langle A_\beta\rangle \\ \lambda \in Y_\beta}} f_{\lambda,\beta}^{-1}(g)$ for all $x \in \bigcup_{\substack{g \in g_\beta\langle A_\beta\rangle \\ \lambda \in Y_\beta}} f_{\lambda,\beta}^{-1}(g)$.

Proof. Let $x \in \bigcup_{\substack{g \in g_\beta\langle A_\beta\rangle \\ \lambda \in Y_\beta}} f_{\lambda,\beta}^{-1}(g)$. Then $x \in G_\lambda$ for some $\lambda \in Y_\beta$ where $f_{\lambda,\beta}(x) \in g_\beta\langle A_\beta\rangle$. Thus we let $f_{\lambda,\beta}(x) = g_\beta a_1^{t_1} a_2^{t_2} \ldots a_m^{t_m}$ where $a_i \in A_\beta$ and $t_i \in \mathbb{Z}$ for all $1 \leq i \leq m$. Assume that $u \in N(x)$, we shall show that $u \in \bigcup_{\substack{g \in g_\beta\langle A_\beta\rangle \\ \lambda \in Y_\beta}} f_{\lambda,\beta}^{-1}(g)$. Consider two cases:

(i) Case $u \in N^+(x)$, which means $(x, u) \in E(Cay(S, A))$. Thus $u = xa$ for some $a \in A$. Since $A \subseteq S$, we assume that $a \in A \subseteq G_\gamma$ for some $\gamma \in Y'$. By the definition of multiplication on S, we obtain $u \in G_{\lambda \wedge \gamma}$. Clearly, $\lambda \wedge \gamma \in Y_\beta$ because $\lambda \in Y_\beta$. Then

$$\begin{aligned}
f_{\lambda \wedge \gamma, \beta}(u) &= f_{\lambda \wedge \gamma, \beta}(f_{\lambda, \lambda \wedge \gamma}(x) f_{\gamma, \lambda \wedge \gamma}(a)) \\
&= f_{\lambda, \beta}(x) f_{\gamma, \beta}(a) \\
&= g_\beta a_1^{t_1} a_2^{t_2} \ldots a_m^{t_m} f_{\gamma, \beta}(a).
\end{aligned}$$

Since $f_{\gamma,\beta}(a) \in A_\beta$, we obtain $a_1^{t_1}a_2^{t_2}\ldots a_m^{t_m}f_{\gamma,\beta}(a) \in \langle A_\beta \rangle$.
Hence $f_{\lambda\wedge\gamma,\beta}(u) = g_\beta a_1^{t_1}a_2^{t_2}\ldots a_m^{t_m}f_{\gamma,\beta}(a) \in g_\beta\langle A_\beta\rangle$. From $\lambda\wedge\gamma \in Y_\beta$ and $f_{\lambda\wedge\gamma,\beta}(u) \in g_\beta\langle A_\beta\rangle$, we conclude that $u \in \bigcup_{h\in g_\beta\langle A_\beta\rangle} f^{-1}_{\lambda\wedge\gamma,\beta}(h) \subseteq \bigcup_{\substack{g\in g_\beta\langle A_\beta\rangle \\ \lambda\in Y_\beta}} f^{-1}_{\lambda,\beta}(g)$.

(ii) Case $u \in N^-(x)$, which means $(u,x) \in E(Cay(S,A))$. Thus $x = ua$ for some $a \in A \cap G_\gamma$ and $\gamma \in Y'$. Assume that $u \in G_\eta$. Clearly, $\eta\wedge\gamma = \lambda$ because $x \in G_\lambda$. First, we will show that $\eta \in Y_\beta$. From $\eta\wedge\gamma = \lambda$, we obtain $\eta\wedge(\bigwedge_{\gamma'\in Y'}\gamma') = (\eta\wedge\gamma)\wedge(\bigwedge_{\gamma'\in Y'}\gamma') = \lambda\wedge(\bigwedge_{\gamma'\in Y'}\gamma') = \beta$. Then $\eta \in Y_\beta$. From $f_{\lambda,\beta}(x) = f_{\lambda,\beta}(f_{\eta,\lambda}(u)f_{\gamma,\lambda}(a)) = f_{\eta,\beta}(u)f_{\gamma,\beta}(a)$, we obtain $f_{\eta,\beta}(u) = f_{\lambda,\beta}(x)(f_{\gamma,\beta}(a))^{-1}$. Since $f_{\gamma,\beta}(a) \in A_\beta$, we conclude that $f_{\gamma,\beta}(a)^{-1} \in \langle A_\beta\rangle$.
Therefore $f_{\eta,\beta}(u) = f_{\lambda,\beta}(x)(f_{\gamma,\beta}(a))^{-1} \in g_\beta\langle A_\beta\rangle$ which implies $u \in \bigcup_{h\in g_\beta\langle A_\beta\rangle} f^{-1}_{\eta,\beta}(h) \subseteq \bigcup_{\substack{g\in g_\beta\langle A_\beta\rangle \\ \lambda\in Y_\beta}} f^{-1}_{\lambda,\beta}(g)$.

Hence $u \in \bigcup_{\substack{g_\beta\in g_\beta\langle A_\beta\rangle \\ \lambda\in Y_\beta}} f^{-1}_{\lambda,\beta}(g_\beta)$, as required. $\square$

Lemma 6. *For each $x \in S$. There exists $\beta \in B$, $\lambda \in Y_\beta$ and $g_\beta\langle A_\beta\rangle \in G_\beta/\langle A_\beta\rangle$ such that $x \in \bigcup_{g\in g_\beta\langle A_\beta\rangle} f^{-1}_{\lambda,\beta}(g)$.*

Proof. Let $x \in S$. Then $x \in G_\lambda$ for some $\lambda \in Y$. By Lemma 2, we obtain $\lambda \in Y_\beta$ for some $\beta \in B$. Thus $f_{\lambda,\beta}(x)$ is defined in G_β which implies there exists $g_\beta\langle A_\beta\rangle \in G_\beta/\langle A_\beta\rangle$ and $g' \in g_\beta\langle A_\beta\rangle$ such that $f_{\lambda,\beta}(x) = g'$. Therefore $x \in \bigcup_{g\in g_\beta\langle A_\beta\rangle} f^{-1}_{\lambda,\beta}(g)$. $\square$

Theorem 1. *Let $\beta \in B$ and $g_\beta\langle A_\beta\rangle \in G_\beta/\langle A_\beta\rangle$. Then $[\bigcup_{\substack{g\in g_\beta\langle A_\beta\rangle \\ \lambda\in Y_\beta}} f^{-1}_{\lambda,\beta}(g)]$ is a maximal connected subdigraph of $Cay(S,A)$.*

Proof. Let $\beta \in B$, $g_\beta\langle A_\beta\rangle \in G_\beta/\langle A_\beta\rangle$ and $g' \in g_\beta\langle A_\beta\rangle$. We first show that, for each $x \in \bigcup_{\substack{g_\beta\in g_\beta\langle A_\beta\rangle \\ \lambda\in Y_\beta}} f^{-1}_{\lambda,\beta}(g_\beta)$, there exists a path from x to g'. Now, let $x \in \bigcup_{\substack{g_\beta\in g_\beta\langle A_\beta\rangle \\ \lambda\in Y_\beta}} f^{-1}_{\lambda,\beta}(g_\beta)$. Then $x \in G_\lambda$ for some $\lambda \in Y_\beta$. From $\lambda \in Y_\beta$, it follows that there exists $\{\gamma_1,\gamma_2,\ldots,\gamma_t\} \subseteq Y_\beta$ such that $\lambda\wedge\gamma_1\wedge\gamma_2\wedge\ldots\wedge\gamma_t = \beta$, and there exists $\{a_1,a_2,\ldots,a_t\} \subseteq A$ where $a_i \in G_{\gamma_i}$ for all $1 \leq i \leq t$, such that $x, xa_1, xa_1a_2, \ldots, xa_1a_2\ldots a_t$ is a path from x to $xa_1a_2\ldots a_t$. Consider

$$xa_1a_2\ldots a_t = (\ldots((f_{\lambda\wedge\gamma_1}(x)f_{\gamma_1,\lambda\wedge\gamma_1}(a_1))a_2)\ldots)a_t$$
$$= (\ldots((f_{\lambda\wedge\gamma_1,(\lambda\wedge\gamma_1)\wedge\gamma_2}(f_{\lambda,\lambda\wedge\gamma_1}(x)f_{\gamma_1,\lambda\wedge\gamma_1}(a_1))f_{\gamma_2,(\lambda\wedge\gamma_1)\wedge\gamma_2}(a_2))\ldots)a_t$$
$$\vdots$$
$$= f_{\lambda\wedge(\bigwedge_{i=1}^{t-1}\gamma_i),\lambda\wedge(\bigwedge_{i=1}^{t-1}\gamma_i)\wedge\gamma_t}(\ldots(f_{\lambda,\lambda\wedge\gamma_1}(x)f_{\gamma_1,\lambda\wedge\gamma_1}(a_1))\ldots)f_{\gamma_t,\lambda\wedge(\bigwedge_{i=1}^{t-1}\gamma_i)\wedge\gamma_t}(a_t)$$
$$= f_{\lambda,\beta}(x)f_{\gamma_1,\beta}(a_1)f_{\gamma_2,\beta}(a_2)\ldots f_{\gamma_t,\beta}(a_t)$$
$$\in f_{\lambda,\beta}(x)\langle A_\beta\rangle.$$

Since $[f_{\lambda,\beta}(x)\langle A_\beta\rangle] \cong Cay(\langle A_\beta\rangle,A_\beta)$, it follows that there exists a path from $xa_1a_2\ldots a_t$ to g'. Thus $[\bigcup_{\substack{g\in g_\beta\langle A_\beta\rangle \\ \lambda\in Y_\beta}} f^{-1}_{\lambda,\beta}(g)]$ is a connected subdigraph of $Cay(S,A)$. Suppose that there exists $x' \in S \setminus \bigcup_{\substack{g \in g_\beta \langle A_\beta \rangle \\ \lambda \in Y_\beta}} f_{\lambda,\beta}^{-1}(g)$ such that $x' \in N(x)$ for some $x \in \bigcup_{\substack{g \in g_\beta \langle A_\beta \rangle \\ \lambda \in Y_\beta}} f_{\lambda,\beta}^{-1}(g)$. By using Lemma 5, we conclude that $x' \in \bigcup_{\substack{g \in g_\beta \langle A_\beta \rangle \\ \lambda \in Y_\beta}} f_{\lambda,\beta}^{-1}(g)$, a contradiction. Therefore $[\bigcup_{\substack{g \in g_\beta \langle A_\beta \rangle \\ \lambda \in Y_\beta}} f_{\lambda,\beta}^{-1}(g)]$ is a maximal connected subdigraph of $Cay(S, A)$, as required. □

From Theorem 1, we have investigated the maximal connected subdigraph of $Cay(S, A)$ and obtained some needed properties. Afterward, we then achieve a characterization for a maximal connected subdigraph of $Cay(S, A)$.

Theorem 2. *A subdigraph C of $Cay(S, A)$ is a maximal connected subdigraph if and only if $C = [\bigcup_{\substack{g \in g_\beta \langle A_\beta \rangle \\ \lambda \in Y_\beta}} f_{\lambda,\beta}^{-1}(g)]$ for some $\beta \in B$ and $g_\beta \langle A_\beta \rangle \in G_\beta / \langle A_\beta \rangle$.*

Proof. Let C be a maximal connected subdigraph of $Cay(S, A)$ and x a vertex of C. By Lemma 6, we obtain $x \in \bigcup_{g \in g_\beta \langle A_\beta \rangle} f_{\lambda,\beta}^{-1}(g)$ for some $\beta \in B$, $\lambda \in Y_\beta$ and $g_\beta \langle A_\beta \rangle \in G_\beta / \langle A_\beta \rangle$, which means $x \in \bigcup_{\substack{g \in g_\beta \langle A_\beta \rangle \\ \lambda \in Y_\beta}} f_{\lambda,\beta}^{-1}(g)$. From Lemma 5 and C is connected, we obtain $V(C) \subseteq \bigcup_{\substack{g \in g_\beta \langle A_\beta \rangle \\ \lambda \in Y_\beta}} f_{\lambda,\beta}^{-1}(g)$. Since $[\bigcup_{\substack{g_\beta \in g_\beta \langle A_\beta \rangle \\ \lambda \in Y_\beta}} f_{\lambda,\beta}^{-1}(g_\beta)]$ is an induced subdigraph and C is maximal connected, we conclude that $C = [\bigcup_{\substack{g_\beta \in g_\beta \langle A_\beta \rangle \\ \lambda \in Y_\beta}} f_{\lambda,\beta}^{-1}(g_\beta)]$.

Conversely, $C = [\bigcup_{\substack{g \in g_\beta \langle A_\beta \rangle \\ \lambda \in Y_\beta}} f_{\lambda,\beta}^{-1}(g)]$ is a maximal connected subdigraph by Theorem 1. □

Example 2. *From the Clifford semigroup $S = [Y; G_{\lambda_i}, f_{\lambda_i,\lambda_j}]$ in an Example 1 and $A = \{\bar{2}_{\lambda_4}, \bar{1}_{\lambda_6}\}$, the $Cay(S, A)$ can be pictured as Figure 2. In addition, we obtain $B = \{\lambda_1, \lambda_2, \lambda_4\}$ and the following:*

(i) Consider $\lambda_1 \in B$. We obtain $[\bigcup_{\substack{g \in g_{\lambda_1} \langle A_{\lambda_1} \rangle \\ \eta \in Y_{\lambda_1}}} f_{\eta,\lambda_1}^{-1}(g)] = [\bigcup_{g \in G_{\lambda_1}} f_{\lambda_1,\lambda_1}^{-1}(g)] = [G_{\lambda_1}]$.

(ii) Consider $\lambda_2 \in B$.
We obtain $[\bigcup_{\substack{g \in \langle A_{\lambda_2} \rangle \\ \eta \in Y_{\lambda_2}}} f_{\eta,\lambda_2}^{-1}(g)] = [(\bigcup_{g \in \langle A_{\lambda_2} \rangle} f_{\lambda_3,\lambda_2}^{-1}(g)) \cup (\bigcup_{g \in \langle A_{\lambda_2} \rangle} f_{\lambda_2,\lambda_2}^{-1}(g))] = [G_{\lambda_3} \cup G_{\lambda_2}]$.

(iii) Consider $\lambda_4 \in B$.
We obtain $[\bigcup_{\substack{g \in \langle A_{\lambda_4} \rangle \\ \eta \in Y_{\lambda_4}}} f_{\eta,\lambda_4}^{-1}(g)] = [(\bigcup_{g \in \langle A_{\lambda_4} \rangle} f_{\lambda_6,\lambda_4}^{-1}(g)) \cup (\bigcup_{g \in \langle A_{\lambda_4} \rangle} f_{\lambda_5,\lambda_4}^{-1}(g)) \cup (\bigcup_{g \in \langle A_{\lambda_4} \rangle} f_{\lambda_4,\lambda_4}^{-1}(g))] = [G_{\lambda_6} \cup G_{\lambda_5} \cup G_{\lambda_4}]$.

We see that, $Cay(S, A)$ is the union of three maximal connected subdigraphs which are $[G_{\lambda_1}]$, $[G_{\lambda_3} \cup G_{\lambda_2}]$ and $[G_{\lambda_6} \cup G_{\lambda_5} \cup G_{\lambda_4}]$.

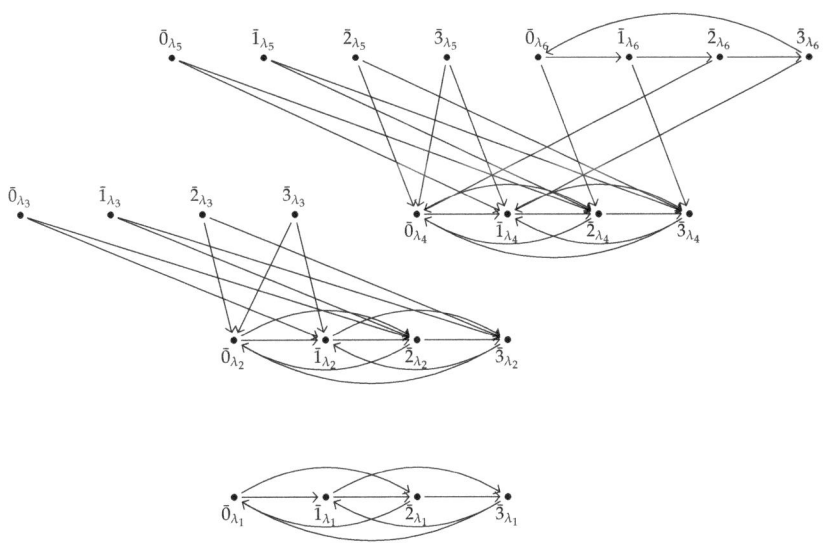

Figure 2. $Cay(S, A)$ where $Y = \{\lambda_1, \lambda_2, \ldots, \lambda_6\}$, $G_{\lambda_i} = \mathbb{Z}_4$ and $A = \{\bar{2}_{\lambda_4}, \bar{1}_{\lambda_6}\}$.

From Theorem 1, we denote by C_{g_β} the maximal connected subdigraph $[\bigcup_{\substack{g \in g_\beta \langle A_\beta \rangle \\ \lambda \in Y_\beta}} f_{\lambda,\beta}^{-1}(g)]$ associate with $\beta \in B$ and $g_\beta \langle A_\beta \rangle \in G_\beta / \langle A_\beta \rangle$. It follows easily that $C_{g_\beta} = C_{g'_\beta}$ if $g'_\beta \in g_\beta \langle A_\beta \rangle$ and $Cay(S, A) \cong \bigcup_{\substack{g \in \mathcal{A}_\beta \\ \beta \in B}} C_{g_\beta}$ where $\mathcal{A}_\beta$ is the set of representatives of all left cosets in $G_\beta / \langle A_\beta \rangle$.

4. Lower and Upper Bounds of the Independence Numbers

In this section, we introduce bounds of the independence number of $Cay(S, A)$. We first denote by $A_{\beta,\lambda}$ the set of all elements of A in which $G_\beta A_{\beta,\lambda} \subseteq G_\lambda$, i.e., $A_{\beta,\lambda} = \{a \in A : G_\beta a \subseteq G_\lambda\}$. Set $Y'_\beta := \{\lambda \in Y \setminus \{\beta\} : \lambda \wedge \gamma = \beta, \exists \gamma \in Y'\}$. For any $\beta \in B$ and $\lambda \in Y_\beta$, we define $M_{g_\beta \lambda} = \begin{cases} \{g_\lambda \langle A_\lambda \rangle \in G_\lambda / \langle A_\lambda \rangle : f_{\lambda,\beta}(g_\lambda) \in g_\beta \langle A_\beta \rangle\}, & \text{if } A_\lambda \neq \emptyset \\ \{g_\lambda \langle e_\lambda \rangle \in G_\lambda / \langle e_\lambda \rangle : f_{\lambda,\beta}(g_\lambda) \in g_\beta \langle A_\beta \rangle\}, & \text{if } A_\lambda = \emptyset. \end{cases}$

Let us denote by $\bigcup M_{g_\beta \lambda}$ the union of all sets in $M_{g_\beta \lambda}$. We here start with the lower bound of the independence number of C_{g_β}.

Lemma 7. $\sum_{\lambda \in Y_\beta} \alpha([\bigcup M_{g_\beta \lambda} - \bigcup_{\eta \in Y'_\lambda} G_\eta A_{\eta,\lambda}]) \leq \alpha(C_{g_\beta})$.

Proof. Let $X_{g_\beta \lambda}$ be an α-set of $[\bigcup M_{g_\beta \lambda} - \bigcup_{\eta \in Y'_\lambda} G_\eta A_{\eta,\lambda}]$. We will show that $\bigcup_{\lambda \in Y_\beta} X_{g_\beta \lambda}$ is an independent set of C_{g_β}. Let $u, v \in \bigcup_{\lambda \in Y_\beta} X_{g_\beta \lambda}$. This gives $u \in X_{g_\beta \eta}$ and $v \in X_{g_\beta \lambda}$ for some $\eta, \lambda \in Y_\beta$. Assume that $(u, v) \in E(C_{g_\beta})$. Then $v = ua$ for some $a \in A$. We consider two cases:

(i) Case $\lambda = \eta$, from $[\bigcup M_{g_\beta \lambda} - \bigcup_{\eta \in Y'_\lambda} G_\eta A_{\eta,\lambda}]$ is an induced subdigraph of $Cay(S, A)$ and $(u, v) \in E(C_{g_\beta})$, we see that (u, v) is an arc in $[\bigcup M_{g_\beta \lambda} - \bigcup_{\eta \in Y'_\lambda} G_\eta A_{\eta,\lambda}]$. Since $u, v \in X_{g_\beta \lambda}$ and $X_{g_\beta \lambda}$ is an independent set of $[\bigcup M_{g_\beta \lambda} - \bigcup_{\eta \in Y'_\lambda} G_\eta A_{\eta,\lambda}]$, we obtain u, v are independent, which is a contradiction.

47

(ii) Case $\lambda \neq \eta$, since $u \in X_{g_\beta \eta} \subseteq G_\eta$ and $v = ua \in X_{g_\beta \lambda} \subseteq G_\lambda$, we have $a \in A_{\eta,\lambda}$. Then we obtain $v = ua \in G_\eta A_{\eta,\lambda} \subseteq \bigcup_{\eta \in Y'_\lambda} G_\eta A_{\eta,\lambda}$ which implies $v \notin X_{g_\beta \lambda} \subseteq \bigcup M_{g_\beta \lambda} - \bigcup_{\eta \in Y'_\lambda} G_\eta A_{\eta,\lambda}$, a contradiction.

Thus we conclude that $\bigcup_{\lambda \in Y_\beta} X_{g_\beta \lambda}$ is an independent set of C_{g_β}. Clearly, $X_{g_\beta \eta} \cap X_{g_\beta \lambda} = \emptyset$ for all $\eta, \lambda \in Y_\beta$ where $\eta \neq \lambda$. Therefore $|\bigcup_{\lambda \in Y_\beta} X_{g_\beta \lambda}| = \sum_{\lambda \in Y_\beta} \alpha([\bigcup M_{g_\beta \lambda} - \bigcup_{\eta \in Y'_\lambda} G_\eta A_{\eta,\lambda}]) \leq \alpha(C_{g_\beta})$. □

The following lemma gives an upper bound of $\alpha(C_{g_\beta})$ obtained by using the fact that if $D = (V, E)$ and $D' = (V, E')$ such that $E' \subseteq E$, then $\alpha(D) \leq \alpha(D')$.

Lemma 8. $\alpha(C_{g_\beta}) \leq \sum_{\lambda \in Y_\beta} \alpha([\bigcup M_{g_\beta \lambda}])$.

Proof. We see that $V(C_{g_\beta}) = V(\bigcup_{\lambda \in Y_\beta} [\bigcup M_{g_\beta \lambda}])$ because

$$u \in V(C_{g_\beta}) \Leftrightarrow u \in \bigcup_{\substack{g \in g_\beta \langle A_\beta \rangle \\ \lambda \in Y_\beta}} f^{-1}_{\lambda,\beta}(g)$$

$$\Leftrightarrow u \in f^{-1}_{\lambda,\beta}(g) \text{ for some } g \in g_\beta \langle A_\beta \rangle \text{ and } \lambda \in Y_\beta$$

$$\Leftrightarrow f_{\lambda,\beta}(u) = g \in g_\beta \langle A_\beta \rangle$$

$$\Leftrightarrow u \langle A_\lambda \rangle \in M_{g_\beta \lambda}$$

$$\Leftrightarrow u \in \bigcup M_{g_\beta \lambda}.$$

Next, we let $(u,v) \in E(\bigcup_{\lambda \in Y_\beta} [\bigcup M_{g_\beta \lambda}])$. Clearly, $u, v \in V(C_{g_\beta})$. Since $[\bigcup M_{g_\beta \lambda}]$ and C_{g_β} are induced subdigraphs of $Cay(S, A)$, we conclude that $(u,v) \in E(C_{g_\beta})$. Thus $E(\bigcup_{\lambda \in Y_\beta} [\bigcup M_{g_\beta \lambda}]) \subseteq E(C_{g_\beta})$ and so $\alpha(C_{g_\beta}) \leq \sum_{\lambda \in Y_\beta} \alpha([\bigcup M_{g_\beta \lambda}])$, as required. □

From C_{g_β} is a maximal connected subdigraph of $Cay(S, A)$ and $Cay(S, A) \cong \bigcup_{\substack{g \in A_\beta \\ \beta \in B}} C_{g_\beta}$, we can directly conclude that

$$\alpha(Cay(S, A)) = \sum_{\substack{g \in A_\beta \\ \beta \in B}} \alpha(C_{g_\beta}).$$

Consequently, a lower(upper) bound of $\alpha(Cay(S, A))$ can be presented in the form of the summation of lower(upper) bounds of each $\alpha(C_{g_\beta})$.

Theorem 3. $\sum_{\beta \in B} (\sum_{\lambda \in Y_\beta} \alpha([\bigcup M_{g_\beta \lambda} - \bigcup_{\eta \in Y'_\lambda} G_\eta A_{\eta,\lambda}])) \leq \alpha(Cay(S, A)) \leq \sum_{\beta \in B} (\sum_{\lambda \in Y_\beta} \alpha([\bigcup M_{g_\beta \lambda}]))$.

Any two elements a and b of a partially ordered set $(P, \leq)$ are called *comparable* (*incomparable*) if either $a \leq b$ or $b \leq a$ (neither $a \leq b$ nor $b \leq a$). A subset X of P is called a *chain* (*anti-chain*) if any two elements of X are comparable (incomparable).

Here, we establish examples to show that the proposed lower and upper bounds are sharp.

Proposition 1. *Let $S = [Y; G_\beta, f_{\lambda,\eta}]$ be a Clifford semigroup in which consists a chain Y with the maximum and minimum elements, namely m' and m, respectively. We put $f_{\lambda,\eta}(x) = e_\eta$ for all*

$x \in G_\lambda$, $\lambda > \eta \in Y$ where e_η is the identity element of G_η. If $A = \{e_\lambda : \lambda \in Y\}$, then C_{e_m} is a maximal connected subdigraph of $Cay(S, A)$ and $\alpha(C_{e_m}) = \sum_{\lambda \in Y_m} \alpha([\bigcup M_{e_m\lambda} - \bigcup_{\eta \in Y'_\lambda} G_\eta A_{\eta,\lambda}])$.

Proof. Let $A = \{e_\lambda : \lambda \in Y\}$. Then $Y' = Y$. From $B = \{\beta \in Y : \beta \wedge \gamma = \beta \text{ for all } \gamma \in Y'\}$, we obtain $B = \{m\}$. Thus C_{e_m} is a maximal connected subdigraph of $Cay(S, A)$. Next, we will show that $\alpha(C_{e_m}) = \sum_{\lambda \in Y_m} \alpha([\bigcup M_{e_m\lambda} - \bigcup_{\eta \in Y'_\lambda} G_\eta A_{\eta,\lambda}]) = 1 + \sum_{\lambda > m}(|G_\lambda| - 1)$. Consider $I := \bigcup_{\lambda > m}(G_\lambda \setminus \{e_\lambda\}) \cup \{e_{m'}\}$, we claim that I is a maximal independent set of C_{e_m}. Let $u, v \in I$ where $u \neq v$. Then $u \in G_\lambda$ and $v \in G_\eta$ for some $\lambda, \eta \in Y \setminus \{m\}$. Assume that $(u, v) \in E(C_{e_m})$. This gives $v = ue_\gamma$ for some $e_\gamma \in A$. By the assumption, we obtain $v = f_{\lambda,\eta}(u) f_{\gamma,\eta}(e_\gamma) = e_\eta e_\eta = e_\eta$ where $\eta \neq m'$. It contradicts to the fact that $e_\eta \notin I$. Thus I is an independent set of C_{e_m}. In addition, by $V(C_{e_m}) \setminus I = \{e_\lambda : \lambda \neq m'\}$ and $(e_\lambda, e_\eta) \in E(C_{e_m})$ for all $\lambda > \eta \in Y$, we obtain I is a maximal independent set of C_{e_m}. Thus $\alpha(C_{e_m}) = 1 + \sum_{\lambda > m}(|G_\lambda| - 1)$.

Now, from the assumption, we have $A_\lambda = \{e_\lambda\}$ for all $\lambda \in Y$. Thus $M_{e_m\lambda} = \{g_\lambda\langle\{e_\lambda\}\rangle \in G_\lambda/\langle\{e_\lambda\}\rangle : f_{\lambda,\beta}(g_\lambda) \in e_m\langle\{e_m\}\rangle\} = G_\lambda$ for all $\lambda \in Y_m$. From $A_{\eta,\lambda} = \{e_\lambda\}$ and $f_{\eta,\lambda}(g_\eta)e_\lambda = e_\lambda e_\lambda = e_\lambda$ for all $g_\eta \in G_\eta$, $\eta \in Y'_\lambda$, we obtain $\bigcup_{\eta \in Y'_\lambda} G_\eta A_{\eta,\lambda} = \{e_\lambda\}$ where $\lambda \neq m'$ and $\bigcup_{\eta \in Y'_{m'}} G_\eta A_{\eta, m'} = \emptyset$. Since $A_\lambda = \{e_\lambda\}$, $E(Cay(G_\lambda, A_\lambda)) = \{(g_\lambda, g_\lambda) : g_\lambda \in G_\lambda\}$. Thus, for each $\lambda \in Y$ where $\lambda \neq m'$, the induced subdigraph $[\bigcup M_{e_m\lambda} - \bigcup_{\eta \in Y'_\lambda} G_\eta A_{\eta,\lambda}]$ is the digraph with vertex set $G_\lambda \setminus \{e_\lambda\}$ and arc set $\{(g_\lambda, g_\lambda) : g_\lambda \in G_\lambda\}$ which implies all vertices in $G_\lambda \setminus \{e_\lambda\}$ are independent. Hence $\alpha([\bigcup M_{e_m\lambda} - \bigcup_{\eta \in Y'_\lambda} G_\eta A_{\eta,\lambda}]) = |G_\lambda| - 1$ for all $\lambda \in Y$ where $\lambda \neq m'$. From $\bigcup_{\eta \in Y'_{m'}} G_\eta A_{\eta,m'} = \emptyset$, we obtain the induced subdigraph $[\bigcup M_{e_m m'} - \bigcup_{\eta \in Y'_{m'}} G_\eta A_{\eta,m'}]$ is the digraph with vertex set $G_{m'}$ and arc set $\{(g_{m'}, g_{m'}) : g_{m'} \in G_{m'}\}$ which implies all vertices in $G_{m'}$ are independent. Hence $\alpha([\bigcup M_{e_m m'} - \bigcup_{\eta \in Y'_{m'}} G_\eta A_{\eta,m'}]) = |G_{m'}|$ and so $\sum_{\lambda \in Y_m} \alpha([\bigcup M_{e_m\lambda} - \bigcup_{\eta \in Y'_\lambda} G_\eta A_{\eta,\lambda}]) = 1 + \sum_{\lambda > m}(|G_\lambda| - 1)$. Therefore $\alpha(C_{e_m}) = \sum_{\lambda \in Y_m} \alpha([\bigcup M_{e_m\lambda} - \bigcup_{\eta \in Y'_\lambda} G_\eta A_{\eta,\lambda}])$, as required. □

Example 3. Let $Y = \{\lambda_1, \lambda_2, \lambda_3, \lambda_4\}$ be a chain such that $\lambda_1 \leq \lambda_2 \leq \lambda_3 \leq \lambda_4$. For $I = \{1, 2, 3, 4\}$, we let $\{G_{\lambda_i} : i \in I\}$ be a family of groups, indexed by Y where $G_{\lambda_i} = \mathbb{Z}_4 = \{\bar{0}_{\lambda_i}, \bar{1}_{\lambda_i}, \bar{2}_{\lambda_i}, \bar{3}_{\lambda_i}\}$ is an additive group of integers modulo 4 for all $i \in I$. Let $f_{\lambda_i, \lambda_j}(\bar{x}_{\lambda_i}) = \bar{0}_{\lambda_j}$ for every $\bar{x}_{\lambda_i} \in G_{\lambda_i}$, $\bar{0}_{\lambda_j} \in G_{\lambda_j}$ and $i > j$. Then $S = [Y; G_{\lambda_i}, f_{\lambda_i, \lambda_j}]$ is a Clifford semigroup. For $A = \{\bar{0}_{\lambda_i} : i \in I\}$, $Cay(S, A)$ can be pictured as in Figure 3.

We now determine the independence number of the maximal connected subdigraph $C_{\bar{0}_{\lambda_1}}$. From $A_{\lambda_1} = \{\bar{0}_{\lambda_1}\}$, we obtain $\bar{0}_{\lambda_1}\langle A_{\lambda_1}\rangle = \{\bar{0}_{\lambda_1}\}$. Since $Y_{\lambda_1} = \{\lambda_1, \lambda_2, \lambda_3, \lambda_4\}$, we obtain the following.

(i) Consider $\lambda_4 \in Y_{\lambda_1}$. We obtain $\alpha([\bigcup M_{\bar{0}_{\lambda_1} \lambda_4} \setminus \bigcup_{\eta \in Y'_{\lambda_4}} G_\eta A_{\eta, \lambda_4}]) = \alpha([\{\bar{0}_{\lambda_4}, \bar{1}_{\lambda_4}, \bar{2}_{\lambda_4}, \bar{3}_{\lambda_4}\}]) = 4$.

(ii) Consider $\lambda_3 \in Y_{\lambda_1}$. We obtain $\alpha([\bigcup M_{\bar{0}_{\lambda_1} \lambda_3} \setminus \bigcup_{\eta \in Y'_{\lambda_3}} G_\eta A_{\eta, \lambda_3}]) = \alpha([\{\bar{1}_{\lambda_3}, \bar{2}_{\lambda_3}, \bar{3}_{\lambda_3}\}]) = 3$.

(iii) Consider $\lambda_2 \in Y_{\lambda_1}$. We obtain $\alpha([\bigcup M_{\bar{0}_{\lambda_1} \lambda_2} \setminus \bigcup_{\eta \in Y'_{\lambda_2}} G_\eta A_{\eta, \lambda_2}]) = \alpha([\{\bar{1}_{\lambda_2}, \bar{2}_{\lambda_2}, \bar{3}_{\lambda_2}\}]) = 3$.

(iv) Consider $\lambda_1 \in Y_{\lambda_1}$. We obtain $\alpha([\bigcup M_{\bar{0}_{\lambda_1}\lambda_1} \setminus \bigcup_{\eta \in Y'_{\lambda_1}} G_\eta A_{\eta,\lambda_1}]) = 0$.

We see that $\alpha(C_{\bar{0}_{\lambda_1}}) = \sum_{\lambda \in Y_{\lambda_1}} \alpha([\bigcup M_{\bar{0}_{\lambda_1}\lambda} - \bigcup_{\eta \in Y'_\lambda} G_\eta A_{\eta,\lambda}]) = 4 + 3 + 3 = 10$.

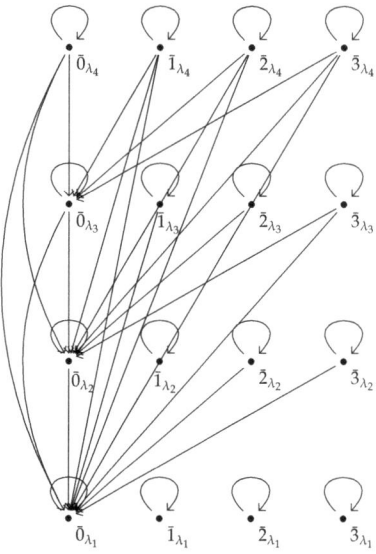

Figure 3. $Cay(S, A)$ where $Y = \{\lambda_1, \lambda_2, \lambda_3, \lambda_4\}$, $G_{\lambda_i} = \mathbb{Z}_4$ and $A = \{\bar{0}_{\lambda_1}, \bar{0}_{\lambda_2}, \bar{0}_{\lambda_3}, \bar{0}_{\lambda_4}\}$.

Proposition 2. *Let $S = [Y; G_\beta, f_{\lambda,\eta}]$ be a Clifford semigroup in which consists a chain Y with the maximum and minimum elements, namely m' and m, respectively. We put $f_{\lambda,\eta}(x) = e_\eta$ for all $x \in G_\lambda$, $\lambda > \eta \in Y$ where e_η is the identity element of G_η. For every $\lambda \in Y$, let $G_\lambda = \langle h_\lambda \rangle$ for some $h_\lambda \in G_\lambda$ such that $h_\lambda \neq e_\lambda$ and $A = \{h_\lambda : \lambda \in Y\}$. Then $\alpha(C_{e_m}) = \sum_{\lambda \in Y_m} \alpha([\bigcup M_{e_m\lambda}])$.*

Proof. Let X_λ be an α-set of the induced subdigraph $[\bigcup M_{e_m\lambda}]$. We then define a set X'_λ by $X'_\lambda := X_\lambda h_\lambda^{-1}$ if $h_\lambda \in X_\lambda$, otherwise $X'_\lambda = X_\lambda$. Consider $X'_\lambda = X_\lambda h_\lambda^{-1}$. If $h_\lambda \in X'_\lambda$, we then obtain $h_\lambda = x_\lambda h_\lambda^{-1}$ for some $x_\lambda \in X_\lambda$. Thus $x_\lambda = h_\lambda h_\lambda$, which implies $(h_\lambda, x_\lambda) \in E([\bigcup M_{e_m\lambda}])$. It contradicts to the fact that X_λ is an independent set of $[\bigcup M_{e_m\lambda}]$ and $x_\lambda, h_\lambda \in X_\lambda$. Hence $h_\lambda \notin X'_\lambda$ for all $\lambda \in Y_m$. Additionally, if $(x_\lambda h^{-1}, y_\lambda h_\lambda^{-1}) \in E([\bigcup M_{e_m\lambda}])$, we obtain $y_\lambda h_\lambda^{-1} = (x_\lambda h^{-1})h_\lambda$ which implies $y_\lambda = x_\lambda h_\lambda$, a contradiction. Thus X'_λ is an independent set of $[\bigcup M_{e_m\lambda}]$ for all $\lambda \in Y$. Now, we claim that $\bigcup_{\lambda \in Y_m} X'_\lambda$ is an independent set of C_{e_m}. Let $x_\lambda h_\lambda^{-1}, x_\eta h_\eta^{-1} \in \bigcup_{\lambda \in Y_m} X'_\lambda$. Assume that $(x_\lambda h_\lambda^{-1}, x_\eta h_\eta^{-1}) \in E(C_{e_m})$ for some $\lambda, \eta \in Y_m$ where $\lambda \neq \eta$. Then $x_\eta h_\eta^{-1} = (x_\lambda h_\lambda^{-1})h_\gamma$ for some $\gamma \in Y$. Because Y is a chain, $\gamma = \eta$. By the assumption, we obtain

$$x_\eta h_\eta^{-1} = f_{\lambda,\eta}(x_\lambda h_\lambda^{-1})f_{\eta,\eta}(h_\eta)$$
$$= f_{\lambda,\eta}(x_\lambda)f_{\lambda,\eta}(h_\lambda^{-1})f_{\eta,\eta}(h_\eta)$$
$$= e_\eta e_\eta h_\eta = h_\eta.$$

It is contradicts to the fact that $h_\lambda \notin X'_\lambda$ for all $\lambda \in Y_m$. Thus $\bigcup_{\lambda \in Y_m} X'_\lambda$ is an independent set of C_{e_m}. Hence we can conclude that $\alpha(C_{e_m}) \geq |\bigcup_{\lambda \in Y_m} X'_\lambda| = \sum_{\lambda \in Y_m} \alpha([\bigcup M_{e_m\lambda}])$. By using the fact that $V(\bigcup_{\lambda \in Y_\beta}[\bigcup M_{g_\beta \lambda}]) = V(C_{e_m})$ and $E(\bigcup_{\lambda \in Y_\beta}[\bigcup M_{g_\beta \lambda}]) \subseteq E(C_{e_m})$, we obtain $\alpha(\bigcup_{\lambda \in Y_\beta}[\bigcup M_{g_\beta \lambda}]) = \sum_{\lambda \in Y_m} \alpha([\bigcup M_{e_m \lambda}]) \geq \alpha(C_{e_m})$. Therefore $\alpha(C_{e_m}) = \sum_{\lambda \in Y_m} \alpha([\bigcup M_{e_m \lambda}])$, as required. □

5. Lower and Upper Bounds of the Weak Independence Numbers

In this section, we present the exact value of the weakly independent number of C_{g_β} that based on the order of $M_{g_\beta \lambda}$ and the independence number of $Cay(\langle A_\lambda \rangle, A'_\lambda)$ where $A'_\lambda := A_\lambda \setminus \{a \in A_\lambda : a^{-1} \notin A_\lambda\}$ for all $\lambda \in Y$. We start with some simple bounds for $\alpha_w(C_{g_\beta})$.

Lemma 9. $\alpha(C_{g_\beta}) \leq \alpha_w(C_{g_\beta}) \leq |V(C_{g_\beta})|$.

Proof. From the fact that every independent set is a weakly independent set. We obtain $\alpha(C_{g_\beta}) \leq \alpha_w(C_{g_\beta})$. For an upper bound, it is obvious that $\alpha_w(C_{g_\beta}) \leq |V(C_{g_\beta})|$. □

By the definition of a Cayley digraphs, we have both (x_λ, y_λ) and (y_λ, x_λ) are belong to $E(Cay(\langle A_\lambda \rangle, A_\lambda))$ if and only if there exists $a, b \in A_\lambda$ such that $y_\lambda = x_\lambda a$ and $x_\lambda = y_\lambda b$. Since G_λ is a group, we obtain $b = a^{-1}$, from that property we can say that, in other words, if $y_\lambda = x_\lambda a$ and $a^{-1} \notin A_\lambda$, then x_λ and y_λ are weakly independent. We now construct an example and then obtain the sharpness of the lower and upper bounds in Lemma 9 as follows;

Proposition 3. Let $S = [Y; G_\beta, f_{\lambda, \eta}]$ be a Clifford semigroup in which consists an ordered set $Y = \{\lambda\}$. Then the following conditions hold:
1. if $A = \{h_\lambda, h_\lambda^{-1}\}$, then $\alpha_w(C_{h_\lambda}) = \alpha(C_{h_\lambda})$;
2. if $|G_\lambda| > 2$ and $A = \{h_\lambda\}$ where $h_\lambda \neq h_\lambda^{-1}$, then $\alpha_w(C_{h_\lambda}) = |V(C_{h_\lambda})|$.

Proof.
1. Let $A = \{h_\lambda, h_\lambda^{-1}\}$. It is easy to check that if $(x_\lambda, y_\lambda) \in E(C_{h_\lambda})$ then $(y_\lambda, x_\lambda) \in E(C_{h_\lambda})$. Thus $\alpha_w(C_{h_\lambda}) = \alpha(C_{h_\lambda})$.
2. Let $A = \{h_\lambda\}$. Let $(x_\lambda, y_\lambda) \in E(C_{h_\lambda})$. Then $y_\lambda = x_\lambda h_\lambda$. Assume that $x_\lambda = y_\lambda h_\lambda$. Thus $x_\lambda h_\lambda = y_\lambda$ which implies $h_\lambda = h_\lambda^{-1}$, a contradiction. We conclude that if $(x_\lambda, y_\lambda) \in E(C_{h_\lambda})$ then $(y_\lambda, x_\lambda) \notin E(C_{h_\lambda})$ for every $x_\lambda, y_\lambda \in V(C_{h_\lambda})$ which implies $V(C_{h_\lambda})$ is weakly independent set. Therefore $\alpha_w(C_{h_\lambda}) = |V(C_{h_\lambda})|$, as required. □

Let G be a group and $\emptyset \neq A \subseteq G$. We next present a result on the weak independence number of $Cay(G, A)$ as follows.

Lemma 10. Let G be a group and $\emptyset \neq A \subseteq G$. Then $\alpha_w(Cay(G, A)) = \alpha_w(Cay(G, A')) = \alpha(Cay(G, A'))$ where $A' := A \setminus \{a \in A : a^{-1} \notin A\}$.

Proof. We first show that $\alpha_w(Cay(G, A)) = \alpha_w(Cay(G, A'))$. Since $A' \subseteq A$, we obtain $E(Cay(G, A')) \subseteq E(Cay(G, A))$. Thus $\alpha_w(Cay(G, A)) \leq \alpha_w(Cay(G, A'))$.

Conversely, we let X' be a weakly independent set of $Cay(G, A')$ and $x, y \in X'$. We claim that X' is a weakly independent set of $Cay(G, A)$. Assume that $(x, y), (y, x) \in E(Cay(G, A))$. Then there exist $a, a^{-1} \in A$ such that $y = xa$ and $x = ya^{-1}$. Thus $a, a^{-1} \in A'$ and it follows that $(x, y), (y, x) \in E(Cay(G, A'))$, a contradiction, because X' is a weakly independent set and $x, y \in X'$. Hence X' is a weakly independent set of $Cay(G, A)$ and then $\alpha_w(Cay(G, A')) \leq \alpha_w(Cay(G, A))$. Therefore $\alpha_w(Cay(G, A')) = \alpha_w(Cay(G, A))$.

Next, we will show that $\alpha_w(Cay(G, A')) = \alpha(Cay(G, A'))$. Clearly, every independent set is a weakly independent set. Thus $\alpha(Cay(G, A')) \leq \alpha_w(Cay(G, A'))$.

Conversely, by the definition of A', we obtain $(x,y) \in E(Cay(G, A'))$ if and only if $(y,x) \in E(Cay(G, A'))$. Let X be a weakly independent set of $Cay(G, A')$. We then obtain x, y are independent for every $x, y \in X$, which implies X is an independent set of $Cay(G, A')$. Hence $\alpha_w(Cay(G, A')) \leq \alpha(Cay(G, A'))$. Thus $\alpha_w(Cay(G, A')) = \alpha(Cay(G, A'))$. □

By the definition of $M_{g_\beta \lambda}$, we then obtain $\left[\bigcup M_{g_\beta \lambda}\right] = \bigcup_{i \in I'} D_i$ where $D_i \cong [g_i \langle A_\lambda \rangle] \cong Cay(\langle A_\lambda \rangle, A_\lambda)$ for all $i \in I'$ where $I' = \{1, 2, \ldots, |M_{g_\beta \lambda}|\}$.

According to the above lemma, we consequently obtain $\alpha_w(Cay(\langle A_\lambda \rangle, A_\lambda)) = \alpha_w(Cay(\langle A_\lambda \rangle, A'_\lambda)) = \alpha(Cay(\langle A_\lambda \rangle, A'_\lambda))$.

We now present the exact value of the weakly independent number of C_{g_β} in the form of the summation of $|M_{g_\beta \lambda}|\alpha_w(Cay(\langle A_\lambda \rangle, A_\lambda))$ for all $\lambda \in Y_\beta$.

Lemma 11. $\alpha_w(C_{g_\beta}) = \sum_{\lambda \in Y_\beta} |M_{g_\beta \lambda}|\alpha_w(Cay(\langle A_\lambda \rangle, A_\lambda))$.

Proof. Let X be an α_w–set of C_{g_β}. We will show that $|X| \leq \sum_{\lambda \in Y_\beta} |M_{g_\beta \lambda}|\alpha_w(Cay(\langle A_\lambda \rangle, A_\lambda))$.

From $\left[\bigcup M_{g_\beta \lambda}\right] = \bigcup_{i \in I'} D_i$ where $D_i \cong [g_i \langle A_\lambda \rangle] \cong Cay(\langle A_\lambda \rangle, A_\lambda)$ for all $i \in I' = \{1, 2, \ldots, |M_{g_\beta \lambda}|\}$, we then obtain $|X \cap (\bigcup M_{g_\beta \lambda})| = \sum_{g_\lambda \langle A_\lambda \rangle \in M_{g_\beta \lambda}} |X \cap g_\lambda \langle A_\lambda \rangle|$ and $|X \cap g_\lambda \langle A_\lambda \rangle| \leq |X_{g_\lambda \langle A_\lambda \rangle}|$ for all $g_\lambda \langle A_\lambda \rangle \in M_{g_\beta \lambda}$ where $X_{g_\lambda \langle A_\lambda \rangle}$ is an α_w–set of $[g_\lambda \langle A_\lambda \rangle]$. Moreover, we conclude that $\sum_{\substack{g_\lambda \langle A_\lambda \rangle \in M_{g_\beta \lambda} \\ \lambda \in Y_\beta}} |X \cap g_\lambda \langle A_\lambda \rangle| \leq \sum_{\substack{g_\lambda \langle A_\lambda \rangle \in M_{g_\beta \lambda} \\ \lambda \in Y_\beta}} |X_{g_\lambda \langle A_\lambda \rangle}|$.

Since $X \subseteq \bigcup_{\lambda \in Y_\beta}(\bigcup M_{g_\beta \lambda})$, we obtain $|X| = |X \cap (\bigcup_{\lambda \in Y_\beta}(\bigcup M_{g_\beta \lambda}))| = \sum_{\substack{g_\lambda \langle A_\lambda \rangle \in M_{g_\beta \lambda} \\ \lambda \in Y_\beta}} |X \cap g_\lambda \langle A_\lambda \rangle| \leq \sum_{\substack{g_\lambda \langle A_\lambda \rangle \in M_{g_\beta \lambda} \\ \lambda \in Y_\beta}} |X_{g_\lambda \langle A_\lambda \rangle}| = \sum_{\lambda \in Y_\beta} |M_{g_\beta \lambda}|\alpha_w(Cay(\langle A_\lambda \rangle, A_\lambda))$. Thus $\alpha_w(C_{g_\beta}) = |X| \leq \sum_{\lambda \in Y_\beta} |M_{g_\beta \lambda}|\alpha_w(Cay(\langle A_\lambda \rangle, A_\lambda))$.

Conversely, we know that $\left[\bigcup M_{g_\beta \lambda}\right]$ is a disjoint union of $[g_\lambda \langle A_\lambda \rangle]$ for all $g_\lambda \langle A_\lambda \rangle \in M_{g_\beta \lambda}$, we obtain $\bigcup_{g_\lambda \langle A_\lambda \rangle \in M_{g_\beta \lambda}} X_{g_\lambda \langle A_\lambda \rangle}$ is a weakly independent set of C_{g_β} where $X_{g_\lambda \langle A_\lambda \rangle}$ is a weakly independent set of $[g_\lambda \langle A_\lambda \rangle]$. From the fact that if $u \in G_\lambda$ and $v \in G_\eta$ where $\lambda \neq \eta$, then u, v are weakly independent, we obtain $\bigcup_{\substack{g_\lambda \langle A_\lambda \rangle \in M_{g_\beta \lambda} \\ \lambda \in Y_\beta}} X_{g_\lambda \langle A_\lambda \rangle}$ is a weakly independent set of C_{g_β}. Since $[g_\lambda \langle A_\lambda \rangle] \cong Cay(\langle A_\lambda \rangle, A_\lambda)$ for all $g_\lambda \langle A_\lambda \rangle \in M_{g_\beta \lambda}$, we obtain $|X_{g_\lambda \langle A_\lambda \rangle}| = \alpha_w(Cay(\langle A_\lambda \rangle, A_\lambda))$ for all $g_\lambda \langle A_\lambda \rangle \in M_{g_\beta \lambda}$ and $\lambda \in Y_\beta$. Hence $\sum_{\substack{g_\lambda \langle A_\lambda \rangle \in M_{g_\beta \lambda} \\ \lambda \in Y_\beta}} |X_{g_\lambda \langle A_\lambda \rangle}| = \sum_{\lambda \in Y_\beta} |M_{g_\beta \lambda}|\alpha_w(Cay(\langle A_\lambda \rangle, A_\lambda))$ and so $\alpha_w(C_{g_\beta}) \geq \sum_{\lambda \in Y_\beta} |M_{g_\beta \lambda}|\alpha_w(Cay(\langle A_\lambda \rangle, A_\lambda))$. □

Example 4. Let $Y = \{\lambda_1, \lambda_2, \lambda_3, \lambda_4\}$ be a semilattice with a partial order that represented by the Hasse diagram in Figure 4. For $I = \{1, 2, 3, 4\}$, we let $\{G_{\lambda_i} : i \in I\}$ be a family of groups, indexed by the semilattice Y where $G_{\lambda_i} = \mathbb{Z}_4 = \{\bar{0}_{\lambda_i}, \bar{1}_{\lambda_i}, \bar{2}_{\lambda_i}, \bar{3}_{\lambda_i}\}$ is an additive group of integers modulo 4 for all $i \in I$. Let $f_{\lambda_i, \lambda_j}(\bar{x}_{\lambda_i}) = \bar{x}_{\lambda_j}$ for every $\bar{x}_{\lambda_i} \in G_{\lambda_i}$, $\bar{x}_{\lambda_j} \in G_{\lambda_j}$ and $i > j$. Then $S = [Y; G_{\lambda_i}, f_{\lambda_i, \lambda_j}]$ is a Clifford semigroup.

Let $A = \{\bar{2}_{\lambda_2}\}$. Then we picture $Cay(S, A)$ in Figure 5. From $A_{\lambda_2} = \{\bar{2}_{\lambda_2}\}$, then $\langle A_{\lambda_2}\rangle = \{\bar{0}_{\lambda_2}, \bar{2}_{\lambda_2}\}$ which implies $G_{\lambda_2}/\langle A_{\lambda_2}\rangle = \{\langle A_{\lambda_2}\rangle, \bar{1}_{\lambda_2}\langle A_{\lambda_2}\rangle\}$. We here consider $C_{\bar{0}_{\lambda_2}}$ and each $\lambda_2, \lambda_4 \in Y_{\lambda_2}$ as follows.

(i) Consider $\lambda_4 \in Y_{\lambda_2}$.
- Since $A = \{\bar{2}_{\lambda_2}\}$, we have $A_{\lambda_4} = \varnothing$. Thus we put $A_{\lambda_4} = \{\bar{0}_{\lambda_4}\}$.
- Then $M_{\bar{0}_{\lambda_2}\lambda_4} = \{g_{\lambda_4}\langle\bar{0}_{\lambda_4}\rangle \in G_{\lambda_4}/\langle\bar{0}_{\lambda_4}\rangle : f_{\lambda_4,\lambda_2}(g_{\lambda_4}) \in \bar{0}_{\lambda_2}\langle A_{\lambda_2}\rangle\}$ $= \{\bar{0}_{\lambda_4}\langle\bar{0}_{\lambda_4}\rangle, \bar{2}_{\lambda_4}\langle\bar{0}_{\lambda_4}\rangle\}$.
- From $A_{\lambda_4} = \{\bar{0}_{\lambda_4}\}$, we obtain $\alpha_w(Cay(\langle A_{\lambda_4}\rangle, A_{\lambda_4})) = \alpha_w(Cay(\{\bar{0}_{\lambda_4}\}, \{\bar{0}_{\lambda_4}\})) = 1$.
- Therefore $|M_{\bar{0}_{\lambda_2}\lambda_4}|\alpha_w(Cay(\{\bar{0}_{\lambda_4}\}, \{\bar{0}_{\lambda_4}\})) = 2$.

(ii) Consider $\lambda_2 \in Y_{\lambda_2}$.
- We have $M_{\bar{0}_{\lambda_2}\lambda_2} = \{g_{\lambda_2}\langle A_{\lambda_2}\rangle \in G_{\lambda_4}/\langle A_{\lambda_4}\rangle : f_{\lambda_2,\lambda_2}(g_{\lambda_2}) \in \bar{0}_{\lambda_2}\langle A_{\lambda_2}\rangle\} = \{\langle A_{\lambda_2}\rangle\}$.
- From $\langle A_{\lambda_2}\rangle = \{\bar{0}_{\lambda_2}, \bar{2}_{\lambda_2}\}$, we obtain $\alpha_w(Cay(\langle A_{\lambda_2}\rangle, A_{\lambda_2})) = 1$.
- Therefore $|M_{\bar{0}_{\lambda_2}\lambda_2}|\alpha_w(Cay(\langle A_{\lambda_2}\rangle, A_{\lambda_2})) = 1$.

Therefore $\alpha_w(C_{\bar{0}_{\lambda_2}}) = |M_{\bar{0}_{\lambda_2}\lambda_4}|\alpha_w(Cay(\{\bar{0}_{\lambda_4}\}, \{\bar{0}_{\lambda_4}\})) + |M_{\bar{0}_{\lambda_2}\lambda_2}|\alpha_w(Cay(\langle A_{\lambda_2}\rangle, A_{\lambda_2}))$ $= 3$. Similarly,

$\alpha_w(C_{\bar{1}_{\lambda_2}}) = |M_{\bar{1}_{\lambda_2}\lambda_4}|\alpha_w(Cay(\{\bar{0}_{\lambda_4}\}, \{\bar{0}_{\lambda_4}\})) + |M_{\bar{1}_{\lambda_2}\lambda_2}|\alpha_w(Cay(\langle A_{\lambda_2}\rangle, A_{\lambda_2})) = 3$,

$\alpha_w(C_{\bar{0}_{\lambda_1}}) = |M_{\bar{0}_{\lambda_1}\lambda_3}|\alpha_w(Cay(\{\bar{0}_{\lambda_3}\}, \{\bar{0}_{\lambda_3}\})) + |M_{\bar{0}_{\lambda_1}\lambda_1}|\alpha_w(Cay(\langle A_{\lambda_1}\rangle, A_{\lambda_1})) = 3$,

$\alpha_w(C_{\bar{1}_{\lambda_1}}) = |M_{\bar{1}_{\lambda_1}\lambda_3}|\alpha_w(Cay(\{\bar{0}_{\lambda_3}\}, \{\bar{0}_{\lambda_3}\})) + |M_{\bar{1}_{\lambda_1}\lambda_1}|\alpha_w(Cay(\langle A_{\lambda_1}\rangle, A_{\lambda_1})) = 3$.

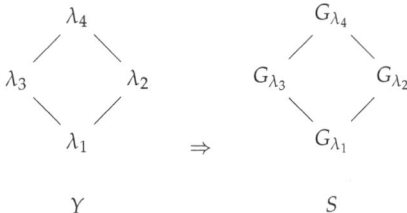

Figure 4. The Hasse diagram of the semilattice $Y = \{\lambda_1, \lambda_2, \lambda_3, \lambda_4\}$ and the family of groups $\{G_{\lambda_i} = \mathbb{Z}_4 : i = 1, 2, 3, 4\}$.

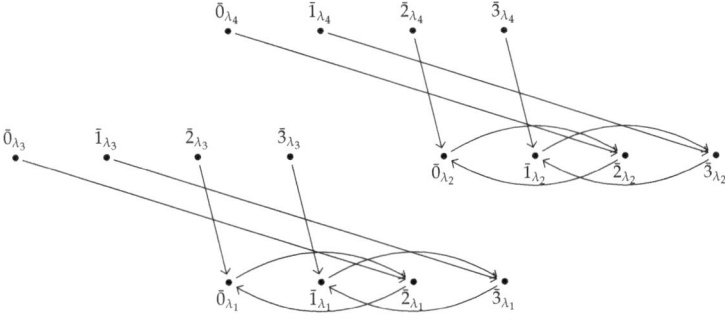

Figure 5. $Cay(S, A)$ where $A = \{\bar{2}_{\lambda_2}\}$.

By Lemma 10, we directly obtain the following corollary.

Corollary 1. $\alpha_w(C_{g_\beta}) = \sum_{\lambda \in Y_\beta} |M_{g_\beta\lambda}|\alpha_w(Cay(\langle A_\lambda\rangle, A'_\lambda)) = \sum_{\lambda \in Y_\beta} |M_{g_\beta\lambda}|\alpha(Cay(\langle A_\lambda\rangle, A'_\lambda))$.

In summary, we now obtain the weak independence number of $Cay(S, A)$, which is presented in terms of $\alpha_w(Cay(\langle A_\lambda \rangle, A_\lambda))$ for all $\lambda \in Y_\beta$.

Theorem 4. $\alpha_w(Cay(S,A)) = \sum\limits_{\substack{g \in A_\beta \\ \beta \in B}} (\alpha_w(C_{g\beta})) = \sum\limits_{\substack{g \in A_\beta \\ \beta \in B}} (\sum\limits_{\lambda \in Y_\beta} |M_{g\beta\lambda}| \alpha_w(Cay(\langle A_\lambda \rangle, A_\lambda)))$.

Example 5. *From the Example 4, $Cay(S, A)$ consists of four components, $C_{\bar{0}_{\lambda_2}}$, $C_{\bar{1}_{\lambda_2}}$, $C_{\bar{0}_{\lambda_1}}$ and $C_{\bar{1}_{\lambda_1}}$. We see that $X = \{\bar{0}_{\lambda_4}, \bar{1}_{\lambda_4}, \bar{2}_{\lambda_4}, \bar{3}_{\lambda_4}, \bar{0}_{\lambda_2}, \bar{1}_{\lambda_2}, \bar{0}_{\lambda_3}, \bar{1}_{\lambda_3}, \bar{2}_{\lambda_3}, \bar{3}_{\lambda_3}, \bar{0}_{\lambda_1}, \bar{1}_{\lambda_1}\}$ is an α_w–set of $Cay(S, A)$. Then $\alpha_w(Cay(S, A)) = \alpha_w(C_{\bar{0}_{\lambda_2}}) + \alpha_w(C_{\bar{1}_{\lambda_2}}) + \alpha_w(C_{\bar{0}_{\lambda_1}}) + \alpha_w(C_{\bar{1}_{\lambda_1}}) = 12 = |X|$.*

6. The Path Independence Numbers

From the fact that, for every $\lambda \in Y$, $Cay(\langle A_\lambda \rangle, A_\lambda)$ is strongly connected. By this information, we can conclude that $\alpha_p(Cay(\langle A_\lambda \rangle, A_\lambda)) = 1$. However, to find the path independence number of $C_{g\beta}$, we need to consider a path between induced subdigraphs $[g_\lambda \langle A_\lambda \rangle]$ and $[h_\eta \langle A_\eta \rangle]$ of $Cay(S, A)$ where $g_\lambda \langle A_\lambda \rangle \in M_{g\beta\lambda}$ and $h_\eta \langle A_\eta \rangle \in M_{g\beta\eta}$.

We here investigate a relation that indicates all paths between $[g_\lambda \langle A_\lambda \rangle]$ and $[h_\eta \langle A_\eta \rangle]$ in $C_{g\beta}$. Let $\tilde{C}_{g\beta} := \bigcup\limits_{\lambda \in Y_\beta} M_{g\beta\lambda}$ and $\tilde{Y}_\eta := \{\lambda \in Y : \lambda \wedge (\bigwedge\limits_{\gamma \in \Gamma_\lambda} \gamma) = \eta \text{ for some } \Gamma_\lambda \subseteq Y'\} \cup \{\eta\}$.
Define a relation $\sim$ on $\tilde{C}_{g\beta}$ by $g_\lambda \langle A_\lambda \rangle \sim h_\eta \langle A_\eta \rangle$ if and only if $f_{\lambda,\eta}(g_\lambda) \in h_\eta \langle A_\eta \rangle$ and $\lambda \in \tilde{Y}_\eta$.

Lemma 12. $(\tilde{C}_{g\beta}, \sim)$ *is a partially ordered set.*

Proof. Let $\beta \in B$. We shall show that $\sim$ is a partial order on $\tilde{C}_{g\beta}$.

(i) Since $f_{\lambda,\lambda}(g_\lambda) \in g_\lambda \langle A_\lambda \rangle$ and $\lambda \in \tilde{Y}_\lambda$, we then obtain $g_\lambda \langle A_\lambda \rangle \sim g_\lambda \langle A_\lambda \rangle$.

(ii) Let $g_\lambda \langle A_\lambda \rangle \sim h_\eta \langle A_\eta \rangle$ and $h_\eta \langle A_\eta \rangle \sim g_\lambda \langle A_\lambda \rangle$. Then $f_{\lambda,\eta}(g_\lambda) \in h_\eta \langle A_\eta \rangle$ and $f_{\eta,\lambda}(h_\eta) \in g_\lambda \langle A_\lambda \rangle$. This gives $\eta \leq \lambda$ and $\lambda \leq \eta$. From Y is a semilattice and $\lambda, \eta \in Y$, we obtain $\lambda = \eta$. Since $h_\eta \langle A_\eta \rangle = h_\lambda \langle A_\lambda \rangle$ and $f_{\eta,\lambda}(h_\eta) = f_{\lambda,\lambda}(h_\lambda) \in g_\lambda \langle A_\lambda \rangle$, it follows that $g_\lambda \langle A_\lambda \rangle = h_\eta \langle A_\eta \rangle$.

(iii) Let $g_\lambda \langle A_\lambda \rangle \sim h_\eta \langle A_\eta \rangle$ and $h_\eta \langle A_\eta \rangle \sim k_\kappa \langle A_\kappa \rangle$. Then $f_{\lambda,\eta}(g_\lambda) \in h_\eta \langle A_\eta \rangle$ and $f_{\eta,\kappa}(h_\eta) \in k_\kappa \langle A_\kappa \rangle$. From Lemma 4, we obtain $f_{\eta,\kappa}(h_\eta \langle A_\eta \rangle) \subseteq f_{\eta,\kappa}(h_\eta) \langle A_\kappa \rangle$. Thus $f_{\eta,\kappa}(h_\eta) \in f_{\eta,\kappa}(h_\eta) \langle A_\kappa \rangle$ and so $f_{\eta,\kappa}(h_\eta) \langle A_\kappa \rangle = k_\kappa \langle A_\kappa \rangle$. Therefore $f_{\lambda,\kappa}(g_\lambda) = f_{\eta,\kappa}(f_{\lambda,\eta}(g_\lambda)) \in f_{\eta,\kappa}(h_\eta \langle A_\eta \rangle) \subseteq f_{\eta,\kappa}(h_\eta) \langle A_\kappa \rangle = k_\kappa \langle A_\kappa \rangle$.
From $\lambda \in \tilde{Y}_\eta$ and $\eta \in \tilde{Y}_\kappa$, there exist two subsets of Y', denoted by Γ_λ and Γ_η, such that $\lambda \wedge (\bigwedge\limits_{\gamma \in \Gamma_\lambda} \gamma) = \eta$ and $\eta \wedge (\bigwedge\limits_{\gamma \in \Gamma_\eta} \gamma) = \kappa$. Then $\lambda \wedge (\bigwedge\limits_{\gamma \in \Gamma_\lambda \cup \Gamma_\eta} \gamma) = \kappa$ and thus $\lambda \in \tilde{Y}_\kappa$.

Therefore $(\tilde{C}_{g\beta}, \sim)$ is a partially ordered set. □

Lemma 13. *Let $x \in g_\lambda \langle A_\lambda \rangle$ and $y \in h_\eta \langle A_\eta \rangle$ where $\lambda \neq \eta$. Then there is a path from x to y if and only if $g_\lambda \langle A_\lambda \rangle \sim h_\eta \langle A_\eta \rangle$.*

Proof. Assume that there exists a path from x to y. Then we let $x = v_1, v_2, \ldots, v_n = y$ be a path from x to y where $(v_i, v_{i+1}) \in E(Cay(S, A))$ for all $i = 1, 2, \ldots n - 1$. It follows that there exist $a_1, a_2, \ldots, a_{n-1} \in A$ and $\gamma_1, \gamma_2, \ldots, \gamma_{n-1} \in Y'$ such that $v_{i+1} = v_i a_i$ and $a_i \in G_{\gamma_i}$ for all $i = 1, 2, \ldots, n - 1$. This gives

$$v_n = (\ldots((v_1 a_1)a_2)\ldots)a_{n-1}$$
$$= (\ldots((xa_1)a_2)\ldots)a_{n-1}$$
$$= (\ldots((f_{\lambda,\lambda\wedge\gamma_1}(x)f_{\gamma_1,\lambda\wedge\gamma_1}(a_1))a_2)\ldots)a_{n-1}$$
$$= (\ldots(((f_{\lambda\wedge\gamma_1,(\lambda\wedge\gamma_1)\wedge\gamma_2}(f_{\lambda,\lambda\wedge\gamma_1}(x)f_{\gamma_1,\lambda\wedge\gamma_1}(a_1))f_{\gamma_2,(\lambda\wedge\gamma_1)\wedge\gamma_2}(a_2))\ldots)a_{n-1}$$
$$\vdots$$
$$= f_{\lambda\wedge(\bigwedge_{i=1}^{n-2}\gamma_i),\lambda\wedge(\bigwedge_{i=1}^{n-2}\gamma_i)\wedge\gamma_{n-1}}(\ldots(f_{\lambda,\lambda\wedge\gamma_1}(x)f_{\gamma_1,\lambda\wedge\gamma_1}(a_1))\ldots)f_{\gamma_{n-1},\lambda\wedge(\bigwedge_{i=1}^{n-2}\gamma_i)\wedge\gamma_{n-1}}(a_{n-1})$$
$$= f_{\lambda,\eta}(x)f_{\gamma_1,\eta}(a_1)f_{\gamma_2,\eta}(a_2)\ldots f_{\gamma_{n-1},\eta}(a_{n-1})$$
$$\in f_{\lambda,\eta}(x)\langle A_\eta\rangle.$$

Since $v_n = y \in h_\eta\langle A_\eta\rangle$, we obtain $f_{\lambda,\eta}(x)\langle A_\eta\rangle = h_\eta\langle A_\eta\rangle$. From Lemma 4, we obtain $f_{\lambda,\eta}(g_\lambda\langle A_\lambda\rangle) = f_{\lambda,\eta}(x\langle A_\lambda\rangle) \subseteq f_{\lambda,\eta}(x)\langle A_\eta\rangle = h_\eta\langle A_\eta\rangle$ which implies $f_{\lambda,\eta}(g_\lambda) \in h_\eta\langle A_\eta\rangle$. Therefore $g_\lambda\langle A_\lambda\rangle \sim h_\eta\langle A_\eta\rangle$.

Conversely, suppose that $g_\lambda\langle A_\lambda\rangle \sim h_\eta\langle A_\eta\rangle$. Then $f_{\lambda,\eta}(g_\lambda) \in h_\eta\langle A_\eta\rangle$ and $\lambda \in \tilde{Y}_\eta$, i.e., there exists $\Gamma_\lambda \subseteq Y'$ such that $\lambda \wedge (\bigwedge_{\gamma\in\Gamma_\lambda}\gamma) = \eta$. Now, we let $\Gamma_\lambda = \{\gamma_1, \gamma_2, \ldots, \gamma_n\}$ and $a_1, a_2, \ldots a_n \in A$. Then $g_\lambda, g_\lambda a_1, g_\lambda a_1 a_2, \ldots, g_\lambda a_1 a_2 \ldots a_n$ is a path from g_λ to $g_\lambda a_1 a_2 \ldots a_n$. Consequently, we conclude that

$$g_\lambda a_1 a_2 \ldots a_n = f_{\lambda,\lambda\wedge(\bigwedge_{i=1}^n\gamma_i)}(g_\lambda)f_{\gamma_1,\lambda\wedge(\bigwedge_{i=1}^n\gamma_i)}(a_{\gamma_1})f_{\gamma_2,\lambda\wedge(\bigwedge_{i=1}^n\gamma_i)}(a_{\gamma_2})\ldots f_{\gamma_n,\lambda\wedge(\bigwedge_{i=1}^n\gamma_i)}(a_{\gamma_n})$$
$$\in f_{\lambda,\eta}(g_\lambda)\langle A_\eta\rangle.$$

Since $f_{\lambda,\eta}(g_\lambda) \in h_\eta\langle A_\eta\rangle$, we obtain $f_{\lambda,\eta}(g_\lambda)\langle A_\eta\rangle = h_\eta\langle A_\eta\rangle$. From the fact that $[g_\lambda\langle A_\lambda\rangle]$ and $[h_\eta\langle A_\eta\rangle]$ are strongly connected, there exist a path from x to g_λ and a path from $g_\lambda a_1 a_2 \ldots a_n$ to y. Therefore there exists a path from x to y, as required. □

By using an anti-symmetric property, we can conclude that if $\lambda \neq \eta$ and there is a path from $x \in g_\lambda\langle A_\lambda\rangle$ to $y \in h_\eta\langle A_\eta\rangle$, then there is no path from y to x. Now, we are ready to give the path independence number of C_{g_β}.

Lemma 14. $\alpha_p(C_{g_\beta}) = max\{|X| : X \text{ is an anti-chain in } (\tilde{C}_{g_\beta}, \sim)\}$.

Proof. Let X' be an α_p-set of C_{g_β} and $x, y \in X'$. Since $x \in g\langle A_\lambda\rangle$ and $y \in h\langle A_\eta\rangle$ for some $g \in G_\lambda, h \in G_\eta$, we obtain $x\langle A_\lambda\rangle \neq y\langle A_\eta\rangle$ because $[x\langle A_\lambda\rangle]$ is strongly connected. By Lemma 13, we have $x\langle A_\lambda\rangle \nsim y\langle A_\eta\rangle$ and $y\langle A_\eta\rangle \nsim x\langle A_\lambda\rangle$. Thus $X = \{g\langle A_\lambda\rangle \in \tilde{C}_{g_\beta} : x \in X'\}$ is an anti-chain in $(\tilde{C}_{g_\beta}, \sim)$ and $|X'| = |X|$. Therefore $\alpha_p(C_{g_\beta}) \leq max\{|X| : X \text{ is an anti-chain in } (\tilde{C}_{g_\beta}, \sim)\}$.

Conversely, we know that for every path independent set X' of C_{g_β}, there exists $X = \{x\langle A_\lambda\rangle \in \tilde{C}_{g_\beta} : x \in X'\}$ where X is an anti-chain in $(\tilde{C}_{g_\beta}, \sim)$, and $|X'| = |X|$. Hence $\alpha_p(C_{g_\beta}) \geq max\{|X| : X \text{ is an anti-chain in } (\tilde{C}_{g_\beta}, \sim)\}$. □

In summary, the path independence number of $Cay(S, A)$ will be obtained in the form of the summation of $max\{|X| : X \text{ is an anti-chain in } (\tilde{C}_{g_\beta}, \sim)\}$ for all $g \in \mathcal{A}_\beta$ and $\beta \in B$.

Theorem 5. $\alpha_p(Cay(S, A)) = \sum_{\substack{g\in\mathcal{A}_\beta \\ \beta\in B}} (\alpha_p(C_{g_\beta})) = \sum_{\substack{g\in\mathcal{A}_\beta \\ \beta\in B}} max\{|X| : X \text{ is an anti-chain in } (\tilde{C}_{g_\beta}, \sim)\}$.

7. The Weak Path Independence Numbers

In this section, a weakly path independent set of C_{g_β} of $Cay(S, A)$ is investigated. By the definition of a weakly path independent set and $[g\langle A_\lambda\rangle] \cong Cay(\langle A_\lambda\rangle, A_\lambda)$ is strongly connected, we can conclude that $\alpha_{wp}([g\langle A_\lambda\rangle])=1$ for every induced subdigraph $[g\langle A_\lambda\rangle]$ of $Cay(S,A)$ and $\beta \in B$.

From the fact that, for all $g \in g_\lambda\langle A_\lambda\rangle$ and $h \in h_\eta\langle A_\eta\rangle$ where $\lambda \neq \eta$, there is no path from h to g if there is a path from g to h. We here obtain the weak path independence number of C_{g_β} and $Cay(S,A)$ as follows.

Lemma 15. $\alpha_{wp}(C_{g_\beta}) = |\bigcup_{\lambda \in Y_\beta} \mathcal{M}_{g_\beta\lambda}|.$

Proof. Let $\mathcal{M}_{g_\beta\lambda}$ be a set of representatives of all cosets in $M_{g_\beta\lambda}$. From the fact that there exists a path either from g to h or from h to g for any different $g, h \in \bigcup_{\lambda \in Y_\beta} \mathcal{M}_{g_\beta\lambda}$. Thus $\bigcup_{\lambda \in Y_\beta} \mathcal{M}_{g_\beta\lambda}$ is a weakly path independent set of C_{g_β} and hence $\alpha_{wp}(C_{g_\beta}) \geq |\bigcup_{\lambda \in Y_\beta} \mathcal{M}_{g_\beta\lambda}| = |\bigcup_{\lambda \in Y_\beta} M_{g_\beta\lambda}|.$

Conversely, let X be an α_{wp}-set of C_{g_β}. We know that $[g\langle A_\lambda\rangle]$ is strongly connected for every $g\langle A_\lambda\rangle \in \bigcup_{\lambda \in Y_\beta} \mathcal{M}_{g_\beta\lambda}$. Hence $|X| \leq |\bigcup_{\lambda \in Y_\beta} \mathcal{M}_{g_\beta\lambda}|$. It follows that $\alpha_{wp}(C_{g_\beta}) \leq |\bigcup_{\lambda \in Y_\beta} \mathcal{M}_{g_\beta\lambda}| = |\bigcup_{\lambda \in Y_\beta} M_{g_\beta\lambda}|$ and so $\alpha_{wp}(C_{g_\beta}) = |\bigcup_{\lambda \in Y_\beta} M_{g_\beta\lambda}|$, as required. □

Now, the weak path independence number of $Cay(S,A)$ will be obtained in the form of the summation of $\alpha_{wp}(C_{g_\beta}) = |\bigcup_{\lambda \in Y_\beta} M_{g_\beta\lambda}|$ as follows.

Theorem 6. $\alpha_{wp}(Cay(S,A)) = \sum_{\substack{g \in \mathcal{A}_\beta \\ \beta \in B}} (\alpha_{wp}(C_{g_\beta})) = \sum_{\substack{g \in \mathcal{A}_\beta \\ \beta \in B}} |\bigcup_{\lambda \in Y_\beta} M_{g_\beta\lambda}|.$

8. Discussion

In this paper, we conducted an in-depth investigation of the independence numbers of the Cayley digraph of the Clifford semigroup. The study focused on a maximal connected subdigraph to analyze its independent sets. Our findings revealed that the independence number of the entire digraph is influenced by the independence numbers of its maximal connected subdigraphs, providing valuable insights into the structural dependencies within the digraph. Although our research aligned with previous studies on the independence numbers of graphs and digraphs, its unique focus on the Cayley digraph of the Clifford semigroup contributes to the theoretical understanding of this specific mathematical structure. As a stepping stone for future research, our study suggests exploring a subdigraph of the Cayley digraphs, which is smaller than a component, to further deepen the understanding of the independence number. In summary, our investigation sheds light on the independence numbers of the Cayley digraph and opens new avenues for future explorations and potential applications in diverse domains.

9. Conclusions

In conclusion, we obtained the characteristic of a maximal connected subdigraph in Cayley digraphs of Clifford semigroups in Section 3. The lower and upper bounds of the independence and the weak independence numbers of Cayley digraphs of Clifford semigroups are presented in Sections 4 and 5. Finally, we have achieved the exact values of the path independence and the weak path independence numbers in Sections 6 and 7, respectively.

Author Contributions: Conceptualization, K.L. and S.P.; methodology, K.L. and S.P.; validation, S.P.; investigation, K.L.; writing—original draft preparation, K.L. and S.P.; writing—review and editing, K.L. and S.P.; visualization, S.P.; supervision, K.L. and S.P.; project administration, S.P.; funding acquisition, S.P. All authors have read and agreed to the published version of the manuscript.

Funding: This research received no external funding.

Institutional Review Board Statement: Not applicable.

Informed Consent Statement: Not applicable.

Data Availability Statement: Not applicable.

Acknowledgments: The authors would like to thank the referees for their useful comments and valuable suggestions on the manuscript. This research was supported by Chiang Mai University.

Conflicts of Interest: The authors declare no conflict of interest.

References

1. Heydemann, M. Cayley graphs and interconnection networks. *Graph Symmetry Algebr. Methods Appl.* **1997**, *497*, 167–224.
2. Xiao, W.; Parhami, B. Some mathematical properties of cayley digraphs with applications to interconnection network design. *Int. J. Comput. Math.* **2005**, *82*, 521–528. [CrossRef]
3. Arworn, S.; Knauer, U.; Na Chiangmai, N. Characterization of digraphs of right (left) zero unions of groups. *Thai J. Math.* **2003**, *1*, 131–140.
4. Hao, Y.; Gao, X.; Luo, Y. On the Cayley graphs of Brandt semigroups. *Commun. Algebra* **2011**, *39*, 2874–2883. [CrossRef]
5. Kelarev, A.V.; Ryan, J.; Yearwood, J.L. Cayley graphs as classifiers for data mining: The influence of asymmetries. *Discret. Math.* **2009**, *309*, 5360–5369. [CrossRef]
6. Khosravi, B. On the Cayley graphs of completely simple semigroups. *Bull. Malays. Math. Sci. Soc.* **2018**, *41*, 741–749. [CrossRef]
7. Panma, S.; Na Chiangmai, N.; Knauer, U.; Arworn, S. Characterizations of Clifford semigroup digraphs. *Discret. Math.* **2006**, *306*, 1247–1252. [CrossRef]
8. Ilić-Georgijević, E. A description of the Cayley graphs of homogeneous semigroups. *Commun. Algebra* **2020**, *48*, 5203–5214. [CrossRef]
9. Harant, J.; Schiermeyer, I. On the independence number of a graph in terms of order and size. *Discret. Math.* **2001**, *232*, 131–138. [CrossRef]
10. Harant, J.; Schiermeyer, I. A Lower bound on the independence number of a graph in terms of degree. *Discuss. Math. Graph Theory* **2006**, *26*, 431–437. [CrossRef]
11. Löwenstein, C.; Pedersen, A.S.; Rautenbach, D.; Regen, F. Independence, odd girth and average degree. *J. Graph Theory* **2011**, *67*, 96–111. [CrossRef]
12. Henning, M.A.; Löwenstein, C. An improved lower bound on the independence number of a graph. *Discret. Appl. Math.* **2014**, *179*, 120–128. [CrossRef]
13. Harant, J. A lower bound on independence in terms of degrees. *Discret. Appl. Math.* **2011**, *159*, 966–970. [CrossRef]
14. Harant, J.; Henning, M.A.; Rautenbach, D.; Regen, F.; Schiermeyer, I. The independence number in graphs of maximum degree three. *Discret. Math.* **2008**, *308*, 5829–5833. [CrossRef]
15. Abay-Asmerom, G.; Hammack, R.; Larson, C.E.; Taylor, D.T. Notes on the independence number in the cartesian product of graphs. *Discuss. Math. Graph Theory* **2011**, *31*, 25–35. [CrossRef]
16. Csizmadia, G. On the independence number of minimum distance graphs. *Discret. Comput. Geom.* **1998**, *20*, 179–187. [CrossRef]
17. Lichiardopol, N. Independence number of iterated line digraphs. *Discret. Math.* **2005**, *293*, 185–193. [CrossRef]
18. Hayat, S.; Siddiqui, H.M.A.; Imran, M.; Ikhlaq, H.M.; Cao, J. On the zero forcing number and propagation time of oriented graphs. *AIMS Math.* **2021**, *6*, 1833–1850. [CrossRef]
19. Panma, S.; Nupo, N. On the Independence number of Cayley digraphs of rectangular groups. *Graphs Comb.* **2018**, *34*, 579–598. [CrossRef]
20. Chartrand, G.; Lesniak, L.; Zhang, P. *Graphs & Digraphs*, 6th ed.; Chapman and Hall/CRC: New York, NY, USA, 2016.
21. Howie, J.M. *Fundamentals of Semigroup Theory*; Clanderon Press: Oxford, UK, 1995.

Disclaimer/Publisher's Note: The statements, opinions and data contained in all publications are solely those of the individual author(s) and contributor(s) and not of MDPI and/or the editor(s). MDPI and/or the editor(s) disclaim responsibility for any injury to people or property resulting from any ideas, methods, instructions or products referred to in the content.

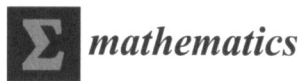

Article

On Edge-Primitive Graphs of Order as a Product of Two Distinct Primes

Renbing Xiao [1], Xiaojiao Zhang [1] and Hua Zhang [2],*

[1] School of Mathematics and Information Science, Nanchang Normal University, Nanchang 330032, China; xiaorenbing@ncnu.edu.cn (R.X.); xiaojiaozhang@ncnu.edu.cn (X.Z.)
[2] School of Mathematics, Yunnan Normal University, Kunming 650091, China
* Correspondence: zhdahua@gmail.com

Abstract: A graph is edge-primitive if its automorphism group acts primitively on the edge set of the graph. Edge-primitive graphs form an important subclass of symmetric graphs. In this paper, edge-primitive graphs of order as a product of two distinct primes are completely determined. This depends on non-abelian simple groups with a subgroup of index pq being classified, where $p > q$ are odd primes.

Keywords: edge-primitive graphs; primitive permutation group; symmetric graphs

MSC: 05E99; 08A99

Citation: Xiao, R.; Zhang, X.; Zhang, H. On Edge-Primitive Graphs of Order as a Product of Two Distinct Primes. *Mathematics* 2023, 11, 3896. https://doi.org/10.3390/math11183896

Academic Editors: Irina Cristea and Alessandro Linzi

Received: 6 June 2023
Revised: 6 August 2023
Accepted: 9 August 2023
Published: 13 September 2023

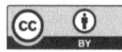

Copyright: © 2023 by the authors. Licensee MDPI, Basel, Switzerland. This article is an open access article distributed under the terms and conditions of the Creative Commons Attribution (CC BY) license (https://creativecommons.org/licenses/by/4.0/).

1. Introduction

Throughout this paper, all graphs considered are assumed to be finite, connected and undirected. Let $\Gamma = (V\Gamma, E\Gamma)$ be a graph with vertex set $V\Gamma$ and edge set $E\Gamma$. The size $|V\Gamma|$ is called the *order* of the graph Γ. Define an *arc* as a pair of ordered adjacent vertices, let $A\Gamma$ be the set of the arcs of Γ. Each edge $\{\alpha, \beta\}$ corresponds to two arcs (α, β) and (β, α).

Let Γ be a graph. For an integer $s \geq 1$, an s-arc in Γ is an (s + 1)-tuple $(v_0, v_1, \cdots, v_s)$ of vertices such that $\{v_i, v_{i+1}\} \in E\Gamma$, and $v_i \neq v_{i+1}$ for $0 \leq i \leq s-1$. A permutation of $V\Gamma$ that preserves the adjacency of Γ is called an *automorphism* of Γ, and all automorphisms of Γ form a group which is called the full automorphism group of Γ, denoted by $\mathrm{Aut}(\Gamma)$. Let G be a subgroup of $\mathrm{Aut}(\Gamma)$, and denoted by $G \leq \mathrm{Aut}(\Gamma)$. Let $G \leq \mathrm{Aut}(\Gamma)$ acting on vertex set $V\Gamma$, $\alpha \in V\Gamma$. We say that G_α as the subgroup of G is a *vertex-stabilizer* if G is fixing the vertex α. (Similarly, let $e = \{\alpha, \beta\} \in E\Gamma$. We may define the *edge-stabilizer* and *arc-stabilizer* of G, denoted by G_e and $G_{\alpha\beta}$, respectively). Moreover, the group $\mathrm{Aut}(\Gamma)$ has a natural action on $E\Gamma$. Then, the graph Γ is said to be G-edge-transitive if $E\Gamma \neq 0$ and for each pair of edges there exists some $g \in G \leq \mathrm{Aut}(\Gamma)$ mapping one of these two edges to the other one. So, the graph Γ is called G-vertex-transitive or G-arc-transitive if $G \leq \mathrm{Aut}(\Gamma)$ is transitive on $V\Gamma$ or $A\Gamma$, respectively. A graph Γ that is a G-arc-transitive graph for some $G \leq \mathrm{Aut}(\Gamma)$ is also known as a *symmetric graph*.

A graph Γ is G-edge-primitive if $G \leq \mathrm{Aut}(\Gamma)$ acts primitively on $E\Gamma$, that is, if G preserves no nontrivial partition of the edge set. A G-edge-transitive graph Γ is G-edge-primitive if some *edge-stabilizer*, the subgroup of its automorphism group which fixes a given edge, is a maximal subgroup of the automorphism [1]. Additionally, Γ is called edge-primitive if it is $\mathrm{Aut}(\Gamma)$-edge-primitive. In this paper, the original motivation was the problem of classifying all edge-primitive graphs of order as a product of two distinct primes. The study of edge-primitive graphs was initiated by R. M. Weiss. In 1973. Weiss [2] confirmed all edge-primitive graphs of valency 3. These graphs are the Heawood graph of order 14, the complete bipartite graph $K_{3,3}$, the Levi graph and the Biggs–Smith cubic distance-transitive graph of order 102. Giudici and Li [3] systematically studied the O'Nan–Scott primitive types of the automorphism groups of edge-primitive graphs, and the G-edge-primitive graphs for G, an almost simple group with socle $\text{PSL}_2(q)$, are classified. We use $\text{soc}(G)$ to denote the socle of a group G, that is, the subgroup of G generated by all minimal normal subgroups of G. In case G is finite, the socle is the product of all minimal normal subgroups of G. A two dimensional projective group is denoted by $\text{PSL}_2(q)$. Li and Zhang [4] annalyzed edge-primitive s-arc-transitive graphs for $s \geq 4$. Guo et al. classified edge-primitive tetravalent and pentavalent graphs in [5] and [6]. Pan et al. discussed edge-primitive graphs of prime valency in [7], and edge-primitive Cayley graphs on abelian groups and dihedral groups in [8]. Lu [9] proved that a finite 2-arc-transitive edge-primitive graph has an almost simple automorphism group if it is neither a cycle nor a complete bipartite graph. Recently, Giudici and King [10] classified edge-primitive 3-arc-transitive graphs.

The work of studying edge-primitive graphs of specific orders is also attractive. Pan et al. studied all edge-primitive graphs of prime power order in [11], and edge-primitive graphs of order twice as a prime power in [12]. The main work of this paper is to classify all edge-primitive graphs of order as a product of two distinct primes.

In this paper, the notations used are standard [1]. For a positive integer n, we usually use K_n and $K_{n,n}$ to denote the complete graph of order n and the complete bipartite graph of order $2n$, respectively. $\mathbb{Z}_n$ is defined as the cyclic group of order n, and D_{2n} as the dihedral group of order $2n$. As in Atlas [13], sometimes we simply use n to denote a cyclic group of order n. For the two groups K and H, we use $K \times H$ and $K : H$ to denote the direct product of K and H and the semidirect product of K by H, respectively. The *general linear group* $\text{GL}_n(q)$ consists of all the $n \times n$ matrices with entries in $\mathbb{F}_q$ that have a non-zero determinant. The *special linear group* $\text{SL}_n(q)$ is the subgroup of all matrices of determinant 1. The *projective general linear group* $\text{PGL}_n(q)$ and *projective special linear group* $\text{PSL}_n(q)$ are the groups obtained from $\text{GL}_n(q)$ and $\text{SL}_n(q)$ on factoring by the scalar matrices contained in those groups. We use $\text{PSU}_n(q)$, $\text{PSp}_n(q)$, and $P\Omega_n(q)$ to denote the *projective special unitary group*, the *projective symplectic group*, and the *projective special orthogonal group*, respectively. See [3] for details.

The classification of graph theory is closely related to the classification of group theory. The application of group theory in graph theory is mainly achieved through the role of groups on graphs. The symmetry of a graph is mainly described by the role of the automorphism group of the graph on each subgraph of the graph, such as the transitivity and primitivity of the automorphism group on the vertex set and edge set of the graph. The edge-primitive graph discussed in this paper is one of them. Specifically, the construction, characterization, and classification of various edge-primitive graphs with additional conditions have become some of the main issues discussed in algebraic graph theory. This paper completes the classification of specific orders in the edge-primitive graph, that is, edge-primitive graphs of order as a product of two distinct primes are completely determined.

The main result of this paper is shown as follows. Some of the graphs that appear in Theorem 1 will be explained in Section 2.

Theorem 1. *Let Γ be a G-edge-primitive graph of order pq, where $G \leq \text{Aut}\Gamma$, and $p > q$ are odd primes. Then, one of the following holds:*

(1) *Γ is a star.*
(2) *Γ, G are listed in Table 1, where for $\alpha \in V\Gamma$ and $e \in E\Gamma$, G_α and G_e is the stabilizer of α and e, respectively.*

Table 1. Edge-primitive graphs of order as a product of two distinct primes.

G	G_e	G_α	$|V\Gamma|$	Remark
M_{22}	M_{10}	$2^4 : A_6$	77	$\mathcal{G}(77,6)$
A_{pq}	S_{pq-2}	A_{pq-1}	pq	$K_{pq}, pq \geq 15$
$\text{PSL}_2(19)$	D_{20}	A_5	57	$\mathcal{G}(57,6)$
$\text{PSL}_2(25)$	D_{24}	S_5	65	$\mathcal{G}(65,10)$

The layout of this paper is as follows. We collect some basic properties of edge-primitive graphs and some examples for edge-primitive graphs in Section 2. The most important theorem was proved in the last section.

2. Preliminary and Examples

The simplest examples of edge-primitive graphs are the stars $K_{1,n}$, the cycles with prime numbers of vertices, and the complete graphs K_n. Following [3], we call an edge-primitive graph *trivial* if it is a star or a cycle. In this paper, non-trivial edge-primitive graphs are our main research object. We first collect some preliminary results of edge-primitive graphs for later use.

Lemma 1 ([3], Lemma 3.4). *Let Γ be a non-trivial G-edge-primitive graph for some $G \leq \mathrm{Aut}(\Gamma)$. Then, Γ is G-arc-transitive.*

Arc transitive graphs can be represented using the group theory method of constructing a *coset graph*. Let G be a finite group, and let $H \leq G$. We say that the set $[G : H]$ is the right coset of H in G if $[G : H] = \{Hx \mid x \in G\}$. For an element $g \in G$ with $g^2 \in H$, $Hx, Hy \in [G : H]$, we say that $\mathrm{Cos}(G, H, HgH)$ is a coset graph of G with respect to H and g if Hx and Hy are adjacent if and only if $yx^{-1} \in HgH$. The graph Γ is connected if and only if $\langle H, g \rangle = G$. Let α be the vertex H of the coset graph. Moreover, the valency of Γ is $|H : H \cap H^g|$, and the stabilizer of the edge $\{H, Hg\}$ is $\langle H \cap H^g, g \rangle$. See [3] for details.

Let $e = \{\alpha, \beta\} \in E\Gamma$, denote by G_α, G_e, and $G_{\alpha\beta}$ as the vertex-stabilizer, edge-stabilizer, and arc-stabilizer of G, respectively.

Lemma 2 ([12], Lemma 2.5). *Let Γ be a graph, $1 \neq N \triangleleft G \leq \mathrm{Aut}\Gamma$, and $e = \{\alpha, \beta\} \in E\Gamma$. Then, the following statements hold.*

(1) *If Γ is G-edge-primitive, then $G_e \cong N_e.(G/N)$. In particular, $|G_e| = |N_e||G : N|$.*
(2) *If Γ is G-arc-transitive, then $G_e \cong G_{\alpha\beta}.\mathbb{Z}_2$.*
(3) *If Γ is G-edge-transitive but not G-arc-transitive, then $G_e \cong G_{\alpha\beta}$.*

The valency of a regular graph Γ is denoted by $\mathrm{val}(\Gamma)$.

Lemma 3. *Let Γ be a nontrivial G-edge-primitive graph and $e = \{\alpha, \beta\} \in E\Gamma$. Then $|G_\alpha| > |G_e|$.*

Proof. It can be easily concluded that Γ is non-trivial, $\mathrm{val}(\Gamma) = |G_\alpha : G_{\alpha\beta}| \geq 3$, and Γ is G-arc-transitive, so $|G_e| = 2 \cdot |G_{\alpha\beta}|$. □

We define a transitive permutation group $G \leq \mathrm{Sym}(\Omega)$ as *quasiprimitive* if every minimal normal subgroup of G is transitive on Ω. Moreover, we say that the group G is *biquasiprimitive* if each of its minimal normal subgroups has at most two orbits, and there is a minimal normal subgroup with exactly two orbits Ω on it.

Let Γ be a G-edge-primitive graph with $G \leq \mathrm{Aut}(\Gamma)$, and let N be a nontrivial normal subgroup of G. If N is transitive on edges, then Γ is either transitive on vertices or Γ is bipartite and N has two orbits on the vertex set. This simple observation leads to the following assertion.

Lemma 4. *Let Γ be a non-trivial G-edge-primitive graph with $G \leq \mathrm{Aut}(\Gamma)$. Then, G is either quasiprimitive or biquasiprimitive on $V\Gamma$.*

Therefore, we need some relevant information for (quasi)primitive permutation groups. Let G be a quasiprimitive group. Utilizing the structure and the action of $\mathrm{soc}(G)$, the quasiprimitive permutation group is divided into eight types by O'Nan–Scott–Praeger theorem, namely HA, HS, HC, AS, SD, CD, PA, and TW. See Praeger [14] for details. As an application of the O'Nan–Scott-Praeger theorem, it is straightforward to obtain the following results.

Lemma 5. *Let G be a quasiprimitive permutation group of degree pq, where $p > q$ are odd primes. Then, G is an almost simple group.*

By Theorem 2.1 of [3], Giudici and Li have classified the groups which act edge-primitively on a complete graph.

Lemma 6 ([8], Lemma 2.4). *Let G be an almost simple group with $\mathrm{soc}(G) = \mathrm{PSL}_n(k)$ and $n \geq 3$. Then, the action of G on a complete graph is not edge-primitive.*

To construct edge-primitive graphs, the most important results are as follows:

Proposition 1 ([3], Proposition 2.5). *Let G be a finite group with a maximal subgroup E. Then, there exists a G-edge-primitive, arc-transitive graph Γ with an edge stabiliser E if and only if E has a subgroup A and $|E : A| = 2$. In addition, G have a core-free subgroup H such that $A < H \neq E$. In this case, $\Gamma = \mathrm{Cos}(G, H, HgH)$ for some $g \in E \backslash A$.*

Example 1. Let $\Gamma = K_{pq}$, where $p > q$ are odd primes. Then, $\mathrm{Aut}\Gamma = S_{pq}$ contains a subgroup $G = A_{pq}$. This subgroup G has a maximal subgroup $E = S_{pq-2}$, and E has a subgroup $A = A_{pq-2}$ of index two. The group G also contains a maximal subgroup isomorphic to $H = A_{pq-1}$, and H contains the subgroup A. So, the graph Γ is G-vertex-primitive, and by Proposition 1, the graph Γ is also G-edge-primitive.

Example 2. Let $T \cong M_{22}$. According to Atlas [13], M_{22} has two maximal subgroups $H \cong 2^4 : A_6$ and $E \cong M_{10}$ such that $H \cap E \cong A_6$. Define a coset graph

$$\mathcal{G}(77, 16) := \mathrm{Cos}(T, H, HgH), \text{ with } g \in E \backslash H \text{ an involution.}$$

By Proposition 1, $\mathcal{G}(77, 16)$ is an T-edge-primitive graph, with valency $|H : H \cap E| = 16$, and $|\mathcal{G}(77, 16)| = |T : H| = 77$. Based on the calculation of the Magma [15], it can be concluded that any T-arc-transitive graph with vertex stabilizer $2^4 : A_6$ and valency 77 is isomorphic to $\mathcal{G}(77, 16)$ and has the automorphism group $M_{22}.\mathbb{Z}_2$. So, $\mathcal{G}(77, 16)$ is G-edge-primitive with $M_{22} \leq G \leq M_{22}.\mathbb{Z}_2$.

Example 3. Let $T \cong \mathrm{PSL}_2(19)$. Then, following Proposition 8.4 of [3], T has a subgroup $H \cong A_5$ and a maximal subgroup $E \cong D_{20}$ of one conjugate class such that $H \cap E \cong D_{10}$. Define a coset graph

$$\mathcal{G}(57, 6) := \mathrm{Cos}(T, H, HgH), \text{ with } g \in E \backslash H \text{ an involution.}$$

By Proposition 1, this graph is T-edge-primitive, with valency $|H : H \cap E| = 6$ and $|\mathcal{G}(57, 6)| = |T : H| = 57$. Furthermore, after calculation in Magma [15], it can be concluded that any T-arc-transitive graph with vertex stabilizer A_5 and valency 57 is isomorphic to $\mathcal{G}(57, 6)$, and has automorphism group $\mathrm{PSL}_2(19).\mathbb{Z}_2$. So $\mathcal{G}(57, 6)$ is G-edge-primitive with $\mathrm{PSL}_2(19) \leq G \leq \mathrm{PGL}_2(19)$.

Example 4. Let $T \cong \mathrm{PSL}_2(25)$. Then, from Proposition 8.4 of [3], T has a subgroup $H \cong S_5$ and of a maximal subgroup $E \cong D_{24}$ of one conjugate class such that $H \cap E \cong D_{12}$. Define a coset graph

$$\mathcal{G}(65, 10) := \mathrm{Cos}(T, H, HgH), \text{ with } g \in E \backslash H \text{ an involution.}$$

By Proposition 1, this graph is T-edge-primitive, with valency $|H : H \cap E| = 10$ and $|\mathcal{G}(65, 10)| = |T : H| = 65$. Furthermore, a computation by Magma [15] shows that any T-arc-transitive graph with vertex stabilizer A_5 and valency 65 is isomorphic to $\mathcal{G}(65, 10)$, and has automorphism group $\mathrm{PSL}_2(25).\mathbb{Z}_2$. So, $\mathcal{G}(65, 10)$ is G-edge-primitive with $\mathrm{PSL}_2(25) \leq G \leq \mathrm{PGL}_2(25)$.

3. Proof of Theorem 1

Let Γ be a non-trivial G-edge-primitive graph for some $G \leq \mathrm{Aut}(\Gamma)$. Further assume that the order of this graph is pq, where $p > q$ are odd primes. By Lemmas 1 and 4, Γ is G-arc-transitive and G is either quasiprimitive or biquasiprimitive on $V\Gamma$.

Therefore, we need to consider two types of cases when G is quasiprimitve on $V\Gamma$. By Lemma 5, G can only be an almost simple group. Thus, $\mathrm{soc}(G) = T$ is non-abelian simple and transitive on $V\Gamma$, so $|T : T_\alpha| = pq$. Non-abelian simple groups with a subgroup of index pq have been classified in [16] (Theorem 1.1) (see also [17] [THEOREM]). The result can be read off as follows.

Lemma 7. *Let T be a non-abelian simple group with a subgroup H of index pq, where $p > q$ are odd primes. Then, the tuple (T, H) is listed in Table 2, where P_1 is the stabilizer of the classical group acting naturally on the 1-subspaces.*

Table 2. Non-abelian simple groups with a subgroups of index pq.

Row	T	H	$\|T:H\|$	Conditions
1	A_5	$\mathbb{Z}_2 \times \mathbb{Z}_2$	$3 \cdot 5$	$\mathbb{Z}_2 \times \mathbb{Z}_2 < A_4$
2	A_7	$\mathrm{PSL}_2(7)$	$3 \cdot 5$	
		$(A_4 \times 3):2$	$5 \cdot 7$	
3	A_8	$2^3 : \mathrm{PSL}_3(2)$	$3 \cdot 5$	
		$2^4 : (S_3 \times S_3)$	$5 \cdot 7$	
4	M_{11}	$M_9 : 2$	$5 \cdot 11$	
5	M_{22}	$2^4 : A_6$	$7 \cdot 11$	
6	M_{23}	$\mathrm{PSL}_3(4):2$	$11 \cdot 23$	
		$2^4 : A_7$	$11 \cdot 23$	
7	$\mathrm{PSL}_2(11)$	A_4	$5 \cdot 11$	
8	$\mathrm{PSL}_2(19)$	A_5	$3 \cdot 19$	
9	$\mathrm{PSL}_2(23)$	S_4	$11 \cdot 23$	
10	$\mathrm{PSL}_2(25)$	S_5	$5 \cdot 13$	
11	$\mathrm{PSL}_2(29)$	A_5	$7 \cdot 29$	
12	$\mathrm{PSL}_2(59)$	A_5	$29 \cdot 59$	
13	$\mathrm{PSL}_2(61)$	A_5	$31 \cdot 61$	
14	$\mathrm{PSL}_5(2)$	$2^6 : (S_3 \times \mathrm{SL}_3(2))$	$5 \cdot 31$	
15	$P\Omega_8^-(2)$	$2^6 : \mathrm{PSU}_4(2)$	$7 \cdot 17$	
16	$P\Omega_{10}^+(2)$	$2^8 : P\Omega_8^+(2)$	$17 \cdot 31$	
17	A_{pq}	A_{pq-1}	pq	$pq \geq 15$
18	A_p	S_{p-2}	$\frac{p-1}{2} \cdot p$	$p \geq 11$, $\frac{p-1}{2}$ prime
19	A_{p+1}	S_{p-1}	$\frac{p+1}{2} \cdot p$	$p \geq 5$, $\frac{p+1}{2}$ prime
20	$\mathrm{PSL}_2(p)$	$D_{p\pm 1}$	$\frac{p\mp 1}{2} \cdot p$	$\frac{p\mp 1}{2}$ odd prime
21	$\mathrm{PSL}_n(k)$	P_1	$\frac{k^d-1}{k-1}$	$n \geq 3$, $\frac{k^d-1}{k-1} = pq$
22	$\mathrm{PSp}_4(2^{2^i})$	P_1	$(2^{2^i}+1)(2^{2^{i+1}}+1)$	$q = 2^{2^i}+1$, $p = 2^{2^{i+1}}+1$
23	$\mathrm{PSU}_3(2^{2^i})$	P_1	$(2^{2^i}+1)(2^{2^{i+1}}-2^{2^i}+1)$	$q = 2^{2^i}+1$, $p = 2^{2^{i+1}}-2^{2^i}+1$
24	$P\Omega_{2(2^i+1)}^+(2)$	P_1	$(2^{2^i}+1)(2^{2^{i+1}}-1)$	$q = 2^{2^i}+1$, $p = 2^{2^{i+1}}-1$
25	$P\Omega_{2^{i+1}}^-(2)$	P_1	$(2^{2^i-1}-1)(2^{2^i}+1)$	$q = 2^{2^i-1}-1$, $p = 2^{2^i}+1$

Lemma 8. *Assume that G is an almost simple quasiprimitive group on $V\Gamma$. Then, Γ and G are listed in Table 1 in Theorem 1.*

Proof. Based on the assumption, $G \cong T.o$, where $o \leq \mathrm{Out}(T)$ and $|T : T_\alpha| = pq$. Hence, the tuple (T, T_α) (as (T, H) there) is listed in Table 2. We analyze each candidate in the following.

Row 1. In this case, $T \cong A_5$, $T_\alpha = \mathbb{Z}_2 \times \mathbb{Z}_2$, $|V\Gamma| = 15$ and $\mathrm{Out}(T) = \mathbb{Z}_2$. Hence, $G \cong A_5$ or $\mathrm{Aut}(A_5) \cong S_5$, and $|G_e| = 4$ or 8, respectively. By Lemma 3, $|G_e| < 4$ or 8. However, by the Atlas [13], A_5 or S_5 have no such maximal subgroup G_e. So, Γ is not edge-primitive in this case.

Row 2. In this case, $T \cong A_7$, if $T_\alpha \cong \text{PSL}(2,7)$, $|V\Gamma| = 15$ and $G \cong T.o$, where $o \leq \text{Out}(A_7) \cong \mathbb{Z}_2$. Then, by [1] (p. 308, TABLE B.2), T is of rank 2 on $V\Gamma$, so one non-trivial suborbit is of lengths 14. Hence, Γ is T-arc-transitive of valency 14. Assume $\text{val}(\Gamma) = 14$, then $|T_{\alpha\beta}| = \frac{|T_\alpha|}{14} = 12$ and $|T_e| = 24$, so $|G_e| = 24|o|$. However, by the Atlas [13], there is no maximum subgroup of order $24|o|$ in group $A_7.o$, which is a contradiction. If $T \cong (A_4 \times 3) : 2$, $|V\Gamma| = 35$, then by Lemma 3, $|G_e| < 72|o|$. However, by the Atlas [13], $G \cong T.o$ has no such maximal subgroup G_e, which is a contradiction.

Row 3. Assume that $T \cong A_8$, if $T_\alpha \cong 2^3 : \text{PSL}_3(2)$, $|V\Gamma| = 15$ and $G \cong T.o$, where $o \leq \text{Out}(A_8) \cong \mathbb{Z}_2$. By [1] (p. 308, TABLE B.2), T is of rank 2 on $V\Gamma$, so one non-trivial suborbit is of lengths 14. Then, Γ is T-arc-transitive of valency 14. Assume $\text{val}(\Gamma) = 14$, then $|T_{\alpha\beta}| = \frac{|T_\alpha|}{14} = 96$ and $|T_e| = 192$, so $|G_e| = 192|o|$. However, by the Atlas [13], there is no maximum subgroup of order $192|o|$ in group $A_8.o$, which is a contradiction. If $T \cong 2^4 : (S_3 \times S_3)$, $|V\Gamma| = 35$, and by Lemma 3, $|G_e| < 576|o|$. By the Atlas [13], $G_e \cong (A_5 \times 3) : 2$ or $S_5 \times S_3$, then $|G_{\alpha\beta}| = \frac{|G_e|}{2} = 360$ or 720. However, a computation by Magma [15] shows that $2^4 : (S_3 \times S_3)$ has no subgroup with order 360 or 720, a contradiction.

Row 4. Assume that $T \cong M_{11}$, $|V\Gamma| = 55$, and $\text{Out}(M_{11}) = 1$. By Lemma 3, $|T_e| < |T_\alpha| = 144$. By the Atlas [13], $T_e \cong S_5$ or $M_8 : S_3$, then $|T_{\alpha\beta}| = \frac{|T_e|}{2} = 120$ or 48. However, according to the calculation in Magma [15], it can be concluded that $T_\alpha \cong M_9 : 2$ has no subgroup with order 120 or 48, which is a contradiction.

Row 5. In this case, T is primitive on $V\Gamma$, $|V\Gamma| = 77$, and $G \cong T.o$, where $o \leq \text{Out}(M_{22}) \cong \mathbb{Z}_2$. By [1] (p. 321, TABLE B.2), T is of rank 3 on $V\Gamma$, and it is easy to compute out that the lengths of its two non-trivial suborbits are 16 and 60. So, Γ is T-arc-transitive of valency 16 and 60. If $\text{val}(\Gamma) = 16$, by Example 2, $\Gamma = \mathcal{G}(77, 16)$. If $\text{val}(\Gamma) = 60$, then $|T_{\alpha\beta}| = \frac{T_\alpha}{val(\Gamma)} = 96$, and by Lemma 6, $|G_e| = |T_e.o| = |T_{\alpha\beta}.\mathbb{Z}_2.o| = 192|o|$, hence, $|G_e| \leq 384$. However, by the Atlas [13], all maximal subgroups of T and $\text{Aut}(T)$ are of order at least 660, which is a contradiction.

Row 6. In this case, $T \cong M_{23}$, if $T_\alpha \cong \text{PSL}_3(4) : 2$, $|V\Gamma| = 253$, and $\text{Out}(M_{23}) = 1$, $G \cong M_{23}$. By Lemma 3, $|G_e| < |G_\alpha| = 40320$. By the Atlas [13], we can see that there are five possibilities for G_e, $2^4 : A_7$, A_8, M_{11}, $2^4 : (3 \times A_5) : 2$, $23 : 11$. Note that only the case $2^4 : (3 \times A_5) : 2$ contains an index two subgroup $2^4 : (3 \times A_5)$, hence $|G_{\alpha\beta}| = 2880$. However, from Magma [15], $G_\alpha \cong \text{PSL}_3(4) : 2$ has no subgroup with order 2880, which is a contradiction. Similarly, for the case $T_\alpha \cong 2^4 : A_7$, we also get a contradiction.

Row 7–13. By [3] (Theorem 1.3), since $|V\Gamma| = pq$, and $p > q$ are odd primes. Now, a direct computation can determine all the possibilities of Γ. If $T \cong \text{PSL}_2(19)$, by Example 3, $\Gamma = \mathcal{G}(57, 6)$. If $T \cong \text{PSL}_2(25)$, by Example 4, $\Gamma = \mathcal{G}(65, 5)$.

Row 14. In this case, $T \cong \text{PSL}_5(2)$, $|V\Gamma| = 155$, and $G \cong T.o$, where $o \leq \text{Out}(\text{PSL}_5(2)) \cong \mathbb{Z}_2$. Using the calculations in Magma [15], it can be concluded that T is of rank 3 on $V\Gamma$, with two non-trivial suborbits of lengths 42 or 112. Hence, val $(\Gamma) = 42$ or 112, and Γ is T-arc-transitive. If val $(\Gamma) = 42$, then $|T_{\alpha\beta}| = \frac{T_\alpha}{val(\Gamma)} = 1536$, by Lemma 2, $|G_e| = |T_e.o| = |T_{\alpha\beta}.\mathbb{Z}_2.o| = 3076|o|$. However, by the Atlas [13], there is no maximum subgroup of order $3076|o|$ in group $\text{PSL}_5(2).o$, which is a contradiction. If val $(\Gamma) = 112$, then $|T_{\alpha\beta}| = \frac{T_\alpha}{val(\Gamma)} = 576$, and $|G_e| = |T_e.o| = |T_{\alpha\beta}.\mathbb{Z}_2.o| = 1152|o|$. By the Atlas [13], there is no maximum subgroup of order $1152|o|$ in group $\text{PSL}_5(2).o$, which is a contradiction.

Row 15. If $T \cong P\Omega_8^-(2)$, $|V\Gamma| = 119$, and $G \cong T.o$, where $o \leq \text{Out}(P\Omega_8^-(2)) \cong \mathbb{Z}_2$. According to the calculation in Magma [15], it can be concluded that T is of rank 3 on $V\Gamma$, with two non-trivial suborbits of lengths 54 or 64. Hence, val $(\Gamma) = 54$ or 64, and Γ is T-arc-transitive. If val $(\Gamma) = 54$, then $|T_{\alpha\beta}| = \frac{T_\alpha}{val(\Gamma)} = 30720$, and $|G_e| = |T_e.o| = |T_{\alpha\beta}.\mathbb{Z}_2.o| = 61440|o|$. However, by Atlas [13], there is no maximum subgroup of order $61440|o|$ in group $P\Omega_8^-(2).o$, which is a contradiction. If val $(\Gamma) = 64$, then $|T_{\alpha\beta}| = \frac{T_\alpha}{val(\Gamma)} = 25920$, and $|G_e| = |T_e.o| = |T_{\alpha\beta}.\mathbb{Z}_2.o| = 51840|o|$. However, by the Atlas [13], there is no maximum subgroup of order $51840|o|$ in group $P\Omega_8^-(2).o$, which is a contradiction.

Row 16. In this case, $T \cong P\Omega_{10}^+(2)$, $|V\Gamma| = 527$, and $G \cong T.o$, where $o \leq \text{Out}(P\Omega_{10}^+(2)) \cong \mathbb{Z}_2$. From Magma [15], a simple computation can determine that the rank of T on $V\Gamma$ is 3, with two non-trivial suborbits of lengths 256 or 270. Hence, val $(\Gamma) = 256$ or 270, and Γ is T-arc-transitive. If val $(\Gamma) = 256$, then $|T_{\alpha\beta}| = \frac{T_\alpha}{val(\Gamma)} = 174182400$, and $|G_e| = |T_e.o| = |T_{\alpha\beta}.\mathbb{Z}_2.o| = 348364800|o|$. However, by Atlas [13], $G \cong T.o$ has no maximal subgroup with order $348364800|o|$, which is a contradiction. Similarly, if val $(\Gamma) = 270$, then $|T_{\alpha\beta}| = \frac{T_\alpha}{val(\Gamma)} = 165150720$, $|G_e| = 330301440|o|$. By the Atlas [13], there is no maximum subgroup of order $330301440|o|$ in group $P\Omega_{10}^+(2).o$, which is a contradiction.

Row 17. In this case, $T \cong A_{pq}$ is 2-transitive on the set of right cosets of A_{pq-1}, where $pq \geq 15$, so $\Gamma = K_{pq}$ and $T_\alpha \cong A_{pq-1}$. Hence, $T_{\alpha\beta} \cong A_{pq-2}$, and $T_e \cong S_{pq-2}$ is maximal in T, so Γ is G-edge-primitive with $G \cong A_{pq}$ and S_{pq}.

Row 18–19. Assume that $T \cong A_p$, $|V\Gamma| = \frac{p-1}{2} \cdot p$, and $G \cong T.o$, where $o \leq \text{Out}(A_p)$. According to the calculation in Magma [15], it can be concluded that T is of rank 3 on $V\Gamma$, with two non-trivial suborbits of lengths $2(p-2)$ or $\frac{(p-2)(p-3)}{2}$. Hence, val $(\Gamma) = 2(p-2)$ or $\frac{(p-2)(p-3)}{2}$, and Γ is T-arc-transitive. If val $(\Gamma) = 2(p-2)$, then $|T_{\alpha\beta}| = \frac{T_\alpha}{val(\Gamma)} = \frac{(p-3)!}{2}$, and $|G_e| = |T_e.o| = |T_{\alpha\beta}.\mathbb{Z}_2.o| = (p-3)!|o|$, By [18] (Theorem 1.1), there exists no subgroup G_e, which is a maximal subgroup of $G \cong T.o$, such that G_e has a subgroup $G_{\alpha\beta}$ of index two. Thus, there is no G-edge-primitive graph arising in this case. If val $(\Gamma) = \frac{(p-2)(p-3)}{2}$. Similarly, $|G_e| = 4(p-4)!|o|$. By [18] (Theorem 1.1), there is no G-edge-primitive graph. Assume that $T \cong A_{p+1}$, similar to the discussion above, $|G_e| = (p-2)!|o|$ or $(p-3)!|o|$, by [18] (Theorem 1.1), there is no G-edge-primitive graph occurring in this case.

Row 20. Then, $T \cong \text{PSL}_2(p)$, $T_\alpha \cong D_{p\pm 1}$. By [3] (Theorem 1.3), no graph Γ exists in this case.

Row 21. Then, $T \cong \text{PSL}_n(k)$ is 2-transitive on $V\Gamma =$ where $n \geq 3$, so Γ is a complete graph, contradicting Lemma 6.

Row 22. In this case, $T \cong \text{PSp}_4(2^{2^i})$, $|V\Gamma| = (2^{2^i} + 1)(2^{2^{i+1}} + 1)$, and $G \cong T.o$ with $o \leq \text{Out}(\text{PSp}_4(2^{2^i}))$. From Magma [15], it can be concluded that T is of rank 3 on $V\Gamma$, with two non-trivial suborbits of lengths $2^{2^i} + 2^{2^{i+1}}$ or $2^{3 \cdot 2^i}$. Hence, val $(\Gamma) = 2^{2^i} + 2^{2^{i+1}}$, and $2^{3 \cdot 2^i}$, and Γ is T-arc-transitive. If val $(\Gamma) = 2^{2^i} + 2^{2^{i+1}}$, then $|T_{\alpha\beta}| = \frac{|P_1|}{val(\Gamma)} = \frac{|\text{PSp}_4(2^{2^i})|}{|V\Gamma| \cdot val(\Gamma)}$, and $|G_e| = |T_e.o| = |T_{\alpha\beta}.\mathbb{Z}_2.o|$, so $|G_e| = \frac{2|\text{PSp}_4(2^{2^i})||o|}{(2^{2^i}+1)(2^{2^{i+1}}+1)(2^{2^i}+2^{2^{i+1}})} = 2^{3 \cdot 2^i+1}(2^{2^i}-1)^2|o|$. Therefore, by [19] (Tables 8.12–8.15), $G \cong T.o$ has no maximal subgroup with order $2^{3 \cdot 2^i+1}(2^{2^i}-1)^2|o|$, which is a contradiction. If val $(\Gamma) = 2^{3 \cdot 2^i}$. Similarly, $|G_e| = \frac{2|\text{PSp}_4(2^{2^i})||o|}{(2^{2^i}+1)(2^{2^{i+1}}+1)(2^{3 \cdot 2^i})} = 2^{2^{i+1}}(2^{2^i}-1)(2^{2^{i+1}}-1)|o|$. By [19] (Tables 8.12–8.15), T has a maximal subgroup $\text{GL}_2(2^{2^i}).\mathbb{Z}_2$ with order $2^{2^{i+1}}(2^{2^i}-1)(2^{2^{i+1}}-1)$. However, $T \cong \text{PSp}_4(2^{2^i})$, so 2^{2^i} is an even number, again a contradiction.

Row 23. In this case, $T \cong \mathrm{PSU}_3(2^{2^i})$, $|V\Gamma| = (2^{2^i}+1)(2^{2^{i+1}} - 2^{2^i} + 1)$, and $G \cong T.o$ with $o \leq \mathrm{Out}(\mathrm{PSU}_3(2^{2^i}))$. From Magma [15], a simple computation can determine that the rank of T on $V\Gamma$ is 2, with one non-trivial suborbit of lengths $2^{3 \cdot 2^i}$. Hence, val $(\Gamma) = 2^{3 \cdot 2^i}$ and Γ is T-arc-transitive. If val $(\Gamma) = 2^{3 \cdot 2^i}$, then $|T_{\alpha\beta}| = \frac{|P_1|}{val(\Gamma)} = \frac{|\mathrm{PSU}_3(2^{2^i})|}{|V\Gamma| \cdot val(\Gamma)}$, and $|G_e| = |T_e.o| = |T_{\alpha\beta}.\mathbb{Z}_2.o|$, so $|G_e| = \frac{2|\mathrm{PSU}_3(2^{2^i})||o|}{(2^{2^i}+1)(2^{2^{i+1}}-2^{2^i}+1)(2^{3 \cdot 2^i})} = 2(2^{2^{i+1}} - 1)|o|$. However, by [19] (Table 8.5–8.6), $G \cong T.o$ has no maximal subgroup with order $2(2^{2^{i+1}} - 1)|o|$, which is a contradiction.

Row 24. In this case, $T \cong P\Omega^+_{2(2^i+1)}(2)$, $|V\Gamma| = (2^{2^i}+1)(2^{2^i+1}-1)$, and $G \cong T.o$ with $o \leq \mathrm{Out}(P\Omega^+_{2(2^i+1)}(2))$. According to the calculation in Magma [15], it can be concluded that T is of rank 3 on $V\Gamma$, with two non-trivial suborbits are of lengths 2^{2^i+1} and $2(2^{2^i}-1)(2^{2^i-1}-1)$. Hence, val $(\Gamma) = 2^{2^i+1}$, and $2(2^{2^i}-1)(2^{2^i-1}-1)$, and Γ is T-arc-transitive. If val $(\Gamma) = 2^{2^i+1}$, then $|T_{\alpha\beta}| = \frac{|P_1|}{val(\Gamma)} = \frac{|P\Omega^+_{2(2^i+1)}(2)|}{|V\Gamma| \cdot val(\Gamma)}$, and $|G_e| = |T_e.o| = |T_{\alpha\beta}.\mathbb{Z}_2.o|$, so $|G_e| = \frac{2|P\Omega^+_{2(2^i+1)}(2)||o|}{(2^{2^i}+1)(2^{2^i+1}-1)(2^{2^i+1})} = 2^{2^{2i}-2^i+1}(2^{2^i}-1)\prod_{j=1}^{2^i-1}(2^{2j}-1)|o|$. However, by [19], $G \cong T.o$ has no maximal subgroup with order $2^{2^{2i}-2^i+1}(2^{2^i}-1)\prod_{j=1}^{2^i-1}(2^{2j}-1)|o|$, which is a contradiction. If val$(\Gamma) = 2(2^{2^i}-1)(2^{2^i-1}-1)$. Similarly, $|G_e| = \frac{2|P\Omega^+_{2(2^i+1)}(2)||o|}{(2^{2^i}+1)(2^{2^i+1}-1)(2(2^{2^i}-1)(2^{2^i-1}-1))} = 2^{2^{2i}+2^i}(2^{2^i-1}-1)\prod_{j=1}^{2^i-2}(2^{2j}-1)|o|$. However, by [19], $G \cong T.o$ has no maximal subgroup with order $2^{2^{2i}+2^i}(2^{2^i-1}-1)\prod_{j=1}^{2^i-2}(2^{2j}-1)|o|$, which is a contradiction.

Row 25. In this last case, $T \cong P\Omega^-_{2^i+1}(2)$, $|V\Gamma| = (2^{2^i-1}-1)(2^{2^i}+1)$, and $G \cong T.o$ with $o \leq \mathrm{Out}(P\Omega^-_{2^i+1}(2))$. After the calculation in Magma [15], it can be concluded that T is of rank 3 on $V\Gamma$, with two non-trivial suborbits of lengths $2(2^{2^i-1}+1)(2^{2^i-2}-1)$ or $2^{2^{i+1}-2}$. Hence, val $(\Gamma) = 2(2^{2^i-1}+1)(2^{2^i-2}-1)$ and $2^{2^{i+1}-2}$, and Γ is T-arc-transitive. If val $(\Gamma) = 2(2^{2^i-1}+1)(2^{2^i-2}-1)$, then $|T_{\alpha\beta}| = \frac{|P_1|}{val(\Gamma)} = \frac{|P\Omega^-_{2^i+1}(2)|}{|V\Gamma| \cdot val(\Gamma)}$, and $|G_e| = |T_e.o| = |T_{\alpha\beta}.\mathbb{Z}_2.o|$, so $|G_e| = \frac{2|P\Omega^-_{2^i+1}(2)||o|}{(2^{2^i-1}-1)(2^{2^i}+1)(2(2^{2^i-1}+1)(2^{2^i-2}-1))} = 2^{2^i}(2^{2^i}-1)(2^{2^i-2}+1)\prod_{j=1}^{2^i-3}(2^{2j}-1)|o|$. However, by [19], $G \cong T.o$ has no maximal subgroup with order $2^{2^i}(2^{2^i}-1)(2^{2^i-2}+1)\prod_{j=1}^{2^i-3}(2^{2j}-1)|o|$, which is a contradiction. If val $(\Gamma) = 2^{2^{i+1}-2}$. Similarly, $|G_e| = \frac{2|P\Omega^-_{2^i+1}(2)||o|}{(2^{2^i-1}-1)(2^{2^i}+1)(2^{2^{i+1}-2})} = 2^{2^{2i}-3 \cdot 2^i+3}(2^{2^i-1}+1)\prod_{j=1}^{2^i-2}(2^{2j}-1)|o|$. However, by [19], $G \cong T.o$ has no maximal subgroup with order $2^{2^{2i}-3 \cdot 2^i+3}(2^{2^i-1}+1)\prod_{j=1}^{2^i-2}(2^{2j}-1)|o|$, which is a contradiction. □

Now, we are ready to complete the proof of Theorem 1.

Proof of Theorem 1. Suppose that the Γ is a G-edge-primitive with order pq, where $G \leq \mathrm{Aut}(\Gamma)$, and $p > q$ are odd primes. Let Γ be a G-edge-primitive graph of order pq, where $G \leq \mathrm{Aut}(\Gamma)$, and $p > q$ are odd primes. Suppose Γ is not a star. By Lemma 4, G is quasiprimitive or biquasiprimitive on $V\Gamma$.

Firstly, suppose that G is quasiprimitive on $V\Gamma$, by Lemma 8, and Γ, G, s are listed in Table 1 in Theorem 1.

Secondly, suppose that G is biquasiprimitive on $V\Gamma$, then G has biparts Δ_1 and Δ_2 with $V\Gamma = \Delta_1 \cup \Delta_2$, so $|\Delta_1| = |\Delta_2| = \frac{pq}{2}$. However, as $p > q$ are odd primes, this is impossible. This completes the proof of Theorem 1. □

4. Conclusions

Currently, the construction, classification, and characterization of various edge-primitive graphs with additional conditions have become some of the main issues discussed in algebraic graph theory. In this paper, edge-primitive graphs of order as a product of two distinct primes are completely determined. This depends on non-abelian simple groups with a subgroup of index pq being classified, where $p > q$ are odd primes. It is meaningful for future research to classify edge-primitive graphs of other specific orders or degrees.

Author Contributions: Writing—original draft, R.X.; Writing—review & editing, X.Z. and H.Z. All authors have read and agreed to the published version of the manuscript.

Funding: This work was supported by the National Natural Science Foundation of China under Grant No. 11564078, the Science and Technology Key Project of Jiangxi Provincial Education Department under grant No. GJJ202602, the Jiangxi Provincial Natural Science Foundation under Grants No. 20161BAB212032, 20232BAB202034, the Natural Science Research Project of Nanchang Normal University under grant No. 23XJZR01.

Data Availability Statement: Not applicable.

Acknowledgments: The authors would like to thank the anonymous referees for many comments and constructive suggestions.

Conflicts of Interest: The authors declare no conflict of interest. The funders had no role in the design of the study; in the writing of the manuscript, or in the decision to publish the results

References

1. Dixon, J.D.; Mortimer, B. *Permutation Groups*; Springer: New York, NY, USA, 1996
2. Weiss, R.M. Kantenprimitive Graphen vom Grad drei. *J. Combin. Theory Ser. B* **1973**, *15*, 269–288. [CrossRef]
3. Giudici, M.; Li, C.H. On finite edge-primitive and edge-quasiprimitive graphs. *J. Combin. Theory Ser. B* **2010**, *100*, 275–298. [CrossRef]
4. Li, C.H.; Zhang, H. The finite primitive groups with soluble stabilizers, and the edge-primitive s-arc transitive graphs. *Proc. Lond. Math. Soc.* **2021**, *103*, 441–472. [CrossRef]
5. Guo, S.T.; Feng, Y.Q.; Li, C.H. The finite edge-primitive pentavalent graphs. *J. Algebr. Comb.* **2013**, *38*, 491–497. [CrossRef]
6. Guo, S.T.; Feng, Y.Q.; Li, C.H. Edge-primitive tetravalent graphs. *J. Combin. Theory Ser. B* **2015**, *38*, 124–137. [CrossRef]
7. Pan, J.M.; Wu, C.X.; Yin, F.G. Finite edge-primitive graphs of prime valency. *Eur. J. Combin.* **2018**, *38*, 61–71. [CrossRef]
8. Pan, J.M.; Wu, C.X.; Yin, F.G. Edge-primitive Cayley graphs on ablian groups and dihedral groups. *Discret. Math.* **2018**, *38*, 3394–3401. [CrossRef]
9. Lu, Z.P. On edge-primitive 2-arc-transitive graphs. *J. Combin. Theory Ser. A* **2020**, *38*, 105172. [CrossRef]
10. Giudici, M.; King, C.S.H. On edge-primitive 3-arc-transitive graphs. *J. Combin. Theory Ser. B* **2021**, *38*, 282–306. [CrossRef]
11. Pan, J.M.; Huang, X.H.; Wu, C.X. Edge-primitive graphs of prime power order. *Graphs Combin.* **2019**, *38*, 249–259. [CrossRef]
12. Pan, J.M.; Wu, C.X. On edge-primitive graphs of order twice a prime power. *Discret. Math.* **2019**, *38*, 11594. [CrossRef]
13. Conway, J.H.; Curtis, R.T.; Norton, S.P.; Parker, R.A.; Wilson, R.A. *Atlas of Finite Groups*; Oxford University Press: London, UK; New York, NY, USA, 1985.
14. Praeger, C.E. An O'Nan-Scott theorem for finite quasiprimitive permutation groups and an application to 2-arc transitive graphs. *J. Lond. Math. Soc* **1992**, *38*, 227–239. [CrossRef]
15. Bosma, W.; Cannon, J.; Playoust, C. The MAGMA algebra system I: The user language. *Symbolic Comput.* **1997**, *38*, 235–265. [CrossRef]
16. Li, C.H.; Li, X.H. On permutation groups of degree a product of two prime-powers. *Comm. Algebra* **2014**, *42*, 4722–4743. [CrossRef]
17. Praeger, C.E.; Xu, M.Y. Vertex-primitive graphs of order a product of two distinct primes. *J. Combin. Theory Ser. B* **1993**, *59*, 245–266. [CrossRef]

18. Zhang, H.; Zhou, S.M. Finite edge-primitive graphs admitting an alternating group. **2023**, *submitted*.
19. Bray, J.N.; Holt, D.F.; Roney-Dougal, C.M. *The Maximal Subgroups of the Low-Dimensional Finite Classical Groups*; Cambrige University Press: New York, NY, USA, 2013.

Disclaimer/Publisher's Note: The statements, opinions and data contained in all publications are solely those of the individual author(s) and contributor(s) and not of MDPI and/or the editor(s). MDPI and/or the editor(s) disclaim responsibility for any injury to people or property resulting from any ideas, methods, instructions or products referred to in the content.

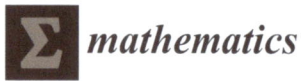

Article

Radio Number for Friendship Communication Networks

Ahmad H. Alkasasbeh [1,*], Elsayed Badr [2,3], Hala Attiya [4] and Hanan M. Shabana [5]

1. Oryx Universal College in Partnership with Liverpool John Moores University, Doha P.O. Box 12253, Qatar
2. Scientific Computing Department, Faculty of Computers and Artificial Intelligence, Benha University, Benha 13518, Egypt; alsayed.badr@fci.bu.edu.eg
3. Data Science Department, Faculty of Computers and Information Systems, Egyptian Chinese University, Cairo 19346, Egypt
4. Basic Science Department, Faculty of Technology and Education, Beni-Suef University, Beni Suef 62511, Egypt; hala.attiya@techedu.bsu.edu.eg
5. Physics and Engineering Mathematics Department, Faculty of Electronic Engineering, Menoufia University, Menouf 32952, Egypt; hanan.magdy@el-eng.menofia.edu.eg
* Correspondence: ahmad.alkasasbeh@oryx.edu.qa

Abstract: This paper investigates the radio labeling of friendship networks ($F_{3,k}$, $F_{4,k}$, $F_{5,k}$, and $F_{6,k}$). In contrast, a mathematical model is proposed for determining the upper bound of radio numbers for ($F_{3,k}$, $F_{4,k}$, $F_{5,k}$, and $F_{6,k}$). A computational investigation is presented to demonstrate that our results are superior to those of the past. In conclusion, the empirical study demonstrates that the proposed results surpass the previous ones in terms of the upper bound of the radio number and the run-time.

Keywords: graph coloring; frequency assignment problem; radio labeling of a graph; integer; programing; span

MSC: 05C78

Citation: Alkasasbeh, A.H.; Badr, E.; Attiya, H.; Shabana, H.M. Radio Number for Friendship Communication Networks. *Mathematics* **2023**, *11*, 4232. https://doi.org/10.3390/math11204232

Academic Editors: Irina Cristea and Alessandro Linzi

Received: 14 August 2023
Revised: 11 September 2023
Accepted: 19 September 2023
Published: 10 October 2023

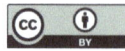

Copyright: © 2023 by the authors. Licensee MDPI, Basel, Switzerland. This article is an open access article distributed under the terms and conditions of the Creative Commons Attribution (CC BY) license (https://creativecommons.org/licenses/by/4.0/).

1. Introduction

Wireless communication includes all techniques and methods of connecting and communicating between devices using a wireless signal and wireless communication technologies and gadgets. Wireless communication network services may appear in many areas, such as satellite communications, internet technology, mobile telephony, military communications, TV and radio broadcasting, and many others. Rapid development in wireless communication services led to a depletion of the most important resources and frequencies in the radio spectrum. Such development affects the economic cost of available frequencies. The reusing of frequencies may give good economies, but on the other hand, it may decrease the quality of the communication service. Using the same frequencies for many wireless communication networks leads to unacceptable interference among signals. This motivated the *frequency assignment problem* (FAP). Given a set of transmitters in a network, the main procedure of FAP is the assignment of frequencies to transmitters, keeping interference at an acceptable level, and making use of the available frequencies in an efficient way. Such constraints of interference are related to the use of the same (or almost the same) frequencies for transmitters within a certain range from each other. The smaller the distance is among transmitters, the stronger the interference is that occurs. Therefore, it is suggested that the difference in frequency assignments should be greater.

The graph theory introduces an effective model for this problem. The interference between transmitters is modeled as a graph, and this graph is called an *interference graph* $G(V, E)$. Every vertex from $V(G)$ stands for a unique transmitter. Any two vertices are adjacent (connected by an edge) if and only if the broadcasting of their corresponding transmitters may interfere. The frequency channels are labeled by positive integers. Hence, the vertex coloring (labeling) problem of the graph G with some constraints on the labeling is equivalent to FAP [1], where it is shown that the propagation of the signal may lead to interference in regions with a large distance from each other. As a result, not only must nearby transmitters be assigned different frequencies but they should be effectively separated. This results in the modeling of FAP as distance-constrained labeling of the graph G. For some services, it is adequate that the transmitters should have distinct frequencies; moreover, the nearby transmitters inquired to use channels with appropriate separation. In this situation, FAP is equivalent to the *radio labeling problem* of the graph G (see ref. [2]). The radio labeling problem of graph G is described as follows. Let $G = (V(G), E(G))$ be a connected graph. For any $u, v \in V(G)$, let $d(u,v)$ denote the distance between two vertices u, v. That is $d(u,v)$ stands for the length of the shortest path between u, v. The maximum distance between any two vertices in G is defined as the diameter of G and denoted as $diam(G)$. Thus, $diam(G) = max\{d(u,v) : u, v \in V(G)\}$. A radio labeling of G is a one-to-one mapping L from $V(G)$ to N, where N is the set of natural number, satisfying the condition

$$|L(u) - L(v)| \geq diam(G) + 1 - d(u,v). \text{ For all } u, \ v \in V(G).$$

The span of a labeling L is the maximum integer (span) that L assigns to a vertex in G. The main objective of the radio labeling problem is to find the minimum span over all such labeling L of the graph G. Such minimum span is denoted as $rn(G)$ or the radio number of G. Saha [3] introduced an algorithm that determines the lower and upper bounds of the radio number of a graph. Badr and Moussa [4] proposed the development of Saha's algorithm and introduced a novel mathematical model for the radio labeling application. The radio labeling problem has been studied for different families of graphs [5–18]. For more details about the mathematical models, the reader can refer to [19–30].

As the number of wireless networks and services increase, this leads to many transmission stations that may be close to each other. Consequently, in most cases, there is at least one transmission station that will overlap with many other stations. This inhibits the ability of the receiver to decipher incoming signals. This concept is illustrated in Figure 1, which shows a typical situation in which the signal of transmission stations A and B overlap in the vicinity of transmission station C as in Figure 1a, while Figure 1b shows the modeling of this interference by path graph. Whenever the number of transmission stations increases, as Figure 2a, every station hopes to increase its coverage area, which leads to more physical overlapping and hence, more radio frequency interference. This situation can be modeled by the friendship graph as shown in Figure 2b.

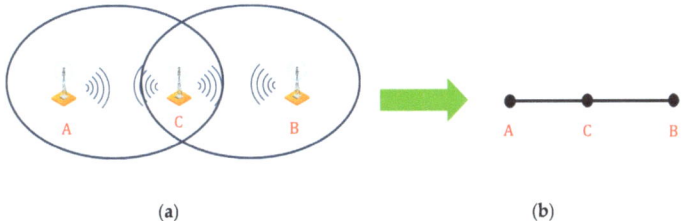

(a)   (b)

Figure 1. Path graph for modeling frequency interference of stations A, B and C. (**a**) Physical frequency interference. (**b**) Path interference graph.

The objective of the present paper is to study the radio labeling of friendship networks ($F_{3,k}$, $F_{4,k}$, $F_{5,k}$, and $F_{6,k}$). On the other hand, a mathematical model is proposed to find the upper bound of $F_{3,k}$, $F_{4,k}$, $F_{5,k}$, and $F_{6,k}$. A computational study is presented to prove the efficiency of our results compared to the previous results. Finally, the empirical study shows that the proposed results outperform the previous results according to the upper bound of the radio number and the running time.

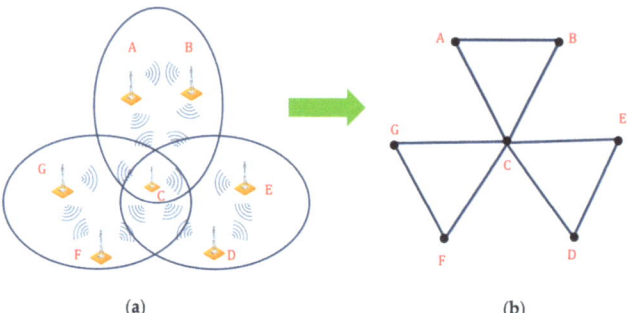

(a) (b)

Figure 2. Friendship graph for modeling frequency interference of stations A, B, C, D, E, F and G. (**a**) Many transmitting stations and more Physical frequency interference. (**b**) Friendship interference graph.

The rest of this paper is organized as follows. Section 2 presents the upper bounds for the radio number of the above-mentioned friendship graphs. The integer linear programming model of radio labeling of such friendship graphs is presented in Section 3. In Section 4, we present an experimental study for comparing results obtained in Sections 2 and 3, and algorithms that solved the same problem from [3,4]. The conclusion of this paper and future work are presented in Section 5.

2. Radio Number of Friendship Graph

In this section, we seek to find the upper bound of $rn(G)$ where G is a friendship graph.

Definition 1. *For the given positive integers k, m, a friendship graph, denoted as $F_{m,k}$, is represented as k cycles (blocks), each of length m, and all have one common vertex. For an illustration, $F_{3,k}$ is shown in Figure 3.*

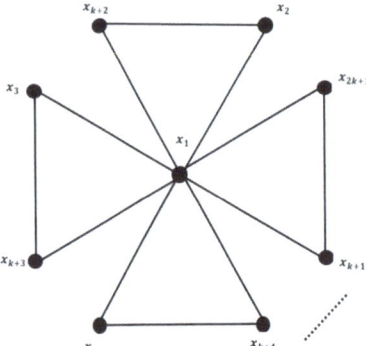

Figure 3. $F_{3,k}$ with labeling of vertices.

Definition 2. *The order of the graph G is the cardinality of its vertex set $V(G)$.*

Theorem 1. *The radio number of the friendship graph $F_{3,k}$ is its order.*

Proof. Following Definition 1 for $F_{3,k}$, we find that $diam(F_{3,k}) = 2$, $|V(F_{3,k})| = 2k+1$, and $d(x_i, x_j) \geq 1$ for any $x_i, x_j \in V(F_{3,k})$ and $i \neq j$. Since any radio labeling L is one-to-one, it follows that

$$rn(F_{3,k}) \geq |V(F_{3,k})| \tag{1}$$

Define the map L with codomain $\{0, 2, 3, \cdots, 2k+1\}$ as follows:

$$L(x_1) = 0;$$
$$L(x_i) = i; 2 \leq i \leq 2k+1$$

Now, we claim to prove that $|L(x_i) - L(x_j)| \geq diam(F_{3,k}) + 1 - d(x_i, x_j)$, that is

$$|L(x_i) - L(x_j)| \geq 3 - d(x_i, x_j) \text{ for all } x_i, x_j \in V(F_{3,k}) \text{ and } i \neq j.$$

Case 1. Let $2 \leq i \leq k+1$ and $2 \leq j \leq k+1$. Then, $|L(x_i) - L(x_j)| = |i - j| \geq 1$. Since $d(x_i, x_j) = 2$, then, $|L(x_i) - L(x_j)| \geq 3 - d(x_i, x_j)$.
Case 2. Let $i = 1, j \in \{2, 3, \cdots, 2k+1\}$. Then, $|L(x_i) - L(x_j)| = |0 - j| = j \geq 2$. Since $d(x_i, x_j) = 1$. Consequently, $|L(x_i) - L(x_j)| \geq 3 - d(x_i, x_j)$.
Case 3. Let $i, j \in \{k+2, k+3, \cdots, 2k+1\}$. Then, $|L(x_i) - L(x_j)| \geq 1$. Since, $d(x_i, x_j) = 2$. Therefore, $|L(x_i) - L(x_j)| \geq 3 - d(x_i, x_j)$.
Case 4. Let $i \in \{2, 3, \cdots, k+1\}, j = k+i$. Then, $|L(x_i) - L(x_j)| = |k+i-i| = k \geq 2$. Since $d(x_i, x_j) = 1$ then $|L(x_i) - L(x_j)| \geq 3 - d(x_i, x_j)$.
Case 5. Let $i \in \{2, 3, \cdots, k+1\}, j \in \{k+2, k+3, \cdots, 2k+1\}$, for every $j \neq k+i$, $|L(x_i) - L(x_j)| = |i - j| \geq k - 1$ where $k \geq 2$. Moreover, $d(x_i, x_j) = 2$.
Hence, $|L(x_i) - L(x_j)| \geq 3 - d(x_i, x_j)$.
Thus, L is a radio labeling of $F_{3,k}$ and

$$rn(F_{3,k}) \leq 2k + 1 \qquad (2)$$

From Formulas (1) and (2), $rn(F_{3,k}) = 2k + 1$. □

For more illustrations, Figure 3 shows $F_{3,k}$ with labeling of vertices.

Theorem 2. *Let $k > 2$ and $G \cong F_{4,k}$ be a friendship graph with blocks each of length 4 and $|V(F_{4,k})| = 3k + 1$ then $rn(F_{4,k}) \leq 7k + 1$.*

Proof. Define the map L as follows:

$$L(x_{jk+i}) = \begin{cases} 0, & i = j = 0 \\ 3 + i - 1, & j = 0, 1 \leq i \leq k \\ k + 1 + 3i, & j = 1, 1 \leq i \leq k \\ 4k + 1 + 3i, & j = 2, 1 \leq i \leq k \end{cases}$$

Since $diam(F_{4,k}) = 4$, we claim to prove that $|L(x_u) - L(x_v)| \geq 5 - d(x_u, x_v)$ for all $x_u, x_v \in V(F_{4,k})$ and $u \neq v$.

Case 1. Let $j = 0, 1 \leq i \leq k$, then $|L(x_0) - L(x_{jk+i})| = |0 - (3 + i - 1)| = 2 + i$. Since $d(x_0, x_{jk+i}) = 2$. Consequently, $|L(x_0) - L(x_{jk+i})| \geq 5 - d(x_0, x_{jk+i})$.
Case 2. Let $j \in \{1, 2\}, 1 \leq i \leq k$, then

$$|L(x_0) - L(x_{jk+i})| = \begin{cases} k + 1 + 3i, & j = 1 \\ 4k + 1 + 3i, & j = 2 \end{cases}$$

Since $d(x_0, x_{jk+i}) = 1$. Consequently, $|L(x_0) - L(x_{jk+i})| \geq 5 - d(x_0, x_{jk+i})$.
Case 3. Let $j \in \{1, 2\}, 1 \leq t \leq k$ and $1 \leq i \leq k$

$$d(x_i, x_{jk+t}) = \begin{cases} 1, & i = t \\ 3 & i \neq t \end{cases}$$

Consequently,

$$\left|L(x_i) - L\left(x_{jk+t}\right)\right| = \begin{cases} 2i+k-1, & j=1 \text{ and } i=t \\ 2i+4k-1, & j=2 \text{ and } i=t \\ 3i-t+k-1, & j=1 \text{ and } i \neq t \\ 3i-t+4k-1, & j=2 \text{ and } i \neq t \end{cases}$$

Therefore, $\left|L(x_i) - L\left(x_{jk+t}\right)\right| \geq \begin{cases} 4, & i=t \\ 2, & i \neq t \end{cases}$

Hence, $\left|L(x_i) - L\left(x_{jk+t}\right)\right| \geq 5 - d\left(x_i, x_{jk+t}\right)$.

Case 4. Let j, m be elements of $\{1,2\}$, $1 \leq t \leq k$ and $1 \leq i \leq k$. Then, $d\left(x_{jk+i}, x_{mk+t}\right) = 2$. Moreover,

$$\left|L\left(x_{jk+i}\right) - L(\,x_{mk+t})\right| = \begin{cases} 3k, & j \neq m \text{ and } i=t \\ 3(i-t), & j=m \text{ and } i \neq t \end{cases}$$

Then, $\left|L\left(x_{jk+i}\right) - L(x_{mk+t})\right| \geq 5 - d\left(x_{jk+i}, x_{mk+t}\right)$.

Case 5. Let $j=0$, $1 \leq i < t \leq k$, then $d\left(x_{jk+i}, x_{jk+t}\right) = 4$ and
$\left|L\left(x_{jk+i}\right) - L\left(x_{jk+t}\right)\right| = |3+i-1-(3+t-1)| = t-i \geq 1$. Therefore,

$$\left|L\left(x_{jk+i}\right) - L\left(x_{jk+t}\right)\right| \geq 5 - d\left(x_{jk+i}, x_{jk+t}\right).$$

From the above cases, the radio condition holds and L is a radio labeling of $F_{4,\,k}$ and

$$rn(F_{4,\,k}) \leq 7k+1. \quad \square$$

The graph $F_{4,\,k}$ with labeling of vertices is presented in Figure 4.

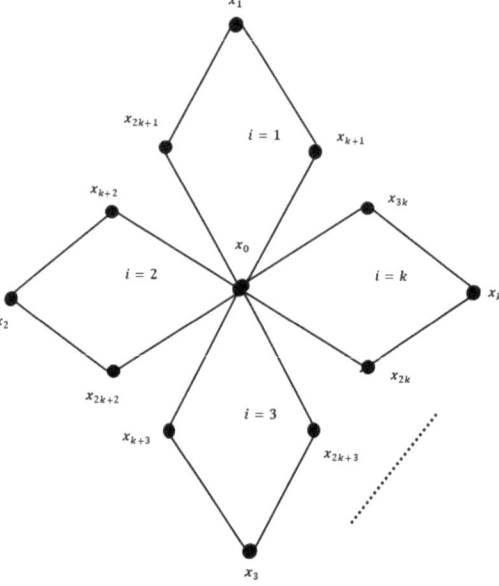

Figure 4. $F_{4,\,k}$ with labeling of vertices.

Theorem 3. *Let $k > 2$ and $G \cong F_{5,k}$ be a friendship graph with blocks each of length 5 and $|V(F_{5,k})| = 4k + 1$ then, $rn(F_{5,k}) \leq 8k + 1$.*

Proof. Define the map L as follows:
Let k be an odd number, and then

$$L\left(x_{jk+i}\right) = \begin{cases} 0, & i = j = 0 \\ 3 + i - 1, & j = 0, 1 \leq i \leq k \\ k + 2(i+1), & j = 1, 1 \leq i \leq k \\ 3k + 2(i+1), & j = 2, 1 \leq i \leq k \\ 5k + 3i + 1, & j = 3, 1 \leq i \leq k \end{cases}$$

while

$$L\left(x_{jk+i}\right) = \begin{cases} 0, & i = j = 0 \\ 3 + i - 1, & j = 0, 1 \leq i \leq k \\ k + 2(i+1), & j = 1, 1 \leq i \leq k \\ 3k + 4, & j = 2, i = 1 \\ 3k + 3 + 2i & j = 2, 2 \leq i \leq k \\ 5k + 5 & j = 3, i = 1 \\ 5k + 1 + 3i & j = 3, 2 \leq i \leq k \end{cases}$$

whenever k is an even number.

Since $diam(F_{5,k}) = 4$, we claim to prove that $|L(x_u) - L(x_v)| \geq 5 - d(x_u, x_v)$ for all $x_u, x_v \in V(F_{5,k})$ and $u \neq v$.

Case 1. Let $j = 0$, $1 \leq i \leq k$, and then, $\left|L(x_0) - L\left(x_{jk+i}\right)\right| = |0 - (3+i-1)| = 2 + i$. Since $d\left(x_0, x_{jk+i}\right) = 2$. Then, $\left|L(x_0) - L\left(x_{jk+i}\right)\right| \geq 5 - d\left(x_0, x_{jk+i}\right)$.

Case 2. Let $j = 1$, $1 \leq i \leq k$, and then $\left|L(x_0) - L\left(x_{jk+i}\right)\right| = |0 - (k+2i+2)| = k + 2i + 2 \geq 3$. Since $d\left(x_0, x_{jk+i}\right) \in \{1, 2\}$. Consequently, $\left|L(x_0) - L\left(x_{jk+i}\right)\right| \geq 5 - d\left(x_0, x_{jk+i}\right)$.

Case 3. Let $j = 2$, $1 \leq i \leq k$ then, $\left|L(x_0) - L\left(x_{jk+i}\right)\right| = |0 - (3k+2i+2)| = 3k + 2i + 2 \geq 3$. Moreover, $d\left(x_0, x_{jk+i}\right) \in \{1, 2\}$. Consequently, $\left|L(x_0) - L\left(x_{jk+i}\right)\right| \geq 5 - d\left(x_0, x_{jk+i}\right)$.

Case 4. Let $j = 3$, $1 \leq i \leq k$, and then $\left|L(x_0) - L\left(x_{jk+i}\right)\right| = |0 - (5k+3i+1)| = 5k + 3i + 1 \geq 3$. Since, $d\left(x_0, x_{jk+i}\right) \in \{1, 2\}$, then, $\left|L(x_0) - L\left(x_{jk+i}\right)\right| \geq 5 - d\left(x_0, x_{jk+i}\right)$.

Case 5. Let $j = 0$, $1 \leq i < t \leq k$, and then $\left|L\left(x_{jk+i}\right) - L\left(x_{jk+t}\right)\right| = |L(x_i) - L(x_t)| = t - i \geq 1$.
Since $d\left(x_{jk+i}, x_{jk+t}\right) = 4$, then $\left|L\left(x_{jk+i}\right) - L\left(x_{jk+t}\right)\right| \geq 5 - d\left(x_{jk+i}, x_{jk+t}\right)$.

Similarly, we can prove that the radio condition holds for every pair of vertices from $V(F_{5,k})$, and L is a radio labeling of $F_{5,k}$ that proved $rn(F_{5,k}) \leq 8k + 1$. □

For more illustrations, $F_{5,k}$ with labeling of vertices is presented in Figure 5.

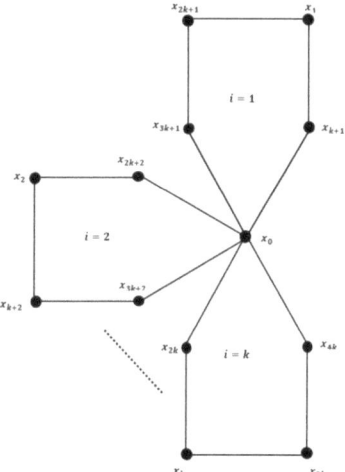

Figure 5. $F_{5,k}$ with labeling of vertices.

Theorem 4. *Let $k > 2$, $F_{6,k}$ be a friendship graph with blocks each of length 6 and $|V(F_{6,k})| = 5k + 1$ and then $rn(F_{6,k}) \leq 17k + 1$.*

Proof. Define the map L as follows:

$$L(x_{jk+i}) = \begin{cases} 0, & i = j = 0 \\ 4 + i - 1, & j = 0, 1 \leq i \leq k \\ k + 6, & j = 1, i = 1 \\ k + 10 + 3(i - 2) & j = 1, 2 \leq i \leq k \\ 4k + 4 + 3i & j = 2, 1 \leq i \leq k \\ 7k + 7 & j = 3, i = 1 \\ 7k + 11 + 5(i - 2) & j = 3, 2 \leq i \leq k \\ 12k + 5i + 1 & j = 3, 2 \leq i \leq k \end{cases}$$

Since $diam(F_{6,k}) = 6$. From the above definition of the labeling function L and Figure 6, one can prove that the radio condition $|L(x_u) - L(x_v)| \geq 7 - d(x_u, x_v)$ holds for all $x_u, x_v \in V(F_{6,k})$ and $u \neq v$. Moreover, $rn(F_{6,k}) \leq 17k + 1$. □

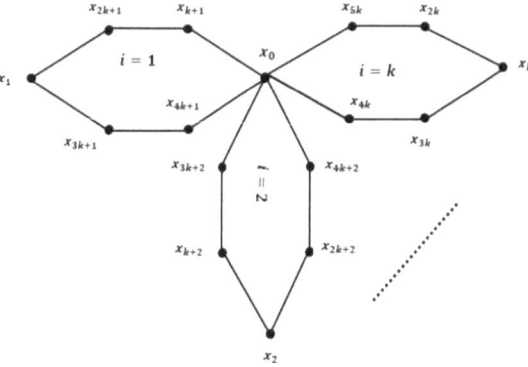

Figure 6. $F_{6,k}$ with labeling of vertices.

A friendship $F_{6,k}$ with labeling of its vertices is shown in Figure 6.

3. Integer Linear Programming Model

A new mathematical formulation for the radio labeling problem is proposed for $F_{3,k}$, $F_{4,k}$, $F_{5,k}$, and $F_{6,k}$. We next describe the problem of finding the radio labeling problem for a graph in terms of an integer programming problem [4]. Let G be a connected graph of order n with $V(G) = \{u_1, u_2, \cdots, u_n\}$ and let $D = [d_{ij}]$ be the distance matrix of G, that is, $d_{ij} = d(u_i, u_j)$ for $1 \leq i, j \leq n$. We suppose that v_i are the labels of the vertices u_i such that $1 \leq i \leq n$. Now, we can introduce the mathematical model for the radio labeling problem as an integer programming model. We define the function F by

$$minF = v_1 + v_2 + \cdots + v_n$$

subject to

$$|v_i - v_j| \geq diam + 1 - d(u_i, u_j) \text{ for } 1 \leq i \leq n-1;\ 2 \leq j \leq n \text{ and } i < j$$

where $v_1, v_2, \cdots, v_n \in \{0, 1\}$

The radio number of the graph $G = max_{1 \leq i \leq n}\{v_i\}$.

4. Computational Study

We carried out a computational study to measure the efficiency of the proposed upper bounds by Theorems 1–4 compared to the results of the algorithms introduced in [3,4]. Moreover, the comparison between the results of those Theorems and the mathematical model introduced in Section 3 is also presented. All of these are compatible with a PC with a Core i7 CPU@2.8 GHz, 8 GB of RAM, and a 64-bit operating system. The computational studies were carried out using MATLAB R2016a and the MS Windows 7 Professional system.

According to the upper bound of the radio number of $F_{3,k}$, Table 1 and Figure 7 show that the proposed results in Theorem 1 outperform the proposed results in [3] for k when it is odd. When k is even, the same results occur. On the other hand, the proposed results in Theorem 1 outperform the proposed results in [4] for every k.

Table 1. A comparison among our results, [3], and integer programming results [4] for $F_{3,k}$.

k	n	Saha [3]		ILPM [4]		Theorem 1
		$rn(F_{3,k})$	CPU Time	$rn(F_{3,k})$	CPU Time	$rn(F_{3,k})$
1	3	4	0.024824	4	0.07009	3
2	5	5	0.026428	7	0.056758	5
3	7	8	0.028891	10	0.060813	7
4	9	9	0.035933	13	0.066483	9
5	11	12	0.035994	16	0.067994	11
6	13	13	0.03913	19	0.07225	13
7	15	16	0.03958	22	0.073795	15
8	17	17	0.041326	25	0.078172	17
9	19	20	0.044408	28	0.078172	19
10	21	21	0.045015	31	0.080299	21
11	23	24	0.047039	34	0.088287	23
12	25	25	0.047221	37	0.102373	25
13	27	28	0.048065	40	0.160287	27
14	29	29	0.04859	43	0.182859	29
15	31	32	0.092601	46	0.272814	31

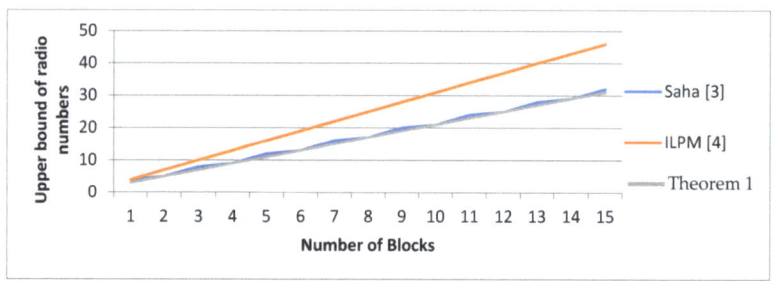

Figure 7. A comparison among our results, the Saha algorithm, Saha, L., et al., 2012 [3]; and integer programming according to the upper bound of the radio number of $F_{3,k}$ from Badr, et al., 2020 [4].

According to the running time, Table 1 and Figure 8 show that the proposed results in Theorem 1 take the constant time complexity $O(1)$, while the proposed results in [3] take $O(n^3)$. On the other hand, the proposed results in Theorem 1 take less time than the proposed results in [4].

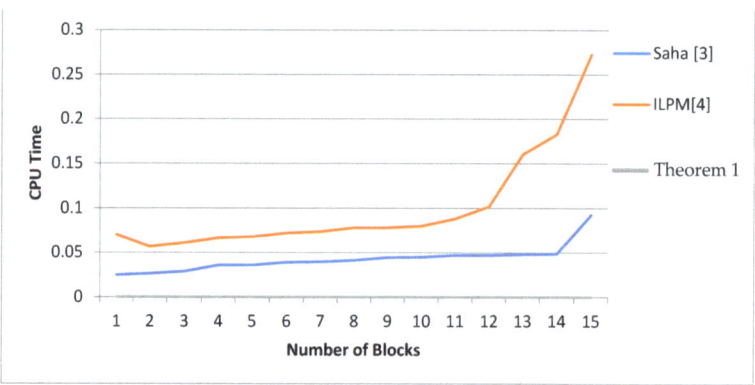

Figure 8. A CPU time comparison among our results, the Saha algorithm, Saha, L., et al., 2012 [3]; and integer programming of $F_{3,k}$ from Badr, et al., 2020 [4].

According to the upper bound of the radio number of $F_{4,k}$, Table 2 and Figure 9 show that the proposed results in Theorem 2 outperform the proposed results in [3] for $k = 1, 2$.

Table 2. A comparison among our results, [3], and integer programming results [4] for $F_{4,k}$.

k	n	Saha [3]		ILPM [4]		Theorem 2
		$rn(F_{4,k})$	CPU Time	$rn(F_{4,k})$	CPU Time	$rn(F_{4,k})$
1	4	10	0.025561	11	0.051869	8
2	7	16	0.027393	17	0.053149	15
3	10	22	0.02758	23	0.055986	22
4	13	29	0.028133	30	0.056235	29
5	16	36	0.030245	37	0.067974	36
6	19	43	0.030387	44	0.067994	43
7	22	50	0.031081	51	0.06921	50
8	25	57	0.031635	58	0.071135	57
9	28	64	0.031749	65	0.07225	64

Table 2. Cont.

k	n	Saha [3]		ILPM [4]		Theorem 2
		$rn(F_{4,k})$	CPU Time	$rn(F_{4,k})$	CPU Time	$rn(F_{4,k})$
10	31	71	0.035689	72	0.073031	71
11	34	78	0.038289	79	0.106774	78
12	37	85	0.043385	86	0.107721	85
13	40	92	0.043505	93	0.160287	92
14	43	99	0.044422	100	0.182859	99
15	46	106	0.054716	107	0.200691	106

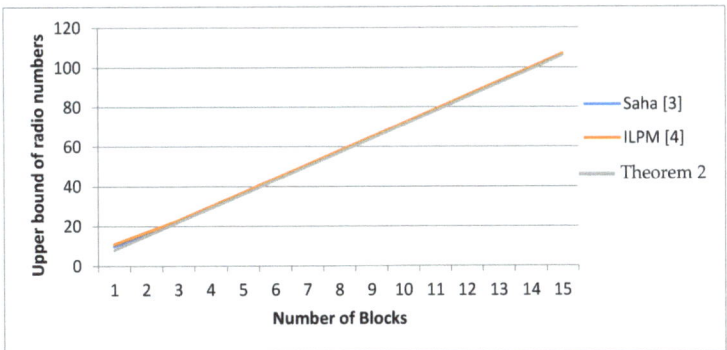

Figure 9. A comparison among our results, the Saha algorithm, Saha, L., et al., 2012 [3]; and integer programming according to the upper bound of the radio number of $F_{4,k}$ from Badr, et al., 2020 [4].

For $k = 3, 4, \ldots, 15$, the same results occur. On the other hand, the proposed results in Theorem 2 outperform the proposed results in [4] for every k.

According to the running time, Table 2 and Figure 10 show that the proposed results in Theorem 2 take the constant time complexity $O(1)$ while the proposed results in [3] take $O(n^3)$. On the other hand, the proposed results in Theorem 2 take less time than the proposed results in [4]

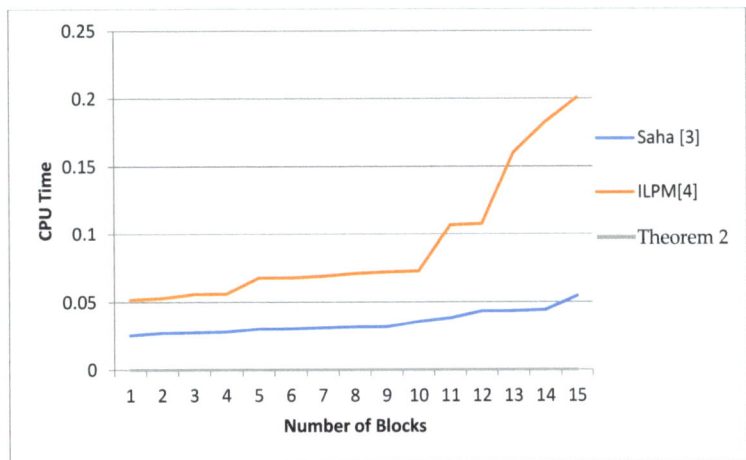

Figure 10. A CPU time comparison among our results, the Saha algorithm, Saha, L., et al., 2012 [3]; and integer programming of $F_{4,k}$ from Badr, et al., 2020 [4].

According to the upper bound of the radio number of $F_{5,k}$, Table 3 and Figure 11 show that the proposed results in Theorem 3 outperform the proposed results in [3] for $k = 1$.

Table 3. A comparison among our results, [3], and integer programming results [4] for $F_{5,k}$.

k	n	Saha [3]		ILPM [4]		Theorem 3
		$rn(F_{5,k})$	CPU Time	$rn(F_{5,k})$	CPU Time	$rn(F_{5,k})$
1	5	12	0.013394	14	0.033658	9
2	9	17	0.013676	24	0.038117	17
3	13	25	0.021828	35	0.048892	25
4	17	33	0.045767	46	0.050592	33
5	21	41	0.159417	57	0.053916	41
6	25	49	0.170631	68	0.057428	49
7	29	57	0.212698	79	0.064091	57
8	33	65	0.248107	90	0.124051	65
9	37	73	0.253468	101	0.133257	73
10	41	81	0.285491	112	0.162882	81
11	45	89	0.286759	123	0.221091	89
12	49	97	0.450209	134	0.23193	97
13	53	105	0.454764	145	0.23485	105
14	57	113	0.604194	156	0.312935	113
15	61	121	0.621928	167	0.317238	121

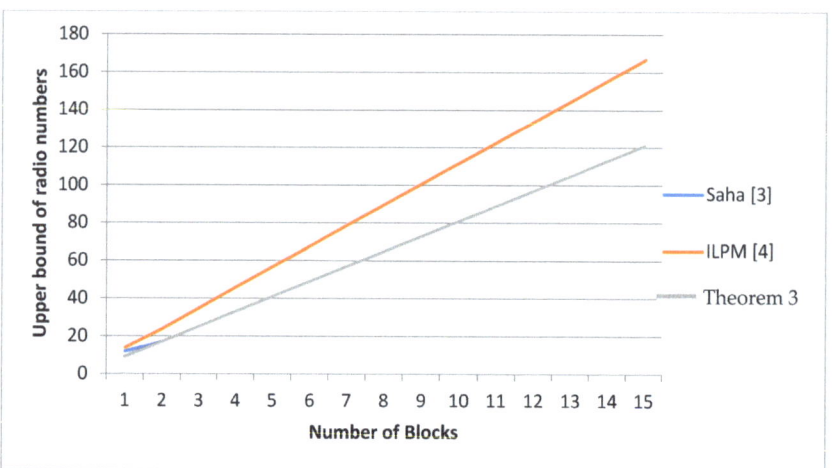

Figure 11. A comparison among our results, the Saha algorithm, Saha, L., et al., 2012 [3]; and integer programming according to the upper bound of the radio number of $F_{5,k}$ from Badr, et al., 2020 [4].

For $k = 2, 3, 4, \cdots, 15$, the same results occur. On the other hand, the proposed results in Theorem 3 outperform the proposed results in [4] for every k.

According to the running time, Table 3 and Figure 12 show that the proposed results in Theorem 3 take the constant time complexity $O(1)$, while the proposed results in [3] take $O(n^3)$. On the other hand, the proposed results in Theorem 3 take less time than the proposed results in [4].

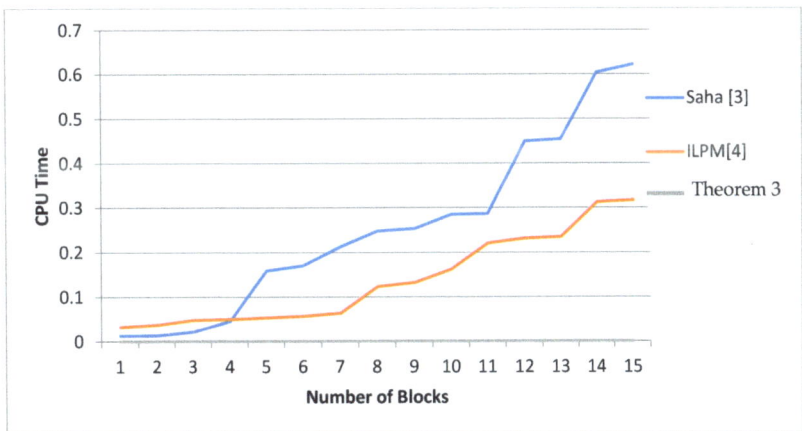

Figure 12. A CPU time comparison among our results, the Saha algorithm, Saha, L., et al., 2012 [3]; and integer programing of $F_{5,k}$ from Badr, et al., 2020 [4].

According to the upper bound of the radio number of $F_{6,k}$, Table 4 and Figure 13 show that the proposed results in Theorem 4 outperform the proposed results in [3] for $k = 1$. For $k = 2, 3, 4, \cdots, 15$, the same results occur. On the other hand, the proposed results in Theorem 4 outperform the proposed results in [4] for every k.

Table 4. A comparison among our results, [3], and integer programming results [4] for $F_{6,k}$.

k	n	Saha [3]		ILPM [4]		Theorem 4
		$rn(F_{6,k})$	CPU Time	$rn(F_{6,k})$	CPU Time	$rn(F_{6,k})$
1	6	22	0.026524	24	0.033143	18
2	11	36	0.029344	44	0.038123	35
3	16	52	0.030768	62	0.040921	52
4	21	69	0.049229	80	0.042084	69
5	26	86	0.092921	98	0.045056	86
6	31	103	0.094403	117	0.046653	103
7	36	120	0.129486	136	0.046656	120
8	41	137	0.258403	155	0.047893	137
9	46	154	0.281746	174	0.04914	154
10	51	171	0.314351	193	0.05036	171
11	56	188	0.417131	212	0.060892	188
12	61	205	0.488938	231	0.06789	205
13	66	222	0.59044	250	0.075292	222
14	71	239	0.703049	269	0.08014	239
15	76	256	1.08618	288	0.09014	256

According to the running time, Table 4 and Figure 14 show that the proposed results in Theorem 4 take the constant time complexity $O(1)$, while the proposed results in [3] take $O(n^3)$. On the other hand, the proposed results in Theorem 4 take less time than the proposed results in [4].

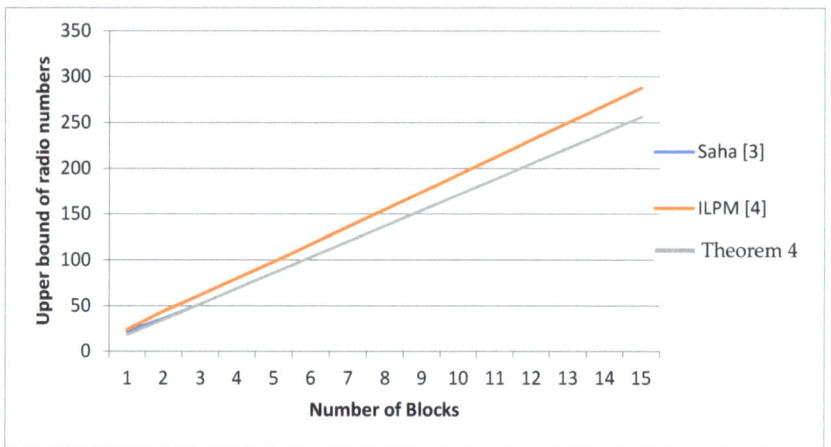

Figure 13. A comparison among our results, the Saha algorithm, Saha, L., et al., 2012 [3]; and integer programming according to the upper bound of the radio number of $F_{6,k}$ from Badr, et al., 2020 [4].

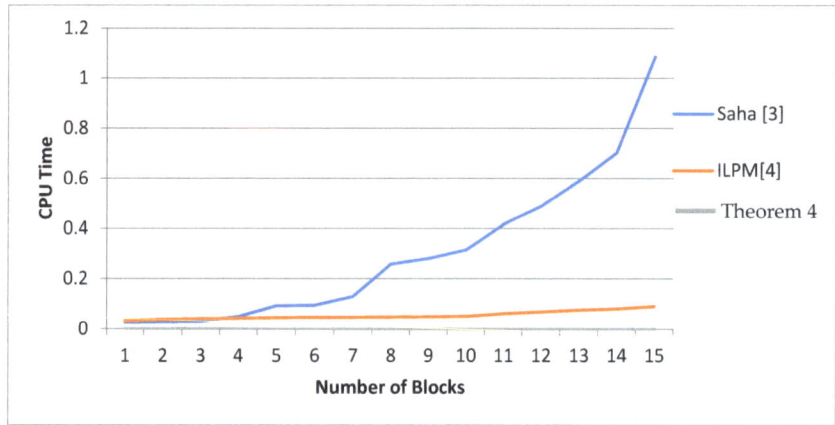

Figure 14. A CPU time comparison among our results, the Saha algorithm, Saha, L., et al., 2012 [3]; and integer programming of $F_{6,k}$ from Badr, et al., 2020 [4].

5. Conclusions

In this paper, the radio labeling of friendship networks ($F_{3,k}$, $F_{4,k}$, $F_{5,k}$, and $F_{6,k}$) are studied. Additionally, a mathematical model is proposed to find the upper bound of ($F_{3,k}$, $F_{4,k}$, $F_{5,k}$, and $F_{6,k}$). A computational study is presented to prove the efficiency of our results compared to the previous results. Finally, the empirical study shows that the proposed results overcome the previous results according to the upper bound of the radio number and the running time. In future work, we will find an upper bound of the radio number of general friendship networks $F_{n,k}$. Moreover, new algorithms and development of known algorithms will be proposed to find the radio numbers of the different radio networks.

Author Contributions: Methodology, A.H.A., E.B., H.A. and H.M.S.; Formal analysis, A.H.A., E.B., H.A. and H.M.S.; Investigation, A.H.A., E.B., H.A. and H.M.S.; Writing—original draft A.H.A., E.B., H.A. and H.M.S.; Writing—review & editing, A.H.A., E.B., H.A. and H.M.S. All authors have read and agreed to the published version of the manuscript.

Funding: Open Access funding provided by the Qatar National Library.

Data Availability Statement: The data used to support the findings of this study are available from the corresponding author upon request.

Acknowledgments: The authors would like to extend their sincere appreciation to the Qatar National Library.

Conflicts of Interest: The authors declare no conflict of interest.

References

1. Hale, W.K. Frequency assignment: Theory; Applications. *Proc. IEEE* **1980**, *68*, 1497–1514. [CrossRef]
2. Chartrand, G.; Erwin, D.; Harary, F.; Zhang, P. Radio labelings of graphs. *Bull. Inst. Combin. Appl.* **2001**, *33*, 77–85.
3. Saha, L.; Panigrahi, P. A graph Radio k-coloring algorithm. *Lect. Notes Comput. Sci.* **2012**, *7643*, 125–129.
4. Badr, E.M.; Moussa, M.I. An upper bound of radio k-coloring problem and its integer linear programming model. *Wirel. Netw.* **2020**, *26*, 4955–4964. [CrossRef]
5. Li, X.; Mak, V.; Zhou, S. Optimal radio labelings of complete m-array trees. *Discret. Appl. Math.* **2010**, *158*, 507–515. [CrossRef]
6. Liu, D.D.-F. Radio number for trees. *Discret. Math.* **2008**, *308*, 1153–1164.
7. Liu, D.D.-F.; Xie, M. Radio number for square of cycles. *Congr. Numer.* **2004**, *169*, 105–125.
8. Liu, D.D.-F.; Xie, M. Radio number for square paths. *Ars Comb.* **2009**, *90*, 307–319.
9. Liu, D.D.-F.; Zhu, X. Multi-level distance labelings for paths and cycles. *SIAM J. Discret. Math.* **2005**, *19*, 610–621. [CrossRef]
10. Morris-Rivera, M.; Tomova, M.; Wyels, C.; Yeager, Y. The radio number of $C_n \times C_n$. *Ars Comb.* **2012**, *103*, 81–96.
11. Ortiz, P.; Martinez, P.; Tomova, M.; Wyels, C. Radio numbers of some generalized rism graphs. *Discuss. Math. Graph Theory* **2011**, *311*, 45–62.
12. Reddy, V.S.; Iyer, V.K. Upper bounds on the radio number of some trees. *Int. J. Pure Appl. Math.* **2011**, *71*, 207–215.
13. Saha, L.; Panigrahi, P. On the Radio number of Toroidal grids. *Aust. J. Comb.* **2013**, *55*, 273–288.
14. Saha, L.; Panigrahi, P. A lower bound for radio *k*-chromatic number. *Discret. Appl. Math.* **2015**, *192*, 87–100. [CrossRef]
15. Zhang, P. Radio labellings of cycles. *Ars Comb.* **2002**, *65*, 21–32.
16. ELrokh, A.; Badr, E.; Al-Shamiri, M.M.A.; Ramadhan, S. Upper bounds of radio number for triangular snake and double triangular snake Graphs. *J. Math.* **2022**, *2022*, 3635499. [CrossRef]
17. Badr, E.; Almotairi, S.; Elrokh, A.; Abdel-Hady, A.; Almutairi, B. An Integer Linear Programming Model for Solving Radio Mean Labeling Problem. *IEEE Access* **2020**, *8*, 162343–162349. [CrossRef]
18. Badr, E.; Nada, S.; Al-Shamiri, M.M.A.; Abdel-Hay, A.; ELrokh, A. A novel mathematical model for radio mean square labeling problem. *J. Math.* **2022**, *2022*, 3303433. [CrossRef]
19. Badr, E.M.; Elgendy, H. A hybrid water cycle—Particle swarm optimization for solving the fuzzy underground water confined steady flow. *Indones J. Electr. Eng. Comput. Sci.* **2020**, *19*, 492–504. [CrossRef]
20. Badr, E.M.; Almotiari, S. On a dual direct cosine simplex type algorithm and its computational behavior. *Math. Probl. Eng.* **2020**, *2020*, 7361092. [CrossRef]
21. Bloom, G.S.; Golomb, S.W. Applications of Numbered Undirected Graphs. *Proc. Ofthe Inst. Electr. Electron. Eng.* **1977**, *65*, 562–570. [CrossRef]
22. Bosck, J. *Cyclic Decompositions, Vertex Labellings and Graceful Graphs*; Decompositions of Graphs; Kluwer Academic Publishers: Dordrecht, The Netherlands, 1990; pp. 57–76.
23. Frucht, R. Graceful Numbering of Wheels and Other Related Graphs. *Ann. N. Y. Acad. Sci.* **1979**, *319*, 219–229. [CrossRef]
24. Frucht, R.; Gallian, J.A. Labeling Prisms. *Ars Comb.* **1988**, *26*, 69–82.
25. Gallian, J.A. A Dynamic Survey of Graph Labeling. *Electron. J. Comb.* **2021**, *24*. [CrossRef]
26. Graham, R.L.; Sloane, N.J.A. On Additive Bases and Harmonious Graphs. *SIAM J. Algebr. Discret. Methods* **1980**, *1*, 382–404. [CrossRef]
27. Golomb, S.W. *How to Number a Graph, Graph Theory and Computing*; Read, R.C., Ed.; Academic Press: Cambridge, MA, USA, 1972; pp. 23–37.
28. Rosa, A. *On Certain Valuations of the Vertices of a Graph, Theory of Graphs*; International Symposium, Rome, Italy, 1966; Gordon and Breach: Philadelphia, PA, USA, 1967; pp. 349–355.
29. Singh, G.S. A Note on Graceful Prisms. *Natl. Acad. Sci. Lett.* **1992**, *15*, 193–194.
30. Acharya, B.D.; Gill, M.K. On the Index of Gracefulness of a Graph and the Gracefulness ofTwo-Dimensional Square Lattice Graphs. *Indian J. Math.* **1981**, *23*, 81–94.

Disclaimer/Publisher's Note: The statements, opinions and data contained in all publications are solely those of the individual author(s) and contributor(s) and not of MDPI and/or the editor(s). MDPI and/or the editor(s) disclaim responsibility for any injury to people or property resulting from any ideas, methods, instructions or products referred to in the content.

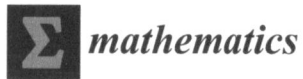

Article

The Structure of Semiconic Idempotent Commutative Residuated Lattices

Wei Chen

School of Mathematics and Statistics, Minnan Normal University, Zhangzhou 363000, China; chenwei6808467@126.com

Abstract: In this paper, we study semiconic idempotent commutative residuated lattices. After giving some properties of such residuated lattices, we obtain a structure theorem for semiconic idempotent commutative residuated lattices. As an application, we make use of the structure theorem to prove that the variety of strongly semiconic idempotent commutative residuated lattices has the amalgamation property.

Keywords: residuated lattices; idempotent semigroup; chain; construction; amalgamation

MSC: 06F05; 20M10

Citation: Chen, W. The Structure of Semiconic Idempotent Commutative Residuated Lattices. *Mathematics* 2024, 12, 179. https://doi.org/10.3390/math12020179

Academic Editor: Irina Cristea

Received: 4 September 2023
Revised: 30 December 2023
Accepted: 4 January 2024
Published: 5 January 2024

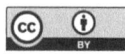

Copyright: © 2024 by the author. Licensee MDPI, Basel, Switzerland. This article is an open access article distributed under the terms and conditions of the Creative Commons Attribution (CC BY) license (https://creativecommons.org/licenses/by/4.0/).

1. Introduction

A *commutative residuated lattice* is defined as an algebra $(L, \wedge, \vee, \cdot, \rightarrow, e)$ of type $(2,2,2,2,0)$ satisfying the following conditions: $(RL1)$ $(L, \wedge, \vee)$ is a lattice; $(RL2)$ $(L, \cdot, e)$ is a commutative monoid with identity e; and $(RL3)$ $(\forall x, y, z \in L)$ $x \cdot y \leq z \iff y \leq x \rightarrow z$, where $\leq$ is the lattice ordering.

Sometimes, commutative residuated lattices are also called *commutative residuated lattice-ordered monoids* and abbreviated by CRLs. It is well known that $(RL3)$ holds if and only if $\leq$ is compatible with $\cdot$ and for all $a, b \in L$, $\{p \in L : a \cdot p \leq b\}$ contains a greatest element (denoted by $a \rightarrow b$).

A CRL **L** is called *idempotent* if for all $a \in L$, $a \cdot a = a$; is called *integral* if for all $a \in L$, $a \leq e$; is called *totally ordered* if for all $a, b \in L$, $a \leq b$ or $a \geq b$; is called *semilinear* when it is a subdirect product of totally ordered CRLs; and is called *conic* if for all $a \in L$, $a \leq e$ or $a \geq e$ (see [1–4]). A semilinear idempotent CRL is said to be an odd Sugihara monoid if for all $a \in L$, $(a \rightarrow e) \rightarrow e = a$. An integral idempotent CRL is said to be a *Brouwerian algebra* if for all $a, b \in L$, $a \cdot b = a \wedge b$. As in [4], a CRL **L** is called *semiconic* when it is a subdirect product of conic CRLs.

Ward and Dilworth were the first to study a class of algebra as a generalization of ideal lattices of rings in [5], which we call commutative residuated lattices. CRLs play an important role in the study of algebraic logic, as they provide an algebraic semantics for substructural logics (see [6]). The multitude of different types of CRLs makes the investigation rather complicated, and at the present moment, large classes of CRLs lack a structural description. The study of constructions is very important in enhancing our understanding of CRLs and, as a result, of substructural logics. Hart, Rafter and Tsinakis were the first to study the structure theory of CRLs in [7]. In [8], the authors extend the main results of [7] to the non-commutative case. More recently, there has been substantial research regarding the structure of some specific classes of CRLs, see, for example, [9–12]. Idempotent CRLs form an important tool both in algebra and logic (see [6]). Among them, semiconic ones make a valuable contribution because they include several important algebraic counterparts of substructural logics (see [13]). Recently, algebra properties for semiconic CRLs have been given by many authors (see [1,2,4,6,14–19]). In [20], the authors obtain a structure theorem for semilinear idempotent CRLs. In this paper, we will study the construction of semiconic idempotent CRLs. From the semigroup algebraic perspective, idempotent CRLs are indeed ordered semigroups (for ordered semigroups, see [21]). The natural partial order plays an important role in the investigation of semigroups (see [22,23]). We will make use of the natural partial order to obtain some important properties and then establish a structure theorem of semiconic idempotent CRLs, which generalizes the main result of [20].

We proceed as follows: in Section 2, we present some definitions and facts used in the sequel. In Section 3, we obtain some properties of semiconic idempotent CRLs. In Section 4, we give a structure theorem for semiconic idempotent CRLs, which generalizes the main result of [20]. In Section 5, we prove that the variety of strongly semiconic idempotent CRLs has the amalgamation property, which generalizes the main result of [10].

2. Preliminaries

In this section, we will list some facts about CRLs.

A monoid $(M, \cdot, e)$ is said to be a *po-monoid* when it is also a poset $(M, \leq)$, and in which $\leq$ is compatible with $\cdot$ in the sense that $(\forall a, b, c \in M)\ a \leq b \implies c \cdot a \leq c \cdot b, a \cdot c \leq b \cdot c$. A po-monoid $(M, \cdot, e, \leq)$ is said to be a *lattice-ordered monoid* when $(M, \leq)$ is a lattice. A lattice-ordered monoid $(M, \cdot, e, \leq)$ is said to be *idempotent* if for all $a \in M$, $a \cdot a = a$; is said to be *commutative* when the monoid reduct $(M, \cdot, e)$ is a commutative monoid; and is said to be *conic*, if for all $a \in M$, $a \leq e$ or $a \geq e$. For convenience, we simply write $a \cdot b$ as ab for $a, b \in M$. The reader is referred to reference [21] for detailed information on lattice-ordered monoids.

We need the following results.

Lemma 1 ([19]). *Let $(M, \cdot, e, \leq)$ be an idempotent lattice-ordered monoid with identity e, and $a, b \in M$.*

(1) $a \wedge b \leq ab \leq a \vee b$.
(2) *If $a, b \geq e$, then $ab = a \vee b$.*
(3) *If $a, b \leq e$, then $ab = a \wedge b$.*
(4) *If $a \leq e \leq ab$, then $ab = b$.*
(5) *If $ab \leq e \leq a$, then $ab = b$.*

Let $(L, \wedge, \vee, \cdot, \to, e)$ be a CRL and $\leq$ shall always denote the lattice order of **L** in this paper.

Lemma 2 ([6,24]). *Let $(L, \wedge, \vee, \cdot, \to, e)$ be a CRL and $a, b, c \in L$.*

(1) $a(b \vee c) = ab \vee ac$.
(2) $a \to (b \wedge c) = (a \to b) \wedge (a \to c)$.
(3) $(b \vee c) \to a = (b \to a) \wedge (c \to a)$.
(4) $b(b \to a) \leq a$.
(5) $e \leq a \to a$.
(6) $((a \to b) \to b) \to b = a \to b$.
(7) $a \to (b \to c) = (ab) \to c$.

From now on, we denote $a \to e$ and $(a \to e) \to e$ by a^* and a^{**}, respectively. Next, we shall present some known facts on conic idempotent CRLs used in later proofs. More details on semiconic residuated lattices can be found in [2,4,25].

Lemma 3 ([4]). *Let **L** be a conic idempotent CRL, and $a, b \in L$.*

(1) *If a and b are incomparable, then $a^* = b^*$.*
(2) *The elements a and b^* are comparable.*
(3) $a \not\leq b$ *if and only if* $a \to b < e$.
(4) *If $a \leq e (a > e)$, then $a^* = a \to a \geq e (a^* < e)$.*
(5) $\{a^* : a \in L\}$ *is a chain in* $(L, \wedge, \vee)$.

3. Some Properties

To begin with, we obtain some properties of conic idempotent commutative lattice-ordered monoids.

Now let $(L, \cdot, e, \leq)$ be a conic idempotent commutative lattice-ordered monoid. Since the monoid reduct of **L** is an idempotent commutative monoid, we define the *natural partial order* on **L** as follows: for $a, b \in L$,

$$a \leq_n b \text{ if and only if } ab = a.$$

It is clear that $(L, \leq_n)$ is a semilattice. For $a, b \in L$, $a \parallel b$ [resp. $a \parallel_n b$] means that a and b are incomparable under $\leq$ [resp. $\leq_n$], and $a \prec b$ [resp. $a \prec_n b$] means that $a < b$ [resp. $a <_n b$]. For any $c \in L$, $a \leq c \leq b$ [resp. $a \leq_n c \leq_n b$] implies either $a = c$ or $b = c$. Let $a \wedge_n b = \max\{c \in L : c \leq_n a, b\}$ and $a \vee_n b = \min\{c \in L : a, b \leq_n c\}$ if it exists in $(L, \leq_n)$.

Proposition 1. *Let* $(L, \cdot, e, \leq)$ *be a conic idempotent commutative lattice-ordered monoid. The following statements are true for* $a, b \in L$:

(1) If $a, b \leq e$, then $a \leq_n b$ if and only if $a \leq b$.
(2) If $a, b \geq e$, then $a \leq_n b$ if and only if $a \geq b$.
(3) $a \parallel b$ if and only if $a \parallel_n b$.
(4) If $a \parallel b$ and $a < e$, then $a \wedge_n b = a \wedge b$.
(5) If $a \parallel b$ and $a > e$, then $a \wedge_n b = a \vee b$.

Proof. (1) Let $a, b \in L$ be such that $a, b \leq e$. Then, by Lemma 1(3), $a \leq_n b \iff ab = a \iff a \wedge b = a \iff a \leq b$.

(2) This is similar to (1).

(3) If $a \parallel b$, then since **L** is conic, $a, b \leq e$ or $a, b \geq e$. If $a, b \leq e$, then by (1), $a \not\parallel_n b$ is impossible. Thus, $a \parallel_n b$. Similarly, if $a, b \geq e$, then $a \parallel_n b$. Conversely, let $a, b \in L$ such that $a \parallel_n b$. Suppose that $a \leq e \leq b$ or $b \leq e \leq a$. Then, since **L** is conic, by Lemma 1(4,5), $ab = a$ or $ab = b$, which implies that $a \leq_n b$ or $b \leq_n a$, a contradiction. Hence, $a, b \leq e$ or $e \leq a, b$. Thus, by (1) and (2), $a \parallel b$.

(4) Let $a, b \in L$ such that $a \parallel b$ and $a < e$. Then, by Lemma 1(3), $a \wedge b = ab$. Let $c \in L$ such that $c \leq_n a$ and $c \leq_n b$. Then, $ca = c$ and $cb = c$, so $cab = cb = c$. Thus, $c \leq_n ab$. Since $ab \leq_n a$ and $ab \leq_n b$, $a \wedge b = ab = a \wedge_n b$.

(5) Let $a, b \in L$ such that $a \parallel b$ and $a > e$. Then, by Lemma 1(2), $ab = a \vee b > a, b > e$. So by (2), $a \vee b \leq_n a$ and $a \vee b \leq_n b$. Let $c \in L$ such that $c \leq_n a$ and $c \leq_n b$. Then, $ca = c$ and $cb = c$, so $cab = cb = c$. Thus, $c \leq_n ab = a \vee b$. Therefore, $a \wedge_n b = a \vee b$. □

Secondly, we obtain some properties of conic idempotent CRLs.

Proposition 2. *Let* **L** *be a conic idempotent* CRL. *The following statements are true for* $a, b \in L$:

(1) If $a < e$, then $a <_n a^*$ and $a^* \not\parallel_n b$.
(2) If $a < e$ and $a <_n b <_n a^*$, then $b < e$.
(3) If $a > e$, then $a^* <_n a$ and $a^* \not\parallel_n b$.
(4) If $a > e$ and $a^* <_n b <_n a$, then $b > e$.
(5) If $a \parallel b$ and $a < e$, then $a \vee_n b = a \vee b$ and $(a \wedge b)^* = a^*$.

Proof. (1) Let $a, b \in L$ such that $a < e$. Then, $ae = a < e$, and so $a < e \leq a \to e = a^*$. Since $a(a \to e) \leq e$ by Lemma 2(4), $a(a \to e) = a$ by Lemma 1(5), which implies that $a <_n a \to e = a^*$. Since by Lemma 3(2), $a^* \not\parallel b$, by Proposition 1(3), $a^* \not\parallel_n b$.

(2) Let $a \in L$ such that $a < e$ and $a <_n b <_n a^* = a \to e$. Then, $ab = a < e$, and so $b \leq a \to e = a^*$. Suppose that $b \geq e$. Then, since by Lemma 3(4), $a^* \geq e$, by Proposition 1(2), $a^* \leq_n b$, contrary to $b <_n a^*$. Thus, $b < e$.

(3) This is similar to (1).

(4) This is similar to (2).

(5) Let $a, b \in L$ such that $a, b < e$ and $a \parallel b$. Since $a, b \leq a \vee b \leq e$, by (1), $a \leq_n a \vee b$ and $b \leq_n a \vee b$. Let $d \in L$ such that $a \leq_n d$ and $b \leq_n d$. Then, $ad = a$ and $bd = b$, so $d(a \vee b) = da \vee db = a \vee b$ by Lemma 2(1). Thus, $a \vee b \leq_n d$. Therefore, $a \vee_n b = a \vee b$. Because $a \wedge b \leq a < e$, $a^* = a \rightarrow e \leq (a \wedge b) \rightarrow e = (a \wedge b)^*$ by Lemma 2(3). Suppose that $a^* < (a \wedge b)^*$. Then, $a \wedge b < a < a^* < (a \wedge b)^*$, so by (2), $a^* < e$. But since $a < e$, $a^* \geq e$ by Lemma 3(4), a contradiction. Thus, $a^* = (a \wedge b)^*$. □

Proposition 3 ([2]). *Let L be a conic idempotent* CRL, *and let* $a, b \in L$ *such that* $a \leq e$. *If* $b < a$ *or* $a \parallel b$, *then* $a \rightarrow b = b$ *or* $a \rightarrow b \parallel a$.

Let $(L, \leq)$ be a join-semilattice, and let $L_\perp = L \cup \{\perp\}$ such that $\perp \leq a$ for all $a \in L$. **L** is said to be an *upper pre-lattice* when **L** is not a lattice and $(L_\perp, \leq)$ is a lattice. Let **L** be a lattice and $C \subseteq L$. **C** is said to be an *upper pre-sublattice of L* if **C** is an upper pre-lattice and there exists $a \in L$ such that $(C \cup \{a\}, \leq)$ is a sublattice of **L**. Similarly, we can define the *lower pre-lattice* and *lower pre-sublattice*.

Let **L** be a conic idempotent CRL. We define the following sets: $L^+ = \{a \in L : a > e\}$, $L^- = \{b \in L : b \leq e\}$, $L^* = \{j \in L : (\exists a \in L)\, j = a^*\}$, $L^{*-} = \{j \in L^* : j \leq e\}$, and $L^{*+} = \{j \in L^* : j > e\} = \{j \in L^* : (\exists i \in L^{*-})\, j = i^*\}$. For every $j \in L^*$, let $L_j = \{c \in L : c^{**} = j\}$. By Lemma 3(4), $L_j \subseteq L^+$ for all $j \in L^{*+}$. Since $a^* <_n a^{**} \leq_n a <_n e$ for all $a > e$ by Proposition 2(1,3) and Lemma 3(4), $a^{**} > e$ by Proposition 2(4). It follows that $L_i \subseteq L^-$ for all $i \in L^{*-}$. Because $L^{*-} \subseteq L^*$ and $(L^*, \leq)$ is a chain by Lemma 3(5), $(L^{*-}, \leq)$ is a chain. It is clear that $L^* = L^{*-} \cup L^{*+}$.

We have the following result, which generalizes ([15] Theorem 3.2).

Theorem 1. *Let L be a conic idempotent* CRL.
(1) *If* $a \in L$, *then* $a \in L^*$ *if and only if* $a^{**} = a$.
(2) *If* $i, l \in L^{*-}$, *then* $i = l$ *if and only if* $i^* = l^*$. *In addition*, $i \prec_n i^*$ *for all* $i \in L^{*-} \setminus \{e\}$.
(3) *If* $j, s \in L^*$ *such that* $j \neq s$, *then* $L_j \cap L_s = \emptyset$.
(4) *If* $i \in L^{*-}$, *then* L_i *is a sublattice of* $(L, \wedge, \vee)$ *and* $(L_i, \wedge, \vee, \cdot, \rightarrow^{L_i}, i)$ *is a Brouwerian algebra, where* $\rightarrow^{L_i}$ *is given by* $x \rightarrow^{L_i} y = (x \rightarrow y) \wedge i$ *for all* $x, y \in L_i$.
(5) *If* $j = i^* \in L^{*+}$, *then* L_j *has a greatest element* j *and is either a sublattice of* **L** *or an upper pre-sublattice of* **L**.
(6) *If* $i, l \in L^{*-}$ *such that* $i \neq l$, $a \in L_i$, $b \in L_l$ *and* $c \in L_{i^*}$, $d \in L_{l^*}$ *then* $i < l \iff a < b \iff c > d$.
(7) *If* $i \in L^{*-}$ *and* $j = i^*$ *such that* L_j *is an upper pre-sublattice of* **L**, *then there exists* $l \in L^{*-}$ *such that* $i \prec l$ *in* L^{*-} *and* $(L_j \cup \{l^*\}, \leq)$ *is a sublattice of* **L** *with a least element* l^*.
(8) *If* **L** *satisfies that* $(x \wedge y)^* = x^* \vee y^*$, *then* L_i *is a sublattice of* **L** *for all* $i \in L^{*+}$.
(9) *If* $i \in L^{*-}$, $l \in L^{*+}$ *and* $a \in L_i$, $b \in L_l$, *then* $i <_n l \iff a <_n b$.
(10) **L** *is finitely subdirectly irreducible if and only if* L_e *is a finitely subdirectly irreducible Brouwerian algebra*.
(11) L^* *is a totally ordered odd Sugihara monoid and subalgebra of* **L**, *that we call its skeleton*.

Proof. (1) We only need to verify the necessity because the sufficiency is clear. Suppose that $a \in L^*$. Then, there exists $c \in L$ such that $c^* = a$. Thus, by Lemma 2(6), $a = c^* = c^{***} = a^{**}$.

(2) We only need to prove the sufficiency because the necessity is obvious. Suppose that $i^* = l^*$. Since $i, l \in L^{*-}$ by assumption, $i = i^{**} = l^{**} = l$ by (1). Let $i \in L^{*-} \setminus \{e\}$. Then, by Proposition 2(1), $i <_n i^*$. Let $a \in L$ such that $i \leq_n a \leq_n i^*$. Suppose that $i <_n a <_n i^*$. If $a \geq e$, then by Proposition 2(2), $a < e$, a contradiction. If $a < e$, then since $i = i^{**} <_n a <_n i^*$, $a > e$ by Proposition 2(4), a contradiction. Consequently, $i \prec_n i^*$.

(3) It is obvious.

(4) Let $i \in L^{*-}$ and let $x, y \in L_i$. Then, $x^{**} = y^{**} = i$, which, together with $(x \vee y)^* = x^* \wedge y^* \in \{x^*, y^*\}$ by Lemmas 2(3) and 3(5), derives that $(x \vee y)^{**} = i$, whence $x \vee y \in L_i$. If $x \leq y$ or $y < x$, then $(xy)^* = (x \wedge y)^* = x^*$ or $(xy)^* = (x \wedge y)^* = y^*$, and so $(xy)^{**} = (x \wedge y)^{**} = i$, which implies that $xy = x \wedge y \in L_i$. If $x \parallel y$, then by

Proposition 2(5), $(xy)^* = (x \wedge y)^* = x^*$, and so $(xy)^{**} = (x \wedge y)^{**} = i$, which implies that $xy = x \wedge y \in L_i$. Thus, L_i is a sublattice of $(L, \wedge, \vee)$. By (1), $i \in L_i$. Let $c \in L_i$. Then, $c \leq (c \to e) \to e = c^* \to e = c^{**} = i$. Thus, i is the greatest element of L_i, and so $(L_i, \cdot, i, \leq)$ is an integral idempotent commutative lattice-ordered monoid with an identity i. We can claim that $\max\{z \in L_i : xz \leq y\} = (x \to y) \wedge i$ for all $x, y \in L_i$. To prove this, we consider the following cases:

- If $x \leq y$, then $i \leq e \leq x \to y$ by Lemma 3(3) and so $\max\{z \in L_i : xz \leq y\} = i = (x \to y) \wedge i$.
- If $x > y$ or $x \parallel y$, then by Proposition 3, $x \to y = y$ or $x \to y \parallel x$. So $(x \to y)^{**} = y^{**} = i$ or $(x \to y)^{**} = x^{**} = i$ by Lemma 3(1). Thus, $x \to y \in L_i$, whence $\max\{z \in L_i : xz \leq y\} = x \to y = (x \to y) \wedge i$

We define $x \to^{L_i} y = (x \to y) \wedge i$ for all $x, y \in L_i$. Thus, $(L_i, \wedge, \vee, \cdot, \to^{L_i}, i)$ is a Brouwerian algebra.

(5) Let $j = i^* \in L^{*+}$. By similar arguments as in the proof of (4), j is the greatest element of L_j and $b \vee c \in L_j$ for all $b, c \in L_j$, so $\mathbf{L}_j$ is a join-semilattice with a greatest element j. Suppose that $\mathbf{L}_j$ is not a sublattice of $\mathbf{L}$. Then, there exists $b, b' \in L_j$ such that $b \parallel b'$ and $d = b \wedge b' \notin L_j$. Hence, $e \leq d < b$ and $d^{**} < b^{**} = j$ by Lemma 2(3). Let $c \in L_j$. Suppose that $c \parallel d$. Then, $d^{**} = c^{**} = j$ by Lemma 3(1), which is contrary to $d^{**} < j$. Assume that $c < d$. Then, $d^{**} > c^{**} = b^{**} = j$ by Lemma 2(3), which is contrary to $d^{**} < j$. Thus, for all $c \in L_j, d < c$. Similarly, if $g, g' \in L_j$ such that $g \wedge g' \notin L_j$, then for all $c \in L_j, g \wedge g' < c$. It follows that $d = g \wedge g'$. Therefore, $(L_j \cup \{d\}, \leq)$ is a sublattice of $\mathbf{L}$. Consequently, $\mathbf{L}_j$ is an upper pre-sublattice.

(6) Let $i, l \in L^{*-}$ such that $i \neq l$ and let $a \in L_i, b \in L_l$. If $i < l$, then by (4), $a \leq i < l$ and $b \leq l$. Suppose that $b \leq i$. Then, $b^{**} \leq i^{**} = i < j$, which is contrary to $b^{**} = j$. Thus, $i < b$ by Lemma 3(2), whence $a < b$. Conversely, if $a < b$, then $a \leq i$ and $a < b \leq l$. Suppose that $l < i$. Then, $a^{**} \leq l^{**} = l < i$, which is contrary to $a^{**} = i$. Thus, $i < l$. Similarly, $i < l \iff c > d$.

(7) Let $i \in L^{*-}$ and $j = i^*$ such that $\mathbf{L}_j$ is an upper pre-sublattice of $\mathbf{L}$. Then, there exists $b, b' \in L_j$ such that $b \parallel b'$ and $d = b \wedge b' \notin L_j$. Let $l = d^*$. Then, $d \in L_{l^*}$. Since $d < b, i < l$ by (6). Let $k \in L^{*-}$ such that $i \leq k \leq l$. Suppose that $i < k < l$. Then, by (6) $d < k^* < b, b'$, contrary to $d = b \wedge b'$. Thus, $i \prec l$ in L^*. We have $dl = dd^* = d(d \to e) \leq e \implies d \leq d^* \to e = d^{**} = l^*$. We claim that $l^* = d$. Otherwise, if $d < l^*$, then since $i < l$, $j = i^* > l^*$ by (6) and so $l^* < b, b'$. It follows that $l^* \leq b \wedge b' = d$. It is a contradiction. Thus, $l^* = d^{**} = d = a \wedge b$. Consequently, $(L_j \cup \{l^*\}, \leq)$ is a sublattice of $\mathbf{L}$ with a least element l^*.

(8) Let $i \in L^{*+}$ and $a, b \in L_i$. Then, $(a \wedge b)^{**} = (a^* \vee b^*)^* = a^{**} \wedge b^{**} = i$, and so $a \wedge b \in L_i$. It follows that $\mathbf{L}_i$ is a sublattice of $\mathbf{L}$.

(9) Since $a \in L_i$ and $b \in L_l$, $a \leq i \leq e < b \leq l$ by (4–5) and $i^* \neq e$. Then, $a \leq_n i$ and $l \leq_n b$ by Proposition 1(1–2). Suppose that $i <_n l$. Then, $a <_n b$. Conversely, assume that $a <_n b$. We claim that $a^* \neq e$. Otherwise if $a^* = e$, then $a <_n b \implies ab = a \leq e \implies b \leq a \to e = a^* = e$, which is contrary to $b > e$. Consequently, $a^* > e$ by Lemma 3(4). By Proposition 2(1,3), $a \leq_n i = a^{**} <_n a^*$ and $b^* <_n l = b^{**} \leq_n b$. Suppose that $l <_n i$. If $a <_n l$, then $a <_n l <_n i = a^{**} <_n a^*$, and so by Proposition 2(2), $l < e$, which is contrary to $l > e$. If $l <_n a$, then $b^* <_n l = b^{**} <_n a <_n b$, and so by Proposition 2(4), $a > e$, which is contrary to $a \leq e$. Consequently, $i <_n l$.

(10) Suppose that $\mathbf{L}$ is finitely subdirectly irreducible, then e is join-irreducible in L. Since $\mathbf{L}_e$ is a sublattice of $\mathbf{L}$, e is join-irreducible in L_e, which implies that $\mathbf{L}_e$ is finitely subdirectly irreducible. Conversely, $\mathbf{L}_e$ is finitely subdirectly irreducible. Then, e is join-irreducible in L_e. By (6), we have that $b < a$ for all $a \in L_e$ and $b \in L_i$ such that $i \in L^{*-} \setminus \{e\}$, which implies that e is join-irreducible in L. Thus, $\mathbf{L}$ is finitely subdirectly irreducible.

(11) By Lemma 3(5), $(L^*, \leq)$ is a totally ordered set, which implies that $\mathbf{L}^*$ is a sublattice of $\mathbf{L}$. Let $a^*, b^* \in L^*$. If $a^*, b^* \leq e$, then $a^*b^* = a^* \wedge b^* \in L^*$. If $a^*, b^* \geq e$, then $a^*b^* = a^* \vee b^* \in L^*$. If $a^* \leq e, b^* > e$ or $a^* > e, b^* \leq e$, then by Lemma 1(4,5), $a^*b^* \in \{a^*, b^*\} \subseteq L^*$. Thus, L^* is closed with respect to multiplication. By Lemma 2(7), we have $a^* \to b^* = $

$a^* \to (b \to e) = (a^*b) \to e \in L^*$. Consequently, $\mathbf{L}^*$ is a subalgebra of $\mathbf{L}$. By Lemma 2(6), $(a^* \to e) \to e = ((a \to e) \to e) \to e = a \to e = a^*$. It follows that $\mathbf{L}^*$ is a totally ordered odd Sugihara monoid. □

Theorem 2. *Let $\mathbf{L}, \mathbf{K}$ be conic idempotent CRLs and $f : L \to K$ be a homomorphism between conic idempotent CRLs.*

(1) *$f(L^*) \subseteq K^*$ and $f(L_i) \subseteq K_{f(i)}$ for all $i \in L^*$.*

(2) *If $i \in L^*$ such that L_i is an upper pre-sublattice of $\mathbf{L}$ and $f(i) \neq e$, then $K_{f(i)}$ is an upper pre-sublattice of $\mathbf{K}$ and there exists $j \in L^*$ such that $j \prec i$ in L^* and $f(j) \prec f(i)$ in K^*.*

Proof. (1) Let $a \in L^*$. Then, there exists $b \in L$ such that $a = b^*$. Since f is a homomorphism, $f(a) = f(b^*) = f(b)^* \in K^*$, which implies that $f(L^*) \subseteq K^*$. Let $i \in L^*$ and $a \in L_i$. Then, $a^{**} = i$, and so $f(a)^{**} = f(a^{**}) = f(i)$, which implies that $f(a) \in K_{f(i)}$. It follows that $f(L_i) \subseteq K_{f(i)}$.

(2) Since L_i is an upper pre-sublattice of $\mathbf{L}$, $i > e$ by Theorem 1(4), and there exists $a, b \in L_i$ such that $a \wedge b \notin L_i$. Let $j = a \wedge b$. By the proof of Theorem 1(7), $e \leq a \wedge b = j \prec i$ in L^*, and so $j < i$ in L. Hence, $i^* < j^*$ by Theorem 1(6). It follows that $i <_n j$ and $i^* <_n j^*$ by Theorem 1(2). We claim that $i <_n j^*$. Otherwise, if $j^* <_n i$, then $i^* <_n j^* <_n i$, and so by Proposition 2(4), $j^* > e$, which is contrary to $j^* = (a \wedge b)^* \leq e$. Thus, $i <_n j^*$. We have $f(a), f(b) \in K_{f(i)}$ and $f(a) \wedge f(b) = f(a \wedge b) = f(j) \in K_{f(j)}$ by (1). Suppose that $f(j) = f(i)$. Then, $f(j) = f(i) = f(ij^*) = f(i)f(j^*) = f(j)f(j)^* = f(j)^*$, and so by Proposition 2(1,3), $f(i) = f(j) = e$, which is contrary to $f(i) \neq e$. Consequently, $f(j) \neq f(i)$. It follows that $K_{f(i)}$ is an upper pre-sublattice of $\mathbf{K}$ and by the proof of Theorem 1(7), $f(j) = f(a \wedge b) = f(a) \wedge f(b) \prec f(i)$ in K^*. □

4. The Construction Theorem

In this section, we shall show how to construct a conic idempotent CRL and then prove that any conic idempotent CRL is isomorphic to some conic idempotent CRL constructed in this way.

To start with, we introduce some new concepts.

Definition 1. *Let $(I, \leq)$ be a chain with a greatest element e. Let $I^+ = \{i^+ : i \in I \setminus \{e\}\}$ such that $I \cap I^+ = \emptyset$ and $i^+ \neq l^+$ for every pair $i, l \in I \setminus \{e\}$ such that $i \neq l$. Let $J = I \cup I^+$. Let $\mathcal{A} = \{(A_j, \leq_{A_j}) : j \in J\}$ be a family of pairwise disjoint nonempty posets indexed by J. $(I, I^+, J; \mathcal{A})$ is called a chain expansion system (abbreviated by CE-system) if the following conditions hold:*

(CE1) *If $i \in I$, then $(A_i, \leq_{A_i})$ is a Brouwerian algebra with a greatest element i.*

(CE2) *If $i^+ \in I^+$, then $(A_{i^+}, \leq_{A_{i^+}})$ is either a lattice with a greatest element i^+ or an upper pre-lattice with a greatest element i^+.*

(CE3) *If $i^+ \in I^+$ such that $(A_{i^+}, \leq_{A_{i^+}})$ is an upper pre-lattice, then there exists $j \in I$ such that $i \prec j$ in I.*

Given a CE-system $(I, I^+, J; \mathcal{A})$, put $L = \bigcup_{j \in J} A_j$. Define a binary relation $\leq$ on the set L as follows. Let $a \in A_j, b \in A_k$. $a \leq b$ in L if one of the following conditions is satisfied:

(P1) $j = k \in J$ and $a \leq_{A_j} b$.

(P2) $j, k \in I$ and $j < k$.

(P3) $j = i_1^+ \in I^+, k = i_2^+ \in I^+$ and $i_2 < i_1$ in I.

(P4) $j \in I$ and $k \in I^+$.

Lemma 4. *$(L, \leq)$ is a lattice.*

Proof. Firstly, we prove that $(L, \leq)$ is a poset. Obviously, $\leq$ is reflexive. Next, we prove that $\leq$ is antisymmetric. To see this, let $a \in A_j, b \in A_k$ such that $a \leq b$ and $b \leq a$. We consider four cases:

- If $j = k \in J$, then by $(P1)$, $a \leq_{A_j} b$ and $b \leq_{A_j} a$. Since $(A_j, \leq_{A_j})$ is a poset, $a = b$.
- Suppose $j \neq k$ and $j, k \in I$. Then, since $a \leq b$ and $b \leq a$, $j < k$ and $k < j$, a contradiction. Thus, $j \neq k$ and $j, k \in I$ is impossible.
- By similar arguments as in the previous case, $j \neq k$, and $j, k \in I^+$ is impossible.
- Similarly, either $j \in I, k \in I^+$ or $k \in I, j \in I^+$ is impossible.

Next, we prove that $\leq$ is transitive. Let $a \in A_j, b \in A_k$, and $c \in A_s$ be such that $a \leq b$ and $b \leq c$. We consider four cases:

- $j = k = s \in J$. Then, by $(P1)$, $a \leq_{A_j} b$ and $b \leq_{A_j} c$. Since $(A_j, \leq_{A_j})$ is a poset, $a \leq_{A_j} c$. Thus, by $(P1)$, $a \leq c$.
- $j = k \neq s$. If $k, s \in I$ and $k < s$, then $j < s$, and so by $(P2)$, $a \leq c$. If $k = i_1^+, s = i_2^+ \in I^+$ such that $i_2 < i_1$ in I, then $j = i_1^+$, and so by $(P3)$, $a \leq c$. If $k \in I$ and $s \in I^+$, then $j \in I$, and so by $(P4)$, $a \leq c$.
- $j \neq k = s$. Then, by similar arguments as in the prior case, $a \leq c$.
- $j \neq k$ and $k \neq s$. If $j, k, s \in I$, then $j < k$ and $k < s$, and so $j < s$, which implies that $a \leq c$ by $(P2)$. If $j \in I$ and $s \in I^+$, then by $(P4)$, $a \leq c$. If $j, k, s \in I^+$ such that $j = i_1^+, k = i_2^+, s = i_3^+$, then $i_3 < i_2$ and $i_2 < i_1$ in I by $(P3)$. Since $(I, \leq)$ is a chain, $i_3 < i_2$, and so by $(P3)$, $a \leq c$.

We conclude $a \leq c$, whence $\leq$ is transitive.

Finally, we will prove that for all $a, b \in L$, $a \vee b$ and $a \wedge b$ exist in L. Let $a \in A_j, b \in A_k$. We consider three cases:

- If $a \leq b$, then $a \vee b = b$ and $a \wedge b = a$ in L.
- If $b \leq a$, then $a \vee b = a$ and $a \wedge b = b$ in L.
- If $a \parallel b$, then by the definition of $\leq$, $j = k$. If $j, k \in I$, then since $(A_j, \leq_{A_j})$ is a Brouwerian algebra, $a \vee^{A_j} b$ exists in A_j. Let $c \in A_s$ such that $a, b \leq c$. If $s = j$, then by $(P1)$, $a \leq_{A_j} c$ and $b \leq_{A_j} c$, and so $a \vee^{A_j} b \leq_{A_j} c$. Thus, by $(P1)$, $a \vee^{A_j} b \leq c$. If $s \neq j$, then since $a \leq c$, either $s \in I$ and $j < s$ or $s \in I^+$, which together with $a \vee^{A_j} b \in A_j$, derives that $a \vee^{A_j} b \leq c$. It follows that $a \vee b = a \vee^{A_j} b$ in L. Similarly, $a \wedge b = a \wedge^{A_j} b$ in L. If $j = k = i^+ \in I^+$, then $(A_{i^+}, \leq_{A_{i^+}})$ is either a lattice or a pre-lattice by (CE2). If $(A_{i^+}, \leq_{A_{i^+}})$ is a lattice or an upper pre-lattice and $a \wedge^{A_{i^+}} b$ exists, then by similar arguments as in the prior case, $a \vee b = a \vee^{A_{i^+}} b$ and $a \wedge b = a \wedge^{A_{i^+}} b$ in L. If $(A_{i^+}, \leq_{A_{i^+}})$ is an upper pre-lattice and $a \wedge^{A_{i^+}} b$ does not exist, then by similar arguments in the prior case, $a \vee b = a \vee^{A_{i^+}} b$ in L. By (CE3), there exists $t \in I$ such that $i \prec t$ in I. We claim that $t^+ = a \wedge b$ in L. Because t^+ is the greatest element of $(A_{t^+}, \leq_{A_{t^+}})$ by (CE2), $t^+ \leq a, b$ by $(P3)$. Let $c \in A_s$ such that $c \leq a, b$. Since $(A_{i^+}, \leq_{A_{i^+}})$ is an upper pre-lattice and $a \wedge^{A_{i^+}} b$ does not exist, $c \notin A_{i^+}$, and so by $(P3 - 4)$, either $s \in I$ or there exists $l \in I$ such that $s = l^+$ and $i < l$ in I, which implies that either $s \in I$ or $s = l^+$ such that $t \leq l$. It follows that $c \leq t^+$ by $(P3 - 4)$. Thus, $a \wedge b = t^+$ in L. □

We define a multiplication $\circ$ on L in the following ways: for $a \in A_j, b \in A_k$,

$$a \circ b = \begin{cases} a \wedge b & \text{if } j, k \in I, \\ a \vee b & \text{if } j, k \in I^+, \\ a & \text{if } j = i^+ \in I^+, k \in I, i < k \text{ or } j \in I, k = l^+ \in I^+, j \leq l, \\ b & \text{if } j = i^+ \in I^+, k \in I, i \geq k \text{ or } j \in I, k = l^+ \in I^+, j > l. \end{cases}$$

Lemma 5. $(L, \wedge, \vee, \circ, e)$ *is a conic lattice-ordered idempotent commutative monoid with identity* e.

Proof. It is clear that $a \circ a = a$ and $a \circ b = b \circ a$ for $a, b \in L$.

Let $a \in A_j$. If $j \in I$, then since e is the greatest of I, $j \leq e$, which together with e is the greatest element of A_e by $(CE1)$, derives that $a \leq e$ and $a \circ e = a$. If $j = i^+ \in I^+$, then $i < e$, so $a > e$ and $a \circ e = a$. Now, we will show that $\circ$ satisfies the associative law. Let $a \in A_j, b \in A_k, c \in A_s$. We consider the following cases:

- If $j, k, s \in I$, then $(a \circ b) \circ c = (a \wedge b) \circ c = a \wedge b \wedge c$ and $a \circ (b \circ c) = a \circ (b \wedge c) = a \wedge b \wedge c$, whence $a \circ (b \circ c) = (a \circ b) \circ c$.
- If $j, k \in I$ and $s = i^+ \in I^+$, then

$$(a \circ b) \circ c = (a \wedge b) \circ c = \begin{cases} a \wedge b & \text{if } j \wedge k \leq i, \\ c & \text{if } i < j \wedge k; \end{cases}$$

and

$$\begin{aligned} a \circ (b \circ c) &= \begin{cases} a \circ b = a \wedge b & \text{if } k \leq i, \\ a \circ c = a = a \wedge b & \text{if } j \leq i < k, \\ c & \text{if } i < j \wedge k; \end{cases} \\ &= \begin{cases} a \wedge b & \text{if } j \wedge k \leq i, \\ c & \text{if } i < j \wedge k. \end{cases} \end{aligned}$$

It follows that $a \circ (b \circ c) = (a \circ b) \circ c$.

- If $j \in I, k = i^+, s = l^+ \in I^+$, then

$$\begin{aligned} (a \circ b) \circ c &= \begin{cases} a \circ c = a & \text{if } j \leq i \wedge l, \\ b \circ c = b \vee c & \text{if } i < j, \\ a \circ c = c & \text{if } l < j \leq i; \end{cases} \\ &= \begin{cases} a & \text{if } j \leq i \wedge l, \\ b \vee c & \text{if } j > i \wedge l; \end{cases} \end{aligned}$$

and

$$a \circ (b \circ c) = a \circ (b \vee c) = \begin{cases} a & \text{if } j \leq i \wedge l, \\ b \vee c & \text{if } j > i \wedge l. \end{cases}$$

However, $a \circ (b \circ c) = (a \circ b) \circ c$.

- If $j, k, s \in I^+$, then $(a \circ b) \circ c = (a \vee b) \circ c = a \vee b \vee c$ and $a \circ (b \circ c) = a \circ (b \vee c) = a \vee b \vee c$, whence $a \circ (b \circ c) = (a \circ b) \circ c$.

Finally, we show that $\leq$ is compatible with $\circ$. Let $a, b \in L$ be such that $a \leq b$. We need only to prove that $a \circ c \leq b \circ c$ for every $c \in L$. Suppose that $a \in A_j, b \in A_k, c \in A_s$. We need to consider the following cases:

(1) If $j, k, s \in I$, then by the definition of $\circ$, $a \circ c = a \wedge c$ and $b \circ c = b \wedge c$. Since $a \leq b$, $a \circ c \leq b \circ c$.

(2) If $j, k \in I$ and $s = i^+ \in I^+$, then $a \leq b < c$ and $j \leq k$. The following subcases need be considered:

- If $i < j$, then $i < k$, and so by the definition of $\circ$, $a \circ c = c$ and $b \circ c = c$, whence $a \circ c \leq b \circ c$.
- If $j \leq i$, then by the definition of $\circ$, $a \circ c = a$ and $b \circ c \in \{b, c\}$. It follows that $a \circ c \leq b \circ c$.

(3) If $j, s \in I$ and $k \in I^+$, then by the definition of $\circ$, $a \circ c = a \wedge c \leq c < b$ and $b \circ c \in \{b, c\}$, whence $a \circ c \leq b \circ c$.

(4) If $j \in I$ and $k, s \in I^+$, then $a < b \leq b \vee c$, so by the definition of $\circ$, $a \circ c \in \{a, c\}$ and $b \circ c = b \vee c$, whence $a \circ c \leq b \circ c$.

(5) If $j = i^+, k = l^+ \in I^+$ and $s \in I$, then since $a \leq b, l \leq i$ in I by (P3). The following subcases need be considered:

- If $s \leq l$, then by the definition of $\circ$, $a \circ c = c$ and $b \circ c = c$, whence $a \circ c \leq b \circ c$.
- If $s > l$, then by the definition of $\circ$, $a \circ c \in \{a, c\}$ and $b \circ c = b$. It follows that $a \circ c \leq b \circ c$.

(6) If $j,k,s \in I^+$, then by the definition of $\circ$, $a \circ c = a \vee c$ and $b \circ c = b \vee c$, whence $a \circ c \leq b \circ c$. □

We may define a binary operation $\to$ on L in the following way: for $a,b \in L$ such that $a \in A_j, b \in A_k$,

$$a \to b = \begin{cases} j^+ & \text{if } j,k \in I \text{ and } a \leq b, \text{ or } j \in I, k = i^+ \in I^+ \text{ and } j \leq i, \\ b & \text{if } j,k \in I \text{ and } j > k, \text{ or } j \in I, k = i^+ \in I^+ \text{ and } j > i, \\ a \to^{A_j} b & \text{if } j = k \in I \text{ such that } a \parallel b \text{ or } a > b, \\ b & \text{if } j,k \in I^+ \text{ and } a \leq b, \text{ or } j = i^+ \in I^+, k \in I \text{ and } i \geq k, \\ i & \text{if } j = i^+, k \in I^+ \text{ and } a \nleq b, \text{ or } j = i^+ \in I^+, k \in I \text{ and } i < k. \end{cases}$$

We denote by $\mathbf{J} \otimes \mathcal{A}$ the above $(L, \wedge, \vee, \circ, \to, e)$.

Theorem 3. *$L = \mathbf{J} \otimes \mathcal{A}$ is a conic idempotent CRL.*

Proof. We need only to prove that for all $a,b \in L, a \to b = \max\{c : a \circ c \leq b\}$. Suppose that $a \in A_j, b \in A_k$. We need to consider the following cases:

Case 1 $j,k \in I$ and $a \leq b$, or $j \in I, k = i^+ \in I^+$ and $j \leq i$. We need only to check the following subcases:

(1) If $j,k \in I$ and $a \leq b$, then by the definition of $\circ$, $a \circ (a \to b) = a \circ j^+ = a \leq b$. Let $c \in A_s \subseteq L$ such that $a \circ c \leq b$. If $s \in I$, then by (P4), $c \leq j^+ = a \to b$. If $s = l^+ \in I^+$, then $b < c$ by (P4), and by the definition of $\circ$, $a \circ c \in \{a,c\}$, which, together with $a \circ c \leq b$, derives that $a \circ c = a$. Thus, $j \leq l$, whence $c \leq j^+ = a \to b$.

(2) If $j \in I, k = i^+ \in I^+$ and $j \leq i$, then by the definition of $\circ$ and (P4), $a \circ (a \to b) = a \circ j^+ = a \leq b$. Let $c \in A_s \subseteq L$ such that $a \circ c \leq b$. If $s \in I$, then by (P4), $c \leq j^+ = a \to b$. If $s = l^+ \in I^+$, then by the definition of $\circ$, $a \circ c \in \{a,c\}$. Assume that $a \circ c = c$. Then, by the definition of $\circ$, $l < j \leq i$, so $b < c = a \circ c$ by (P3), which is contrary to $a \circ c \leq b$. Thus, $a \circ c = a$, which implies that $j \leq l$, and so $c \leq j^+$ by (P1) and (P3).

Case 2 $j,k \in I$ and $j > k$, or $j \in I, k = i^+ \in I^+$ and $j > i$. We need only to check the following subcases:

(1) If $j,k \in I$ and $j > k$, then $a > b$ by (P2), and so by the definition of $\circ$, $a \circ (a \to b) = a \circ b = a \wedge b = b$. Let $c \in A_s \subseteq L$ such that $a \circ c \leq b$. Suppose that $s \in I^+$. Then, $c > b$ by (P4), and by the definition of $\circ$, $a \circ c \in \{a,c\}$, which implies that $a \circ c > b$, a contradiction. Suppose that $s \in I$ such that $s \geq j$. Then, $a \circ c = a \wedge c \in A_j$, which implies that $a \circ c > b$, a contradiction. Thus, $s \in I$ and $s < j$, whence $c = a \wedge c = a \circ c \leq b = a \to b$.

(2) If $j \in I, k = i^+ \in I^+$ and $j > i$, then by the definition of $\circ$, $a \circ (a \to b) = a \circ b = b$. Let $c \in A_s \subseteq L$ such that $a \circ c \leq b$. If $s \in I$, then $c \leq b = a \to b$ by (P4). If $s = l^+ \in I^+$ such that $l \geq j$, then $l > i$, and so $c \leq b = a \to b$ by (P3). If $s = l^+ \in I^+$ such that $l < j$, then by the definition of $\circ$, $c = a \circ c \leq b = a \to b$.

Case 3 $j = k \in I$ such that $a \parallel b$ or $a > b$. Then, by the definition of $\circ$ and (CE1), $a \circ (a \to b) = a \circ (a \to^{A_j} b) = a \wedge (a \to^{A_j} b) = a \wedge^{A_j} (a \to^{A_j} b) \leq_{A_j} b$, which implies that $a \circ (a \to b) \leq b$. Let $c \in A_s \subseteq L$ such that $a \circ c \leq b$. Suppose that $s \in I^+$ or $s \in I$ such that $s > j$. Then, $c > b$ by (P2,4), and by the definition of $\circ$, $a \circ c \in \{a,c\}$, which implies that $a \circ c \nleq b$, a contradiction. If $s \in I$ such that $s < j$, then $c \leq a \to^{A_j} b = a \to b$ by (P2). If $s \in I$ such that $s = j$, then by the definition of $\circ$, $a \wedge^{A_j} c = a \wedge c = a \circ c \leq b$, which implies that $a \wedge^{A_j} c \leq_{A_j} b$, so $c \leq_{A_j} a \to^{A_j} b$ by (CE1). Thus, $c \leq a \to^{A_j} b = a \to b$.

Case 4 $j,k \in I^+$ and $a \leq b$, or $j = i^+ \in I^+, k \in I$ and $i \geq k$. We need only to check the following subcases:

(1) If $j,k \in I^+$ and $a \leq b$, then by the definition of $\circ$, $a \circ (a \to b) = a \circ b = a \vee b = b$. Let $c \in A_s \subseteq L$ such that $a \circ c \leq b$. If $s \in I$, then by (P4), $c \leq b$. If $s \in I^+$, then by the definition of $\circ$, $c \leq a \vee c = a \circ c \leq b = a \to b$.

(2) If $j = i^+ \in I^+, k \in I$ and $i \geq k$, then by the definition of $\circ$, $a \circ (a \to b) = a \circ b = b$. Let $c \in A_s \subseteq L$ such that $a \circ c \leq b$. Suppose that $s \in I^+$. Then, by the definition of $\circ$,

$a \circ c = a \vee c > b$, a contradiction. If $s \in I$, then by the definition of $\circ$, $a \circ c \in \{a, c\}$, which together with $a > b$, derives that $c = a \circ c \leq b = a \to b$.

Case 5 $j = i^+, k \in I^+$ and $a \not\leq b$, or $j = i^+ \in I^+, k \in I$ and $i < k$. We need only to check the following subcases:

(1) If $j = i^+, k \in I^+$ and $a \not\leq b$, then by the definition of $\circ$ and (P4), $a \circ (a \to b) = a \circ i = i \leq b$. Let $c \in A_s \subseteq L$ such that $a \circ c \leq b$. Suppose that $s \in I^+$. Then, $a \circ c = a \vee c \not\leq b$, a contradiction. If $s \in I$, then by the definition of $\circ$, $a \circ c \in \{a, c\}$, which together with $a \not\leq b$, derives that $c = a \circ c \leq b$.

(2) If $j = i^+ \in I^+, k \in I$ and $i < k$, then by the definition of $\circ$ and (P2), $a \circ (a \to b) = a \circ i = i \leq b$. Let $c \in A_s \subseteq L$ such that $a \circ c \leq b$. Suppose that $s \in I^+$. Then, by the definition of $\circ$, $a \circ c = a \vee c > b$, a contradiction. If $s \in I$, then by the definition of $\circ$, $a \circ c \in \{a, c\}$, which together with $a > b$, derives that $a \circ c = c$. Thus, $s \leq i$, whence $c \leq i$. □

Next we shall prove that any conic idempotent CRL is isomorphic to some $\mathbf{J} \otimes \mathcal{A}$. Suppose that $\mathbf{L} = (L, \wedge, \vee, \cdot, \to, e)$ is a conic idempotent CRL. Let $L^* = \{j \in L : (\exists a \in L) j = a^*\}$, $I = \{i \in L^* : i \leq e\} = L^{*-}$ and $I^* = \{i^* : i \in I \setminus \{e\}\} = L^{*+}$. Let $\mathcal{Y} = \{(L_j, \leq) : j \in L^*\}$. By Proposition 2, for all $i \in I \setminus \{e\}$, $i^* > e$, so $I^* \cap I = \emptyset$. If $i, l \in I$ such that $i \neq l$, then there exists $a, b \in L$ such that $a^* = i$ and $b^* = l$, so $i^{**} = a^{***} = a^* = i \neq l = b^* = b^{***} = l^{**}$. Thus, $i^* \neq l^*$.

Lemma 6. $(I, I^*, L^*; \mathcal{Y})$ is a CE-system.

Proof. By Theorem 1(1–5,7), $(I, I^*, L^*; \mathcal{Y})$ is a CE-system. □

Theorem 4. $\mathbf{L}$ is equal to $\mathbf{L}^* \otimes \mathcal{Y}$.

Proof. For convenience, we denote by $\leq_1$ the imposed ordering on $L^* \otimes \mathcal{Y}$. We need only to prove that for all $a, b \in L$, $\leq = \leq_1$ and $a \cdot b = a \circ b$.

We now prove $\leq = \leq_1$. Let $a, b \in L$. Assume that $a \leq b$. We need to consider three cases:

(1) If $a \leq e, b \leq e$, then $a^{**}, b^{**} \in I$ by Lemma 3(4), and by Theorem 1(6), $a^{**} \leq b^{**}$, which, together with $a \in L_{a^{**}}$ and $b \in L_{b^{**}}$, derives that $a \leq_1 b$ by (P1 − 2).

(2) If $a \geq e, b \geq e$, then $a^*, b^* \in I$, which, together with $a \in L_{a^{**}}$ and $b \in L_{b^{**}}$, derives that $a^* \geq b^*$ by Theorem 1(6). Thus, by (P3), $a \leq_1 b$.

(3) If $a \leq e$ and $b > e$, then by Lemma 3(4), $a^{**} \leq e$ and $b^{**} > e$, so $a^{**} \in I$ and $b^{**} \in I^*$, whence by (P4), $a \leq_1 b$.

Thus, $\leq \subseteq \leq_1$.

Suppose that $a \leq_1 b$. We need to consider four cases:
(1) If $a^{**} = b^{**} \in I$, then $a \leq b$ by (P1).
(2) If $a^{**}, b^{**} \in I$ such that $a^{**} < b^{**}$, then by Theorem 1(6), $a \leq b$.
(3) If $a^{**}, b^{**} \in I^*$ such that $a^* > b^*$, then by Theorem 1(6), $a \leq b$.
(4) If $a^{**} \in I$ and $b^{**} \in I^*$, then by Lemma 3(4), $a \leq e$ and $b > e$, so $a \leq b$.
Thus, $\leq_1 \subseteq \leq$, whence $\leq_1 = \leq$

It remains to be verified that $a \cdot b = a \circ b$ for all $a, b \in L$. For this, we need to consider three cases:

(1) If $a \leq e, b \leq e$, then by Lemma 1(3), $a \cdot b = a \wedge b$. On the other hand, by the definition of $\circ$ and $\leq = \leq_1$, $a \circ b = a \wedge b$, whence $a \cdot b = a \circ b$.

(2) If $a > e, b > e$, then by similar arguments as in (1), $a \cdot b = a \circ b$.

(3) $a > e$ and $b \leq e$.

- If $b \leq a^*$, then $a^*, b^{**} \in I$ by Lemma 3(4) and $b^{**} \leq a^{***} = a^*$ by Lemma 2(3), which together with $a \in L_{(a^*)^*}$ and $b \in L_{b^{**}}$ derives $a \circ b = b$ by the definition of $\circ$. On the other hand, $a \cdot b = a \cdot a^* \cdot b = a^* \cdot b = b$ by Proposition 2(3). Hence, $a \cdot b = b = a \circ b$.

- If $b > a^*$, then $a^*, b^{**} \in I$ by Lemma 3(4), and $b^{**} \geq b > a^{***} = a^*$ by Theorem 1(4), which, together with $a \in L_{(a^*)^*}$ and $b \in L_{b^{**}}$, derives $a \circ b = a$ by the definition of $\circ$. Suppose that $a \cdot b = b$. Then, $a^* <_n b <_n a$, so by Proposition 2(4), $b > e$, a contradiction. Thus, $a \cdot b = a$ by Lemma 1(4,5). Hence, $a \cdot b = a = a \circ b$. □

By Theorem 4, we have the following result, which generalizes ([20] Theorem 20).

Theorem 5. *Let* $\mathbf{L} = (L, \wedge, \vee, \cdot, \rightarrow, e)$ *be a CRL. The following conditions are equivalent:*

(I) $\mathbf{L}$ *is a subdirectly irreducible idempotent semiconic CRL.*

(II) *There exists a CE-system* $(I, I^+, J; \mathcal{A})$ *such that*

(1) A_e *is a nontrivial subdirectly irreducible Brouwerian algebra or* $A_e = \{e\}$, *and there exists* $i \in I$ *such that* $i \prec e$ *in* I;

(2) $\mathbf{L} \cong J \otimes \mathcal{A}$.

Proof. Let $\mathbf{L}$ be a subdirectly irreducible semiconic idempotent CRL. Then, since semiconic idempotent CRL is the variety generated by conic idempotent CRLs, $\mathbf{L}$ is conic. By Theorem 4, $\mathbf{L} \cong \mathbf{L}^* \otimes \mathcal{Y}$, where $(I, I^*, L^*; \mathcal{Y})$ is a CE-system. Because $\mathbf{L}$ is a subdirectly irreducible CRL, the set $\{a \in L : a < e\}$ has a greatest element. Let $i = \max\{a \in L : a < e\}$. If $i \in L_e$, then $i = \max\{a \in L_e : a < e\}$, so by Theorem 1(4), $\mathbf{L}_e$ is a nontrivial subdirectly irreducible Brouwerian algebra. If $i \notin L_e$, then since $L_e \subseteq L^-$, $L_e = \{e\}$ and $i \prec e$, so $i^{**} < e$, which implies that $i^{**} \leq i$. On the other hand, by Proposition 2(1), $ii^* = i \leq e$, so $i \leq i^* \rightarrow e = i^{**}$. Thus, $i = i^{**}$, whence $i \in I$ by Theorem 1(1).

Conversely, let $(I, I^+, J; \mathcal{A})$ be a CE-system such that (1) and (2). Then, by Theorem 3, $\mathbf{L}$ is a conic idempotent CRL. If A_e is a nontrivial subdirectly irreducible Brouwerian algebra, then $\max\{a \in A_e : a < e\}$ exists, and so $\max\{a \in A_e : a < e\} = \max\{a \in L : a < e\}$, which implies that $\mathbf{L}$ is a subdirectly irreducible semiconic idempotent CRL. If $A_e = \{e\}$ and there exists $i \in I$ such that $i \prec e$, then by $(P1, 2)$, $\max\{a \in L : a < e\} = i$, which implies that $\mathbf{L}$ is a subdirectly irreducible semiconic idempotent CRL. □

5. The Amalgamation Property

In this section, we will use the structure theorem of conic idempotent CRLs to give some new result about the amalgamation property of the variety of semiconic idempotent CRLs, which generalizes the main results of [10].

Let $\mathbf{K}$ be a class of algebras. A *span* is a pair of embeddings $\langle i_1 : \mathbf{A} \hookrightarrow \mathbf{B}, i_2 : \mathbf{A} \hookrightarrow \mathbf{C} \rangle$ between algebras $\mathbf{A}, \mathbf{B}, \mathbf{C} \in \mathbf{K}$. The class $\mathbf{K}$ is said to have the *amalgamation property* if for every span of $\mathbf{K}$, there exists an *amalgam* $\mathbf{D} \in \mathbf{K}$ and embeddings $j_1 : \mathbf{B} \hookrightarrow \mathbf{D}$ and $j_2 : \mathbf{C} \hookrightarrow \mathbf{D}$ such that $j_1 \circ i_1 = j_2 \circ i_2$.

Example 1. *Let* $A = \{a_2, a_1, e, a_{-1}, a_{-2}\}$. *We define an order relation* $\leq_A$ *on A by* $a_{-2} <_A a_{-1} <_A e <_A a_1 <_A a_2$, *see Figure 1a. We can define a multiplication operation on A by the following: for all* $i, j \in \{1, 2, -1, -2\}$,

$$a_i a_j = a_j a_i = \begin{cases} a_i & \text{if } |j| < |i|, \\ a_i & \text{if } i = j, \\ a_i & \text{if } i = -j < 0; \end{cases}$$

and $ae = ea = a$ *for all* $a \in A$. *Let* $B = \{x_{-2}, x_{-1}, e, x_1, y_2, z_2, x_2\}$. *We define an order relation* $\leq_B$ *on B by* $x_{-2} <_B x_{-1} <_B e <_B x_1 <_B y_2, z_2 <_B x_2$, *see Figure 1b. We can define a multiplication operation on B by for all* $i, j \in \{1, 2, -1, -2\}$ *and* $b \in \{y, z\}$,

$$x_i x_j = x_j x_i = \begin{cases} x_i & \text{if } |j| < |i|, \\ x_i & \text{if } i = j, \\ x_i & \text{if } i = -j < 0; \end{cases}$$

$$x_i b_2 = b_2 x_i = \begin{cases} b_2 & \text{if } |i| < 2, \\ x_i & \text{if } |i| = 2; \end{cases}$$

$y_2 z_2 = z_2 y_2 = x_2$ and $ce = ec = c$ for all $c \in B$. Let $C = \{m_{-3}, m_{-2}, m_{-1}, e, m_1, m_2, n_3, k_3, m_3\}$. We define an order relation $\leq_C$ on C by $m_{-3} <_C m_{-2} <_C m_{-1} <_C e <_C m_1 <_C m_2 <_C n_3, k_3 <_C m_3$, see Figure 1c. We can define a multiplication operation on C by for all $i, j \in \{1, 2, 3, -1, -2, -3\}$ and $b \in \{n, k\}$,

$$m_i m_j = m_j m_i = \begin{cases} m_i & \text{if } |j| < |i|, \\ m_i & \text{if } i = j, \\ m_i & \text{if } i = -j < 0; \end{cases}$$

$$m_i b_3 = b_3 m_i = \begin{cases} b_3 & \text{if } |i| < 3, \\ m_i & \text{if } |i| = 3; \end{cases}$$

$n_3 k_3 = k_3 n_3 = m_3$ and $ce = ec = c$ for all $c \in C$. We define a division operation on P by $a \to b = \max\{p \in P \mid ap \leq b\}$ for all $a, b \in P$, where $P \in \{A, B, C\}$. It is easy to see that A, B and C are subdirectly irreducible semiconic idempotent CRLs. We define two maps as follows. $\varphi_1 : A \longrightarrow B; e \mapsto e$ and $a_i \mapsto x_i$ for $i \in \{-2, -1, 1, 2\}$. $\varphi_2 : A \longrightarrow C; e \mapsto e, a_i \mapsto m_i$ for $i \in \{-1, 1\}; a_2 \mapsto m_3$ and $a_{-2} \mapsto m_{-3}$. It is clear that φ_1 and φ_2 are embeddings of A into B, C, respectively. We claim that there are no amalgams in $\mathbf{K}$ where $\mathbf{K}$ is the class of all conic idempotent CRLs. Suppose that there exists an amalgam $D \in \mathbf{K}$ and embeddings $\psi_1 : B \hookrightarrow D$ and $\psi_2 : C \hookrightarrow D$ such that $\psi_1 \varphi_1 = \psi_2 \varphi_2$. Then, $\psi_1(x_1) = \psi_1 \varphi_1(a_1) = \psi_2 \varphi_2(a_1) = \psi_2(m_1)$ and $\psi_1(x_2) = \psi_1 \varphi_1(a_2) = \psi_2 \varphi_2(a_2) = \psi_2(m_3)$. Hence, by Theorem 2, $\psi_2(m_1) = \psi_1(x_1) \prec \psi_1(x_2) = \psi_2(m_3)$ in D^*. But $\psi_2(m_1) < \psi_2(m_2) < \psi_2(m_3)$ in D^*. It is a contradiction. We conclude that the span $\langle \varphi_1 : A \longrightarrow B, \varphi_2 : A \longrightarrow C \rangle$ has no amalgam in $\mathbf{K}$.

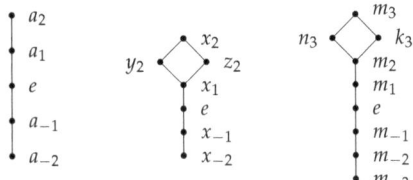

(**a**) $(A, \leq_A)$ (**b**) $(B, \leq_B)$ (**c**) $(C, \leq_C)$

Figure 1. We define an order relation $\leq_A$ on A by $a_{-2} <_A a_{-1} <_A e <_A a_1 <_A a_2$, in (**a**), an order relation $\leq_B$ on B by $x_{-2} <_B x_{-1} <_B e <_B x_1 <_B y_2, z_2 <_B x_2$, in (**b**) and order relation $\leq_C$ on C by $m_{-3} <_C m_{-2} <_C m_{-1} <_C e <_C m_1 <_C m_2 <_C n_3, k_3 <_C m_3$ in (**c**).

An immediate consequence of Example 1 is the following.

Proposition 4. *The class of all conic idempotent CRLs and the class of subdirectly irreducible semiconic idempotent CRLs do not have the amalgamation property.*

Proof. By Example 1, there exists a span of (subdirectly irreducible) conic idempotent CRLs such that it has no amalgam in the class of all (subdirectly irreducible) conic idempotent CRLs. It follows that the class of all conic idempotent CRLs and the class of subdirectly irreducible semiconic idempotent CRLs do not have the amalgamation property. □

We introduce the following concept.

Definition 2. *The variety of strongly semiconic idempotent* CRLs *consists of the semiconic idempotent* CRLs *that satisfy* $(x \wedge y)^* = x^* \vee y^*$.

A consequence of Theorem 1 is the following.

Proposition 5. *A conic idempotent* CRL **L** *is a strongly semiconic idempotent* CRL *if and only if* L_i *is a lattice for all* $i \in L^*$.

Proof. Let **L** be a conic idempotent CRL. Suppose that **L** is a strongly semiconic idempotent CRL. Then, **L** satisfies $(x \wedge y)^* = x^* \vee y^*$. Hence, by Theorem 1(4,8), L_i is a sublattice of CRL for all $i \in L^*$, and so L_i is a lattice for all $i \in L^*$. Conversely, suppose that L_i is a lattice for all $i \in L^*$. Let $a, b \in L$. If $a < b$, then by Lemma 2(3), $b^* \leq a^*$, so $(a \wedge b)^* = a^* = a^* \vee b^*$. Similarly, if $b < a$, then $(a \wedge b)^* = a^* \vee b^*$. If $a \parallel b$, then by Lemma 3(1), $a^* = b^*$, so $a^{**} = b^{**}$. Hence, there exists $i \in L^*$ such that $a, b \in L_i$. Since L_i is a lattice, by Theorem 1(4,5), L_i is a sublattice of L. Hence, $a \wedge b \in L_i$. Thus, $(a \wedge b)^* = (a \wedge b)^{***} = i^* = i^* \vee i^* = a^{***} \vee b^{***} = a^* \vee b^*$. Consequently, **L** satisfies $(x \wedge y)^* = x^* \vee y^*$. It follows that **L** is a strongly semiconic idempotent CRL. □

Let **L** be a CRL. A lattice filter F of **L** is called *normal* if it contains e and it is closed under multiplication. A normal filter F of **L** is said to be *prime* if it is prime in the usual lattice theoretic sense; that is, whenever $x \vee y \in F$, then $x \in F$ or $y \in F$. Let F and Θ be a normal filter and a congruence of **L** respectively. It is well known that $\Theta_F = \{(x, y) \in L^2 \mid (x \to y) \wedge (y \to x) \in F\}$ is a congruence of **L** and the upper set $F_\Theta = \uparrow [e]_\Theta$ of the equivalence class $[e]_\Theta$ is a normal filter. Moreover, we have the following.

Lemma 7 ([8]). *The lattice $\mathcal{NF}(L)$ of normal filters of a* CRL **L** *is isomorphic to its congruence lattice* Con(**L**). *The isomorphism is given by the mutually inverse maps* $F \mapsto \Theta_F$ *and* $\Theta \mapsto \uparrow [e]_\Theta$.

Lemma 8 ([8]). *Let **L** be a* CRL, *and let F be a normal filter of* **L**. *Then,* $[e]_{\Theta_F} = \{x \mid x \wedge (x \to e) \wedge e \in F\} = \{x \mid \exists a \in F^-, a \leq x \leq a \to e\}$.

In what follows, if F is a normal filter of **L**, **L**/F shall always denote the quotient algebra **L**/Θ_F. Given an element $x \in L$, we write $[x]_F$ or $[x]$ if there is no confusion for the equivalence class of x in L/F.

Lemma 9. *Let **L** be a semiconic* CRL, *and let F be a normal filter of* **L**. *Then, the following statements are equivalent:*

(1) F *is prime.*

(2) *For all* $a, b \in L^-$, *whenever* $a \vee b \in F$, *then* $a \in F$ *or* $b \in F$.

(3) **L**/F *is a finitely subdirectly irreducible conic* CRL.

Proof. (1) $\Rightarrow$ (2) By specialization.

(2) $\Rightarrow$ (3) Suppose that (2) holds, and let $a \in L$. Since **L** is semiconic, $(a \wedge e) \vee (a \to e \wedge e) = e \in F$. It follows that either $a \wedge e \in F$ or $a \to e \wedge e \in F$. If $a \wedge e \in F$, then by Lemma 8, $[a \wedge e] = [e] \Longrightarrow [a] \wedge [e] = [e] \Longrightarrow [a] \geq [e]$. If $a \to e \wedge e \in F$, then $[a \to e \wedge e] = [e] \Longrightarrow [a] \to [e] \wedge [e] = [e] \Longrightarrow [a] \to [e] \geq [e] \Longrightarrow [a] \leq [e]$. Thus, **L**/$F$ is a conic CRL. Let $a, b \in L$ such that $[a] \vee [b] = [e]$. Then, since **L** is conic, $([a] \vee [b]) \wedge [e] = [e] \Longrightarrow ([a] \wedge [e]) \vee ([b] \wedge [e]) = [e] \Longrightarrow [(a \wedge e) \vee (b \wedge e)] = [e]$, which implies that $(a \wedge e) \vee (b \wedge e) \in F$. Hence, $a \wedge e \in F$ or $b \wedge e \in F$, which derives that $[a \wedge e] = [e]$ or $[b \wedge e] = [e]$. Since $[a \vee b] = [e], [a] \leq [e]$ and $[b] \leq [e]$. It follows that $[a] = [a] \wedge [e] = [a \wedge e] = [e]$ or $[b] = [b] \wedge [e] = [b \wedge e] = [e]$. Consequently, **L**/$F$ is a finitely subdirectly irreducible conic CRL.

(3) $\Rightarrow$ (1) Assume that (3) holds, and let $a, b \in L$ such that $a \vee b \in F$. Then, $(a \vee b) \wedge e = (a \wedge e) \vee (b \wedge e) \in F$. It follows that $[(a \wedge e) \vee (b \wedge e)] = [e] \Longrightarrow [a \wedge e] \vee [b \wedge e] = $

$[e] \implies [a \wedge e] = [e]$ or $[b \wedge e] = [e] \implies a \wedge e \in F$ or $b \wedge e \in F \implies a \in F$ or $b \in F$. Thus, F is prime. □

Lemma 10 ([8]). *Let L be a residuated lattice and $\{a_i \mid 1 \leq i \leq n\}$, $\{b_j \mid 1 \leq j \leq m\} \subseteq L^-$ be finite subsets of the negative cone of L with the property that $a_i \vee b_j = e$ for any i and j. Then, $(\prod_{i=1}^n a_i) \vee (\prod_{j=1}^m b_j) = e$.*

Lemma 11 ([26]). *Let U be a subclass of variety V satisfying the following conditions:*

(i) *Every subdirectly irreducible member of V is in U.*

(ii) *U is closed under isomorphisms and subalgebras.*

(iii) *For any algebra $B \in V$ and subalgebra A of B, if $\Theta \in Con(A)$ and $A/\Theta \in U$, then there exists $\Phi \in Con(B)$ such that $\Phi \cap A^2 = \Theta$ and $B/\Phi \in U$.*

(iv) *Every span in U has an amalgam in V.*

Then, V has the amalgamation property.

We have the following result, which generalizes [26] (Theorem 49) in the commutative case.

Theorem 6. *Let V be a variety of semiconic CRLs, and suppose that the class of finitely subdirectly irreducible conic CRLs in V has the amalgamation property. Then, V has the amalgamation property.*

Proof. It is well known that every subdirectly irreducible semiconic CRL is a finitely subdirectly irreducible conic CRL. It is clear that the class of finitely subdirectly irreducible conic CRLs is closed under isomorphisms and subalgebras. By Lemma 11, we need only to prove that for any $B \in V$, any subalgebra A of B, and $P \in \mathcal{NF}(A)$ such that A/P is a finitely subdirectly irreducible conic CRL, there is $Q \in \mathcal{NF}(B)$ such that $Q \cap A = P$ and B/Q is a finitely subdirectly irreducible conic CRL. Since V has the congruence extension property, there is a normal filter F of B such that $P = F \cap A$. Let $\mathcal{X}$ denote the poset under set-inclusion of all set-inclusions of all normal filters of B whose intersection with A is P. Since $F \in \mathcal{X}$, $\mathcal{X} \neq \emptyset$. By Zorn's lemma, we have element Q. Next, we shall show that Q is a prime normal filter of B. Suppose otherwise, and let $x, y \in B^-$ be such that $x \vee y \in Q$ but $x \notin Q$ and $y \notin Q$. Let Q_x and Q_y be the normal filters of B generated by $Q \cup \{x\}$ and $Q \cup \{y\}$, respectively. Then, by the maximality of Q, P is a proper subset of the normal filters $Q_x \cap A$ and $Q_y \cap A$ of A, and so there exist elements $c, d \in A \setminus P$, $q, r \in Q^-$ and $n, m \in \mathbb{Z}^+$ such that $qx^n \leq c \leq e$, and $ry^m \leq d \leq e$. Hence, by Lemma 8, $[q]_Q = [r]_Q = [e]_Q$ and $x \vee y \in Q \cap B^- \implies [x \vee y]_Q = [e]_Q$. Thus, by Lemma 10, $[e]_Q = [x^n]_Q \vee [y^m]_Q = [q]_Q[x^n]_Q \vee [r]_Q[y^m]_Q = [qx^n]_Q \vee [ry^m]_Q = [qx^n \vee ry^m]_Q \leq [c \vee d]_Q \leq [e]_Q$. It follows that $[c \vee d]_Q = [e]_Q$. Since $P = Q \cap A$, the map $\varphi : A/P \to B/Q$ is an embedding, which together with $c \vee d \in A$ derives that $[c]_P \vee [d]_P = [c \vee d]_P = [e]_P$. Because A/P is a finitely subdirectly irreducible conic CRL, $[c]_P = [e]_P$ or $[d]_P = [e]_P$. Then, by Lemma 8, $c \in P$, or $d \in P$. But $c, d \notin P$, which is a contradiction. Thus, Q is a prime normal filter of B, and by Lemma 9, B/Q is a finitely subdirectly irreducible conic CRL. The proof of the theorem is complete. □

Lemma 12 ([10]). *The class of totally ordered Sugihara monoids has the amalgamation property.*

The following result is essentially due to Maksimova (see [27] Chapter 6).

Lemma 13. *(Maksimova) The variety of all Brouwerian algebras has the amalgamation property and the class of finitely subdirectly irreducible Brouwerian algebras has the amalgamation property.*

Theorem 7. *The class of finitely subdirectly irreducible strongly conic idempotent CRLs has the amalgamation property.*

Proof. Let $\langle i_1 : \mathbf{A} \hookrightarrow \mathbf{B}, i_2 : \mathbf{A} \hookrightarrow \mathbf{C}\rangle$ be a span of finitely subdirectly irreducible strongly conic idempotent CRLs, assuming, without loss of generality, that i_1 and i_2 are inclusion maps and that $B \cap C = A$. Then, using Theorem 1(11), we also have inclusions between their skeletons $\mathbf{A}^* \hookrightarrow \mathbf{B}^*$ and $\mathbf{A}^* \hookrightarrow \mathbf{C}^*$. Since by Theorem 1(11), these skeletons are totally ordered odd Sugihara monoids, Lemma 12 yields an amalgam J for this span that is also a totally ordered odd Sugihara monoid. Moreover, we may assume that $J = B^* \cup C^*$. Let $J^- = \{j \in J \mid j \leq e\}$ and $J^+ = \{j \in J \mid j > e\}$.

Consider $i \in A^*$. Recalling that $A_i = \{x \in A \mid x^{**} = i\}$, clearly $A_i \subseteq B_i = \{x \in B \mid x^{**} = i\}$ and $A_i \subseteq C_i = \{x \in C \mid x^{**} = i\}$. If $i = e$, then by Theorem 1(10), $\mathbf{A}_e$, $\mathbf{B}_e$ and $\mathbf{C}_e$ are finitely subdirectly irreducible Brouwerian algebras, and by Theorem 2, $\mathbf{A}_e$ is a subalgebra of $\mathbf{B}_e$ and $\mathbf{C}_e$. Hence, by Lemma 13, there exists a finitely subdirectly irreducible Brouwerian algebra $\mathbf{D}_e$ as an amalgam with $D_e = B_e \cup C_e$. If $i < e$, then by Lemma 13, there exists a Brouwerian algebra $\mathbf{D}_i$ as an amalgam with $D_i = B_i \cup C_i$. If $i > e$, then by Proposition 5, each of $\mathbf{B}_i$ and $\mathbf{C}_i$ is a lattice. It is well known that the class of lattices has the amalgamation property. It follows that there exists a lattice $\mathbf{D}_i$ as an amalgam with $D_i = B_i \cup C_i$. Since i is the greatest element of A_i, B_i and C_i, it is also the greatest element of D_i. Now, for all $j \in B^* \setminus A^*$ and $k \in C^* \setminus A^*$, let $D_j = B_j$ and $D_k = C_k$. Let $\mathcal{X} = \{(D_j, \leq_{D_j}) \mid j \in J\}$. By construction, $(J^-, J^+, J; \mathcal{X})$ is a CE-system. Thus, $\mathbf{D} = \mathbf{J} \otimes \mathcal{X}$ is a conic idempotent CRL. Since $\mathbf{D}_e$ is a finitely subdirectly irreducible Brouwerian algebra, $\mathbf{D} = \mathbf{J} \otimes \mathcal{X}$ is a finitely subdirectly irreducible conic idempotent CRL. By Proposition 5, $\mathbf{D} = \mathbf{J} \otimes \mathcal{X}$ is a strongly finitely subdirectly irreducible conic idempotent CRL. To show that $\mathbf{D}$ is an amalgam of the original span, it suffices to check that $\mathbf{B}$ and $\mathbf{C}$ are subalgebras of $\mathbf{D}$. Consider $x, y \in B$ with $x \in B_i, y \in B_j$. Then, $i, j \in J$. If $i < j$ in $B^* \subseteq J$, then $x \leq_B y$ and $x \leq_D y$, so $x \vee^D y = y = x \vee^B y$ and $x \wedge^D y = x = x \wedge^B y$. If $i = j \in B^{*+} \subseteq J^+$, then since $\mathbf{D}_i$ is a lattice and $\mathbf{B}_i$ is a sublattice of $\mathbf{D}_i$, $x \vee^D y = x \vee^{D_i} y = x \vee^{B_i} y = x \vee^B y$ and $x \wedge^D y = x \wedge^{D_i} y = x \wedge^{B_i} y = x \wedge^B y \in B$. If $i = j \in B^{*-} \subseteq J^-$, then since $\mathbf{D}_i$ is a Brouwerian algebra and $\mathbf{B}_i$ is a subalgebra of $\mathbf{D}_i$, $x \vee^D y = x \vee^{D_i} y = x \vee^{B_i} y = x \vee^B y$ and $x \wedge^D y = x \wedge^{D_i} y = x \wedge^{B_i} y = x \wedge^B y$. Thus, $\mathbf{B}$ is a sublattice of $\mathbf{D}$. By the definition of $\mathbf{D}$, we have

$$x \circ^B y = \begin{cases} x \wedge^B y & \text{if } i, j \in B^{*-} \subseteq J^-, \\ x \vee^B y & \text{if } i, j \in B^{*+} \subseteq J^+, \\ x & \text{if } i \in B^{*+} \subseteq J^+, j \in B^{*-} \subseteq J^-, i^* <_{B^*} j \text{ or } i \in B^{*-} \subseteq J^-, j \in B^{*+} \subseteq J^+, i \leq_{B^*} j^*, \\ y & \text{if } i \in B^{*+} \subseteq J^+, j \in B^{*-} \subseteq J^-, i^* \geq_{B^*} j \text{ or } i \in B^{*-} \subseteq J^-, j \in B^{*+} \subseteq J^+, i >_{B^*} j^*. \end{cases}$$

and

$$x \circ^D y = \begin{cases} x \wedge^D y & \text{if } i, j \in J^-, \\ x \vee^D y & \text{if } i, j \in J^+, \\ x & \text{if } i \in J^+, j \in J^-, i^* <_J j \text{ or } i \in J^-, j \in J^+, i \leq_J j^*, \\ y & \text{if } i \in J^+, j \in J^-, i^* \geq_J j \text{ or } i \in J^-, j \in J^+, i >_J j^*. \end{cases}$$

Thus, $x \circ^D y = x \circ^B y$.

By similar arguments, we have $x \to^D y = x \to^B y$.

The proof that $\mathbf{C}$ is a subalgebra of $\mathbf{D}$ is symmetrical. □

Since every variety of commutative residuated lattices has the congruence extension property, by Theorem 6, we have the following result, which generalizes [10] (Theorem 5.6).

Theorem 8. *The variety of strongly semiconic idempotent CRLs has the amalgamation property.*

Funding: This research was funded by the NSF of China (grant number 11571158), and the NSF of Fujian Province (grant number 2020J01799, 2022J02046).

Data Availability Statement: No new data were created or analyzed in this study. Data sharing is not applicable to this article.

Acknowledgments: The author is extremely grateful to the referees for their careful reading and valuable suggestions which lead to a substantial improvement of this paper. Supported by the Institute of Meteorological Big Data-Digital Fujian and Fujian Key Laboratory of Data Science and Statistics.

Conflicts of Interest: The author declares no conflicts of interest.

References

1. Chen, W. On semiconic idempotent commutative residuated lattices. *Algebra Universalis* **2020**, *81*, 36. [CrossRef]
2. Chen, W.; Chen, Y. Variety generated by conical residuated lattice-ordered idempotent monoids. *Semigroup Forum* **2019**, *98*, 431–455. [CrossRef]
3. Galatos, N.; Olson, J.; Raftery, J.G. Irreducible residuated semilattices and finitely based varieties. *Rep. Math. Log.* **2008**, *43*, 85–108.
4. Hsieh, A.; Raftery, J.G. Semiconic idempotent residuated structures. *Algebra Universalis* **2009**, *61*, 413–430. [CrossRef]
5. Ward, M.; Dilworth, R.P. Residuated Lattices. *Trans. Am. Math. Soc.* **1939**, *45*, 335–354. [CrossRef]
6. Galatos, N.; Jipsen, P.; Kowalski, T.; Ono, H. *Residuated Lattices: An Algebraic Glimpse at Substructural Logics*; Studies in Logics and the Foundations of Mathematics; Elsevier: Amsterdam, The Netherlands, 2007.
7. Hart, J.B.; Rafter, L.; Tsinakis, C. The structure of commutative residuated latttices. *Int. J. Algebra Comput.* **2002**, *12*, 509–524. [CrossRef]
8. Blount, K.; Tsinakis, C. The structure of residuated lattices. *Int. J. Algebra Comput.* **2003**, *13*, 437–461. [CrossRef]
9. Aglianó, P.; Ugolini, S. Projectivity in (bounded) commutative integral residuated lattices. *Algebra Universalis* **2023**, *84*, 2. [CrossRef]
10. Gil-Férez, J.; Jipsen, P.; Metcalfe, G. Structure theorems for idempotent residuated lattices. *Algebra Universalis* **2020**, *81*, 28. [CrossRef]
11. Jenei, S. Group representation for even and odd involutive commutative residuated chains. *Stud. Log.* **2022**, *110*, 881–922. [CrossRef]
12. Jipsen, P.; Tuyt, O.; Valota, D. The structure of finite commutative idempotent involutive residuated lattices. *Algebra Universalis* **2021**, *82*, 57. [CrossRef]
13. Olson, J.S.; Raftery, J.G. Positive Sugihara monoids. *Algebra Universalis* **2007**, *57*, 75–99. [CrossRef]
14. Chen, W.; Zhao, X. The structure of idempotent residuated chains. *Czechoslov. Math. J.* **2009**, *59*, 453–479. [CrossRef]
15. Galatos, N.; Raftery, J.G. Idempotent residuated structures: Some category equivalences and their applications. *Trans. Am. Math. Soc.* **2015**, *367*, 3189–3223. [CrossRef]
16. Galatos, N.; Raftery, J.G. A category equivalence for odd Sugihara monoids and its applications. *J. Pure Appl. Algebra* **2012**, *216*, 2177–2192. [CrossRef]
17. Olson, J.S. The subvariety lattice for representable idempotent commutative residuated lattices. *Algebra Universalis* **2012**, *67*, 43–58. [CrossRef]
18. Olson, J.S. Free representable idempotent commutative residuated lattices. *Int. J. Algebra Comput.* **2008**, *18*, 1365–1394. [CrossRef]
19. Stanovský, D. Commutative idempotent residuated lattices. *Czechoslov. Math. J.* **2007**, *57*, 191–200. [CrossRef]
20. Raftery, J.G. Representable idempotent commutative residuated lattices. *Trans. Amer. Math. Soc.* **2007**, *359*, 4405–4427. [CrossRef]
21. Birkhoff, G. *Lattice Theory*; American Mathematical Society: Providence, RI, USA, 1967.
22. Howie, J.M. *Fundamentals of Semigroup Theory*; Oxford University Press Inc.: New York, NY, USA, 1996.
23. Mitsch, H. A natural partial order for semigroups. *Proc. Am. Math. Soc.* **1986**, *97*, 384. [CrossRef]
24. Jipsen, P.; Tsinakis, C. A survey of residuated lattices. In *Ordered Algebraic Structures*; Martinez, J., Ed.; Kluwer Academic Publishers: Dordrecht, The Netherlands, 2002; pp. 19–56.
25. Hsieh, A. Some locally tabular logics with contraction and mingle. *Rep. Math. Log.* **2010**, *45*, 143–159.
26. Metcalfe, G.; Montagna, F.; Tsinakis, C. Amalgamation and interpolation in ordered algebras. *J. Algebra* **2014**, *402*, 21–82. [CrossRef]
27. Gabbay, D.M.; Maksimova, L. *Interpolation and Definability: Modal and Intuitionistic Logics*; Oxford Logic Guides; The Clarendon Press Oxford University Press: Oxford, UK, 2005; Volume 46.

Disclaimer/Publisher's Note: The statements, opinions and data contained in all publications are solely those of the individual author(s) and contributor(s) and not of MDPI and/or the editor(s). MDPI and/or the editor(s) disclaim responsibility for any injury to people or property resulting from any ideas, methods, instructions or products referred to in the content.

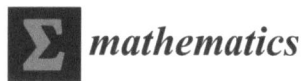

Article

Classifying Seven-Valent Symmetric Graphs of Order $8pq$

Yingbi Jiang, Bo Ling *, Jinlong Yang and Yun Zhao

School of Mathematics and Computer Science, Yunnan Minzu University, Kunming 650031, China; yingbijiang2727@163.com (Y.J.); 041761@ymu.edu.cn (J.Y.); yunzhao_ynni@163.com (Y.Z.)
* Correspondence: boling@ynni.edu.cn

Abstract: A graph is symmetric if its automorphism group is transitive on the arcs of the graph. Guo et al. determined all of the connected seven-valent symmetric graphs of order $8p$ for each prime p. We shall generalize this result by determining all of the connected seven-valent symmetric graphs of order $8pq$ with p and q to be distinct primes. As a result, we show that for each such graph of Γ, it is isomorphic to one of seven graphs.

Keywords: normal quotient; symmetric graph; automorphism group

MSC: 05C25

1. Introduction

We assume that the graphs in this paper are finite, simple, connected and undirected. For undefined terminologies of groups and graphs, we refer the reader to [1,2].

Let Γ be a graph. We denote $V\Gamma$, $E\Gamma$, $A\Gamma$ and $\mathrm{Aut}\Gamma$ as a vertex set, edge set, arc set and full automorphism group of the graph Γ, respectively. We define that the graph Γ is *vertex-transitive* if $\mathrm{Aut}\Gamma$ is transitive on the vertex set $V\Gamma$ of Γ, and Γ is an *arc-transitive* graph if $\mathrm{Aut}\Gamma$ is transitive on the arc set $A\Gamma$ of Γ. An arc-transitive graph is also called a *symmetric* graph.

Let G be a group, and let S be a subset of G such that $S = S^{-1} := \{s^{-1} | s \in S\}$. The Cayley graph $\mathrm{Cay}(G, S)$ is defined to have a vertex set G and edge set $\{\{g, sg\} \| g \in G, s \in S\}$. Now, we denote the following Cayley graphs of dihedral groups by $\mathcal{CD}_{2pq}^k$.

Set $\mathcal{CD}_{2pq}^k = \mathrm{Cay}(G, \{b, ab, a^{k+1}b, \ldots, a^{k^5+k^4+\cdots+k+1}b\})$, where $G = \langle a, b | a^{pq} = b^2 = 1, a^b = a^{-1}\rangle \cong D_{2pq}$, and k is a solution of the equation $x^6 + x^5 + \cdots + x + 1 \equiv 0 \pmod{pq}$.

There are many graph parameters to characterize the reliability and vulnerability of an interconnection network, such as spectral characterization, main eigenvalues, distance characteristic polynomials, and arc-transitivity. Among these parameters, the spectral characterizations, main eigenvalues, and distance characteristic polynomials are the better ones to measure the stability of a network; see [3–7], for example. For arc-transitivity, see [8], as an example. In this paper, we study the arc-transitivity of graphs.

Let p and q be distinct primes. By [9–11], symmetric graphs of orders p, $2p$, and $3p$ have been classified. Furthermore, Praeger et al. determined symmetric graphs of order pq in [12,13].

Recently, the classification of symmetric graphs with certain valency and with a restricted order has attracted much attention. For example, all cubic symmetric graphs of an order up to 768 have been determined by Conder and Dobcsa ń yi [14]. Tetravalent s-transitive graphs of order $6p$, $6p^2$, $8p$, $8p^2$, $10p$ or $10p^2$ were classified in [15–17]. More recently, a large number of papers on seven-valent symmetric graphs have been published. The classification of seven-valent symmetric graphs of order $8p$, $12p$, $16p$, $24p$ or $2pq$ were presented in [18–22]. We shall generalize these results by determining all connected seven-valent symmetric graphs of the order $8pq$.

In this paper, the main result we obtain is the following theorem.

Citation: Jiang, Y.; Ling, B.; Yang, J.; Zhao, Y. Classifying Seven-Valent Symmetric Graphs of Order $8pq$. *Mathematics* **2024**, *12*, 787. https://doi.org/10.3390/math12060787

Academic Editors: Irina Cristea and Alessandro Linzi

Received: 3 February 2024
Revised: 2 March 2024
Accepted: 5 March 2024
Published: 7 March 2024

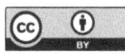

Copyright: © 2024 by the authors. Licensee MDPI, Basel, Switzerland. This article is an open access article distributed under the terms and conditions of the Creative Commons Attribution (CC BY) license (https://creativecommons.org/licenses/by/4.0/).

Theorem 1. *Let $p < q$ be primes and let Γ be a seven-valent symmetric graph of the order $8pq$. Then, Γ is isomorphic to one of the graphs in Table 1.*

Table 1. seven-valent symmetric graphs of order $8pq$.

Γ	AutΓ	(p,q)
$\mathcal{C}_{48}$	PGL$(2,7) \times$ D$_8$	$(2,3)$
$\mathcal{C}_{112}$	$(\mathbb{Z}_2^3 \times$ D$_{14})$:F$_{21}$	$(2,7)$
$\mathcal{C}_{120}$	S$_7$	$(3,5)$
$\mathcal{C}_{312}^i$	PGL$(2,13) \times \mathbb{Z}_2$	$(3,13), i = 1,2,3,4$
$\mathcal{C}_{312}^5$	(PSL$(2,13) \times \mathbb{Z}_2$):$\mathbb{Z}_2$	$(3,13)$
$\mathcal{C}_{312}^6$	PSL$(2,13)$:D$_8$	$(3,13)$
$\mathcal{C}_{(2^3,2q)}$	$(\mathbb{Z}_2^3 \times$ D$_{2q})$:$\mathbb{Z}_7$	$(2,7 \mid q-1)$

Some of the properties in Table 1 are obtained with the help of the Magma system [23]. The method of proving Theorem 1 is to reduce the automorphism groups of the graphs to some nonabelian simple groups. To make this method effective, we need to know the classification result of stabilizers of symmetric graphs. If the valency is a prime p, the method may still work. However, we need information about the stabilizers of prime-valent symmetric graphs and a more detailed discussion. Additionally, the term symmetric graph that is used in this paper has been also used for a different type of symmetry in other research works; see [24], for example. It studied the symmetry of graphs through characteristic polynomials, which is more interesting and detailed.

2. Preliminary Results

In this section, we will provide some necessary preliminary results to be used in later discussions.

For a graph Γ and its full automorphism group AutΓ, let G be a vertex-transitive subgroup of AutΓ and let N be an intransitive normal subgroup of G on $V\Gamma$. We use V_N to denote the set of N-orbits in $V\Gamma$. The *normal quotient graph* Γ_N is a graph that satisfies the vertex set of V_N and two N-orbits B, and $C \in V_N$ are adjacent in Γ_N if and only if some vertex of B is adjacent in Γ to some vertex of C. The following Lemma ([25] Theorem 9) provides a basic method for studying our seven-valent symmetric graphs.

Lemma 1. *Let Γ be an G-arc-transitive graph of the prime valency p, where $p > 2$ and $G \leq$ AutΓ, and let N be a normal subgroup of G and have at least three orbits on $V\Gamma$. Then, the following statements hold.*
(i) *N is semi-regular on $V\Gamma$ and $G/N \leq$ AutΓ_N, and Γ is a normal cover of Γ_N;*
(ii) *Γ is (G,s)-transitive if and only if Γ_N is $(G/N,s)$-transitive, where $1 \leq s \leq 5$ or $s = 7$.*

By ([26] Theorem 3.4) and ([27] Theorem 1.1), we have the following lemma, which describes the vertex stabilizers of symmetric seven-valent graphs.

Lemma 2. *Let Γ be a seven-valent (G,s)-transitive graph, where $G \leq$ AutΓ and $s \geq 1$ are integers. Let $\alpha \in V\Gamma$. Then, $s \leq 3$ and one of the following holds, where F$_{14}$, F$_{21}$ and F$_{42}$ denote the Frobenius group of order 14, 21 and 42, respectively.*
(i) *If G_α is soluble, then $|G_\alpha| \mid 2^2 \cdot 3^2 \cdot 7$. Further, the couple (s, G_α) lie in the following table.*

s	1	2	3
G_α	$\mathbb{Z}_7$, F$_{14}$, F$_{21}$, F$_{14} \times \mathbb{Z}_2$, F$_{21} \times \mathbb{Z}_3$	F$_{42}$, F$_{42} \times \mathbb{Z}_2$, F$_{42} \times \mathbb{Z}_3$	F$_{42} \times \mathbb{Z}_6$

(ii) *If G_α is insoluble, then $|G_\alpha| \mid 2^{24} \cdot 3^4 \cdot 5^2 \cdot 7$. Further, the couple (s, G_α) lie in the following table.*

s	2	3
G_α	PSL(3,2), ASL(3,2), ASL(3,2) $\times \mathbb{Z}_2$, A_7, S_7	PSL(3,2) $\times S_4$, $A_7 \times A_6$, $S_7 \times S_6$, $(A_7 \times A_6) : \mathbb{Z}_2$, $\mathbb{Z}_2^6 : (\text{SL}(2,2) \times \text{SL}(3,2))$, $[2^{20}]$: (SL(2,2) $\times$ SL(3,2))
$\|G_\alpha\|$	$2^3 \cdot 3 \cdot 7, 2^6 \cdot 3 \cdot 7, 2^7 \cdot 3 \cdot 7,$ $2^3 \cdot 3^2 \cdot 5 \cdot 7, 2^4 \cdot 3^2 \cdot 5 \cdot 7$	$2^6 \cdot 3^2 \cdot 7, 2^6 \cdot 3^4 \cdot 5^2 \cdot 7, 2^8 \cdot 3^4 \cdot 5^2 \cdot 7,$ $2^7 \cdot 3^4 \cdot 5^2 \cdot 7, 2^{10} \cdot 3^2 \cdot 7, 2^{24} \cdot 3^2 \cdot 7$

To construct seven-valent symmetric graphs, we need to introduce the Sabidussi coset graph. Let G be a finite group, and H is a core-free subgroup of G. Suppose D is a union of some double cosets of H in G, such that $D^{-1} = D$. The Sabidussi *coset graph* $\text{Cos}(G, H, D)$ of G with respect to H and D is defined to have a vertex set $V\Gamma = [G : H]$ (the set of right cosets of H in G), and the edge set $E\Gamma = \{\{Hg, Hdg\} | g \in G, d \in D\}$ [28,29].

Proposition 1 ([30] Proposition 2.9). *Let Γ be a graph and let G be a vertex-transitive subgroup of $\text{Aut}(\Gamma)$. Then, Γ is isomorphic to a Sabidussi coset graph $\text{Cos}(G, H, D)$, where $H = G_\alpha$ is the stabilizer of $\alpha \in V\Gamma$ in G and D consists of all elements of G with a map of α to one of its neighbors. Further,*

(i) *Γ is connected if and only if D generates the group G;*
(ii) *Γ is G-arc-transitive if and only if D is a single double coset. In particular, if $g \in G$ interchanges α and one of its neighbors, then $g^2 \in H$ and $D = HgH$;*
(iii) *The valency of the graph Γ is equal to $|D|/|H| = |H : H \cap H^g|$.*

In the following lemmas, we provide classification information of seven-valent symmetric graphs of order $8p$ and $2pq$, where p and q are two distinct primes. By [19], we obtain the classification of seven-valent symmetric graphs of order $8p$.

Lemma 3. *Let Γ be a seven-valent symmetric graph of order $8p$. Then $\Gamma \cong K_{8,8} - 8K_2$ or $\mathcal{C}_{24}$.*

By [22], we can describe seven-valent symmetric graphs of order $2pq$.

Lemma 4. *Let $3 \leq p < q$ be primes and let Γ be a seven-valent symmetric graph of order $2pq$. Then, the following statements hold:*

(i) *$\Gamma \cong \mathcal{CD}_{2pq}^k$, where k is a solution of the equation $x^6 + x^5 + \cdots + x + 1 \equiv 0 (\text{mod } pq)$, and $\text{Aut}\Gamma \cong D_{2pq} : \mathbb{Z}_7$, where $p \mid q - 1$.*
(ii) *Γ lies in Table 2.*

Table 2. Seven-valent symmetric graphs of order $2pq$.

Γ	AutΓ	(p,q)
$\mathcal{C}_{78}^1$	PGL(2,13)	(3,13)
$\mathcal{C}_{78}^2$	PSL(2,13)	(3,13)
$\mathcal{C}_{310}$	PSL(5,2).$\mathbb{Z}_2$	(5,31)
$\mathcal{C}_{30}$	S_8	(3,5)

Next, we need some information about nonabelian simple groups. The first one has information about maximal subgroups of PSL(2, t) and PGL(2, t), where t is an odd prime; refer to ([31] Section 239) and ([32] Theorem 2).

Lemma 5. *Let $G = \text{PSL}(2,t)$ or $\text{PGL}(2,t)$, where $t \geq 5$ is a prime, and let M be a maximal subgroup of G.*

(i) *If $G = \text{PSL}(2,t)$, then $M \in \{D_{t-1}, D_{t+1}, \mathbb{Z}_2 : \mathbb{Z}_{(t-1)/2}, A_4, S_4, A_5\}$;*
(ii) *If $G = \text{PGL}(2,t)$, then $M \in \{D_{2(t-1)}, D_{2(t+1)}, \mathbb{Z}_2 : \mathbb{Z}_{t-1}, S_4, \text{PSL}(2,t)\}$.*

The next proposition is about nonabelian simple groups of order that are divisible by at most seven primes. By [2] (pp. 134–136), we have the following proposition.

Proposition 2. *Let T be a nonabelian simple group, such that $28pq \mid |T|$ and $|T| \mid 2^{27} \cdot 3^4 \cdot 5^2 \cdot 7 \cdot p \cdot q$, where $5 \leq p < q$ are primes. Then, T is one of the groups in Table 3.*

Table 3. Simple group T with order dividing $2^{27} \cdot 3^4 \cdot 5^2 \cdot 7 \cdot p \cdot q$.

T	$|T|$	(p,q)	T	$|T|$	(p,q)
M_{22}	$2^7 \cdot 3^2 \cdot 5 \cdot 7 \cdot 11$	$(5,11)$	$PSL(3,8)$	$2^9 \cdot 3^2 \cdot 7^2 \cdot 73$	$(7,73)$
M_{23}	$2^7 \cdot 3^2 \cdot 5 \cdot 7 \cdot 11 \cdot 23$	$(11,23)$	$PSL(3,16)$	$2^{12} \cdot 3^2 \cdot 5^2 \cdot 7 \cdot 13 \cdot 17$	$(13,17)$
M_{24}	$2^{10} \cdot 3^3 \cdot 5 \cdot 7 \cdot 11 \cdot 23$	$(11,23)$	$PSL(2,5^3)$	$2^2 \cdot 3^2 \cdot 5^3 \cdot 7 \cdot 31$	$(5,31)$
J_1	$2^3 \cdot 3 \cdot 5 \cdot 7 \cdot 11 \cdot 19$	$(11,19)$	$PSL(2,7^2)$	$2^4 \cdot 3 \cdot 5^2 \cdot 7^2$	$(5,7)$
HS	$2^9 \cdot 3^2 \cdot 5^3 \cdot 7 \cdot 11$	$(5,11)$	$PSL(4,4)$	$2^{12} \cdot 3^4 \cdot 5^2 \cdot 7 \cdot 17 \cdot 17$	$(5,17)$
A_{11}	$2^7 \cdot 3^4 \cdot 5^2 \cdot 7 \cdot 11$	$(5,11)$	$PSL(5,2)$	$2^{10} \cdot 3^2 \cdot 5 \cdot 7 \cdot 31$	$(5,31)$
$Sz(8)$	$2^6 \cdot 5 \cdot 7 \cdot 13$	$(5,13)$	$PSL(6,2)$	$2^{15} \cdot 3^4 \cdot 5 \cdot 7^2 \cdot 31$	$(7,31)$
$PSp(4,8)$	$2^{12} \cdot 3^4 \cdot 5 \cdot 7^2 \cdot 13$	$(7,13)$	$^3D_4(2)$	$2^{12} \cdot 3^4 \cdot 7^2 \cdot 13$	$(7,13)$
$PSL(2,2^6)$	$2^6 \cdot 3^2 \cdot 5 \cdot 7 \cdot 13$	$(5,13)$	$^2D_4(2)$	$2^{12} \cdot 3^4 \cdot 5 \cdot 7 \cdot 17$	$(5,17)$
$PSL(2,2^9)$	$2^9 \cdot 3^2 \cdot 7 \cdot 19 \cdot 73$	$(19,73)$	$G_2(4)$	$2^{12} \cdot 3^3 \cdot 5^2 \cdot 7 \cdot 13$	$(5,13)$
$PSL(2,q)$	$\frac{q(q+1)(q-1)}{2}$				

Proof. Suppose T is a sporadic simple group, by [2] (pp.135–136), $T = M_{22}, M_{23}, M_{24}, J_1$, or HS. Suppose $T = A_n$ is an alternating group. Then, $T = A_{11}$ is the limitation of $|T|$.

Let X be one type of the Lie group, and let $t = r^f$ be a prime power. Now, suppose that $T = X(t)$ is a simple group of the Lie type, as T contains at most four 3-factors, three 5-factors, and two 7-factors [2] (p.135), and $T = PSL(2,q), PSL(2,5^3)$ or $PSL(2,7^2)$.

Similarly, if $r = 2$, then $T = Sz(8), PSp(4,8), PSL(2,2^6), PSL(2,2^9), PSL(3,8), PSL(3,16)$, $PSL(4,4), PSL(5,2), PSL(6,2), {}^3D_4(2), {}^2D_4(2)$ or $G_4(2)$. □

3. The Proof of Theorem 1

We will prove Theorem 1 through a series of lemmas in this section. To prove Theorem 1, we need information on seven-valent symmetric graphs of order $4pq$. Therefore, we first prove the following lemma.

Lemma 6. *Let $p < q$ be primes and let Γ be a seven-valent symmetric graph of order $4pq$. Then, $\Gamma \cong C_{24}, C_{60}, SG^i_{156}$ or CG^j_{156}, where $i = 1,2,3,4,5$ and $j = 1,2,3,4$.*

Proof. Let Γ be a seven-valent symmetric graph of the order $4pq$, where $p < q$ are primes. Let $A = \text{Aut}\Gamma$. In Lemma 2, $|A| \mid 2^{26} \cdot 3^4 \cdot 5^2 \cdot 7 \cdot p \cdot q$ is $|A_\alpha| \mid 2^{24} \cdot 3^4 \cdot 5^2 \cdot 7$, where $\alpha \in V\Gamma$. If $p = 2$, then Γ has the order $8q$; in Lemma 3, we have $q = 3$ and $\Gamma \cong C_{24}$. If $p = 3$, then Γ has the order $12q$, and in [18,33], we have $q = 5$ or 13 and $\Gamma \cong C_{60}, SG^i_{156}$ or CG^j_{156}, where $i = 1,2,3,4,5$ and $j = 1,2,3,4$. Therefore, we only need to prove that there is no seven-valent symmetric graph of order $4pq$ for $5 \leq p < q$, and the Lemma 6 is proved.

Now, we assume $5 \leq p < q$. By ([33] Theorem 1.1), we have $A \cong PSL(2,r) \times \mathbb{Z}_2$, $PGL(2,r) \times \mathbb{Z}_2, PSL(2,r)$ or $PGL(2,r)$, where $r \equiv \pm 1 \pmod{7}$ is a prime. If $A \cong PSL(2,r) \times \mathbb{Z}_2$ or $PGL(2,r) \times \mathbb{Z}_2$, then A has a normal subgroup $N \cong \mathbb{Z}_2$. It follows that Γ_N is a seven-valent symmetric graph of order $2pq$ and $A/N \leq \text{Aut}\Gamma_N$. Since A/N is isomorphic to $PSL(2,r)$ or $PGL(2,r)$ for $5 \leq p < q$, there exists no such graph in Lemma 4. Hence, A is not isomorphic to $PSL(2,r) \times \mathbb{Z}_2$ or $PGL(2,r) \times \mathbb{Z}_2$.

If $A \cong PSL(2,r)$ or $PGL(2,r)$, then A has a normal subgroup $N \cong PSL(2,r)$. Assume that N has t orbits on the vertex set of Γ, $t \geq 3$. Then, N is semi-regular on $V\Gamma$ in Lemma 1 and thus $|N|$ divides $4pq$, contradicting with $N \cong PSL(2,r)$ and $5 \leq p < q$. Hence, $N_\alpha \neq 1$, N has, at most, two orbits on $V\Gamma$ and $2pq \mid |N : N_\alpha|$. Note that Γ is connected, $N \trianglelefteq A$, and $N_\alpha \neq 1$. Then, we have $1 \neq N_\alpha^{\Gamma(\alpha)} \trianglelefteq A_\alpha^{\Gamma(\alpha)}$. This implies that $7 \mid |N_\alpha|$; thus, we have that $14pq \mid |N|$. And, $|N| \mid 2^{26} \cdot 3^4 \cdot 5^2 \cdot 7 \cdot p \cdot q$ is $|N| \mid |A|$. Since $|A : N| \leq 2$, we have

$|A_\alpha : N_\alpha| \leq 2$. If A_α is insoluble, then N_α is also insoluble as $|A_\alpha : N_\alpha| \leq 2$. In Lemma 5, $N_\alpha = A_5$ (the alternating group on $\{1,2,3,4,5\}$), which contradicts with $7 \mid |N_\alpha|$. Therefore, A_α is soluble. It follows that $|A_\alpha| \mid 252$ in Lemma 2; thus, $|N_\alpha|$ divides 252. This implies that $|N| \mid 1008 \cdot p \cdot q$.

We claim that $r = q$, since $|V\Gamma| = |A|/|A_\alpha| = 4pq$ and $|A_\alpha| \mid 252$. Then, we have $4pq = \dfrac{r(r-1)(r+1)}{2|A_\alpha|}$ or $\dfrac{r(r-1)(r+1)}{|A_\alpha|}$. Since $r \equiv \pm 1 \pmod 7$ is a prime and $|A_\alpha| \mid 252$, we have $r = p$ or q. Assume that $r = p$. Then, $4q = \dfrac{(r-1)(r+1)}{2|A_\alpha|}$ or $\dfrac{(r-1)(r+1)}{|A_\alpha|}$. This implies that $q = r+1$ as $q > p$, which is impossible because $r+1$ is not a prime. Thus, $r = q$ and $|N| = \dfrac{q(q-1)(q+1)}{2}$. Note that $(\dfrac{q+1}{2}, \dfrac{q-1}{2}) = 1$. Assume that $p \mid \dfrac{q-1}{2}$. Then, $q+1 \mid 1008$. And then, we have $q = 7, 11, 13, 17, 23, 41, 47, 71, 83, 167, 251$ or 503. Assume that $p \mid \dfrac{q+1}{2}$. Then, $q-1 \mid 1008$. And then, we have $q = 7, 13, 17, 19, 29, 37, 43, 73, 113, 127, 337$ or 1009. Note that $14pq \mid |N|$, $|N| \mid 2^{26} \cdot 3^4 \cdot 5^2 \cdot 7 \cdot p \cdot q$ and $5 \leq p < q$. Therefore, N is one of the groups in the following table:

N	Order	N	Order
PSL(2,29)	$2^2 \cdot 3 \cdot 5 \cdot 7 \cdot 29$	PSL(2,41)	$2^3 \cdot 3 \cdot 5 \cdot 7 \cdot 41$
PSL(2,43)	$2^2 \cdot 3 \cdot 7 \cdot 11 \cdot 43$	PSL(2,71)	$2^3 \cdot 3^2 \cdot 5 \cdot 7 \cdot 71$
PSL(2,83)	$2^2 \cdot 3 \cdot 7 \cdot 41 \cdot 83$	PSL(2,113)	$2^4 \cdot 3 \cdot 7 \cdot 19 \cdot 113$
PSL(2,167)	$2^3 \cdot 3 \cdot 7 \cdot 83 \cdot 167$	PSL(2,251)	$2^2 \cdot 3^2 \cdot 5^3 \cdot 7 \cdot 251$
PSL(2,337)	$2^4 \cdot 3 \cdot 7 \cdot 13^2 \cdot 337$	PSL(2,503)	$2^3 \cdot 3^2 \cdot 7 \cdot 251 \cdot 503$
PSL(2,1009)	$2^4 \cdot 3^2 \cdot 5 \cdot 7 \cdot 101 \cdot 1009$		

Assume that $q = 29, 71, 113, 251$ or 1009. Note that $|N : N_\alpha| = 2pq$ or $4pq$. N has no subgroup of index $2pq$ or $4pq$ in Lemma 5, which is a contradiction.

Assume that $q = 337$. Then, $N = \text{PSL}(2,337)$, contradicting with $|N| \mid 2^{26} \cdot 3^4 \cdot 5^2 \cdot 7 \cdot p \cdot q$.

Assume that $q = 41$. Then, $N = \text{PSL}(2,41)$ and $(p,q) = (5,41)$. Since N has no subgroup of index $2pq$ in Lemma 5, we have that N is transitive on $V\Gamma$, and thus $|N_\alpha| = 42$. Hence, $N_\alpha = F_{42}$ in Lemma 2. In Proposition 1, $\Gamma = \text{Cos}(N, N_\alpha, N_\alpha g N_\alpha)$, where g is a 2-element in N such that $g^2 \in N_\alpha$ and $\langle N_\alpha, g \rangle = N$. In Magma [23], there is no such $g \in N$, which is a contradiction.

Finally, assume that $q = 43$. Then, $N = \text{PSL}(2,43)$ and $(p,q) = (11,43)$. If N has two orbits on $V\Gamma$, then $A = \text{PGL}(2,43)$ and $A_\alpha = F_{42}$ in Lemma 2. This is impossible, as $\text{PGL}(2,41)$ has no subgroup isomorphic to F_{42}. Therefore, N is transitive on $V\Gamma$ and in Lemma 2, $N_\alpha = F_{21}$. In Lemma 5, $\text{PSL}(2,41)$ has no subgroup isomorphic to F_{21}, which is a contradiction. Similarly, $q \neq 83, 167$ or 503. This completes the proof. □

Now, let Γ be a seven-valent symmetric graph of the order $8pq$, where $p < q$ are primes. Let $A := \text{Aut}\Gamma$. Take $\alpha \in V\Gamma$. In Lemma 2, $|A_\alpha| \mid 2^{24} \cdot 3^4 \cdot 5^2 \cdot 7$, and hence $|A| \mid 2^{27} \cdot 3^4 \cdot 5^2 \cdot 7 \cdot p \cdot q$.

If $p = 2$, then Γ has the order $16q$; by [20], we have $q = 3, 7$ or $7 \mid q-1$, and Γ is isomorphic to $\mathcal{C}_{48}$, $\mathcal{C}_{112}$ or $\mathcal{C}_{(2^3,2q)}$. If $p = 3$, then Γ has the order $24q$; in [21], we have $q = 5$ or 13, and Γ is isomorphic to $\mathcal{C}_{120}$, $\mathcal{C}_{312}^i$ with $i = 1,2,3,4$, $\mathcal{C}_{312}^5$ or $\mathcal{C}_{312}^6$. Therefore, we only need to prove that there is no seven-valent symmetric graph of the order $8pq$ for $5 \leq p < q$, and the Theorem 1 is proved. For the remainder of this paper, we let $5 \leq p < q$.

In the next lemma, we deal with the case where there is a soluble minimal normal subgroup of A.

Lemma 7. *Assume that A has a soluble minimal normal subgroup. Then, there exists no seven-valent symmetric graph of order $8pq$ for $5 \leq p < q$.*

Proof. Assuming N is a soluble minimal normal subgroup of the full automorphism group A. Then, N is an elementary abelian group. Since $|V\Gamma| = 8pq$, we have $N \cong \mathbb{Z}_2, \mathbb{Z}_2^2, \mathbb{Z}_2^3, \mathbb{Z}_p$ or $\mathbb{Z}_q$. It is easy to prove that N has more than two orbits on $V\Gamma$; if not, we have $4pq \mid |N|$, a contradiction. Therefore, in Lemma 1, $|N_\alpha| = 1$, and the quotient graph Γ_N of Γ relative to N is a seven-valent symmetric graph, with A/N as an arc-transitive subgroup of the automorphism of Γ_N.

If $N \cong \mathbb{Z}_2^3$, then Γ_N is a seven-valent symmetric graph of the order pq (pq is an odd number), which is a contradiction, as symmetric graphs of the odd order odd valent do not exist. If $N \cong \mathbb{Z}_2$, then Γ_N is a seven-valent symmetric graph of the order $4pq$. In Lemma 6, we note that $5 \leq p < q$, Γ_N does not exist, which is a contradiction. If $N \cong \mathbb{Z}_p$, then Γ_N is a seven-valent symmetric graph of the order $8q$. Γ_N does not exist in Lemma 3, which is a contradiction. Similarly, we obtain that $N \not\cong \mathbb{Z}_q$.

If $N \cong \mathbb{Z}_2^2$, then Γ_N is a seven-valent symmetric graph of the order $2pq$. In Lemma 4, $\Gamma_N \cong \mathcal{C}_{310}$ or $\mathcal{CD}_{2pq}^k$, where k is a solution of the equation $x^6 + x^5 + \cdots + x + 1 \equiv 0 \pmod{pq}$ and $p \mid q - 1$.

Let $\Gamma_N \cong \mathcal{C}_{310}$. Then, $A/N \leq \mathrm{Aut}\mathcal{C}_{310} = \mathrm{PSL}(5,2).\mathbb{Z}_2$. Furthermore, A/N is arc-transitive on $V\Gamma_N$. By Magma [23], $\mathrm{Aut}\Gamma_N$ has a minimal arc-transitive subgroup, which is isomorphic to $\mathrm{PSL}(5,2)$. Thus, $\mathrm{PSL}(5,2) \leq A/N \leq \mathrm{PSL}(5,2).\mathbb{Z}_2$. Since the Schur Multiplier of $\mathrm{PSL}(5,2)$ is trivial, $A = \mathbb{Z}_2^2 \times \mathrm{PSL}(5,2)$ or $(\mathbb{Z}_2^2 \times \mathrm{PSL}(5,2)).\mathbb{Z}_2$. For the former case, in Proposition 1, $\Gamma = \mathrm{Cos}(A, A_\alpha, A_\alpha g A_\alpha)$, where g is a 2-element in A such that $g^2 \in A_\alpha$ and $\langle A_\alpha, g \rangle = A$. By Magma [23], there is no such $g \in A$, which is a contradiction. For the latter case, A/N has a normal subgroup, $M \cong \mathrm{PSL}(5,2)$. It is obvious that M has at most two orbits on $V\Gamma$. Since M has no subgroup of order 16128, M is transitive on $V\Gamma$, implying that $|M_\alpha| = 8064$; this is impossible in Lemma 2.

Let $\Gamma_N \cong \mathcal{CD}_{2pq}^k$, where k is a solution of the equation $x^6 + x^5 + \cdots + x + 1 \equiv 0 \pmod{pq}$. Note that A/N is an arc-transitive subgroup of $\mathrm{Aut}(\Gamma_N) = D_{2pq} : \mathbb{Z}_7$. Hence, $2pq \cdot 7 \mid |A/N|$. This implies that $A/N = D_{2pq} : \mathbb{Z}_7$. Let H be a normal subgroup of the order pq of D_{2pq} and Q be a Sylow q-subgroup of H. Then, in the Sylow Theorem, Q char H and thus $Q \trianglelefteq D_{2pq}$ is $H \trianglelefteq D_{2pq}$. Note that Q is also a Sylow q-subgroup of D_{2pq}. Then, Q char D_{2pq} and thus $Q \trianglelefteq A/N$ is $D_{2pq} \trianglelefteq A/N$. Then, $5 \leq p < q$ and $p \mid q - 1$. Then, $q \geq 11$. Hence, Q is also a Sylow q-subgroup of A/N. Let $Q = G/N$. Then, $G/N \cong \mathbb{Z}_q$ and $|G| = 2^2 \cdot q$. In the Sylow Theorem, the Sylow q-subgroup of G is normal, at say L. Then, $L \cong \mathbb{Z}_q$, and thus $G = \mathbb{Z}_2^2 \times \mathbb{Z}_q = N \times L$. Hence, $L \trianglelefteq A$ is $G \trianglelefteq A$. Then, the normal quotient graph Γ_L of Γ relative to L is a seven-valent symmetric graph of order $8p$. In Lemma 3, there exists no graph for this case, which is a contradiction.

Thus, we complete the proof of Lemma 7. □

Now we move on to the case where there is no soluble minimal normal subgroup of A. Then, we have the following lemma.

Lemma 8. *Assume that A has no soluble minimal normal subgroup. Then, there exists no seven-valent symmetric graph of order $8pq$ for $5 \leq p < q$.*

Proof. Let N be an insoluble minimal normal subgroup of A, and let $C = C_A(N)$ be the centralizer of N in A. Then, N is isomorphic to T^d, where $d \geq 1$ and T are non-abelian simple groups. Assume that N has t orbits on the vertex set of Γ. If $t \geq 3$, then $N_\alpha = 1$ by Lemma 1 and thus $|N| = |T|^d \mid 8pq$, since N is insoluble. Then, $|N| = 4pq$ or $8pq$. Thus, N has two orbits or an orbit on $V\Gamma$, which is a contradiction. Hence, N has at most two orbits on $V\Gamma$, and it follows that $4pq \mid |N|$.

If $N_\alpha = 1$, then $|N| = 4pq$ or $8pq$, since $q \mid |N|$ and $q^2 \nmid |N|$. Then, $N = T$. Note that $5 \leq p < q$ [34]; no such simple group exists, and this is a contradiction. Hence, $N_\alpha \neq 1$. Since Γ is connected to $N \trianglelefteq A$ and $N_\alpha \neq 1$, we have $1 \neq N_\alpha^{\Gamma(\alpha)} \trianglelefteq A_\alpha^{\Gamma(\alpha)}$. It follows that 7 divides $|N_\alpha|$. Then, we have that $28pq \mid |N|$.

Now, we claim that $d = 1$. Otherwise, $d \geq 2$, and thus $7^2 \mid |N|$. We have $d = 2$ as $|N| \mid 2^{27} \cdot 3^4 \cdot 5^2 \cdot 7 \cdot p \cdot q$. So $p = 7$ or $q = 7$. If $p = 7$, then $q > 7$ and $q^2 \mid |T|^2$, which contradicts with $|N| \mid 2^{27} \cdot 3^4 \cdot 5^2 \cdot 7 \cdot p \cdot q$. If $q = 7$, then $p = 5$. This implies that $|T| \mid 2^{13} \cdot 3^2 \cdot 5 \cdot 7$. Note that $35 \mid |T|$. By checking the nonabelian simple group of an order less than $2^{13} \cdot 3^2 \cdot 5 \cdot 7$, we have that $T = A_7$, A_8 or $\mathrm{PSL}(3,4)$, and $N = A_7{}^2$, $A_8{}^2$ or $\mathrm{PSL}(3,4)^2$ as $d = 2$. On the other side of the coin, $C \trianglelefteq A$, $C \cap N = 1$ and thus $\langle C, N \rangle = C \times N$. Because $|C \times N| \mid 2^{27} \cdot 3^4 \cdot 5^2 \cdot 7 \cdot p \cdot q$ and $|N| = |T|^2 = 2^6 \cdot 3^4 \cdot 5^2 \cdot 7^2$ or $2^{12} \cdot 3^4 \cdot 5^2 \cdot 7^2$, C is a $\{2, p\}$-group, and hence soluble, where $p = 5$. So, $C = 1$ as A contains no soluble minimal normal subgroup. This implies $A = A/C \leq \mathrm{Aut}(N) \cong \mathrm{Aut}(T)wr\mathbb{Z}_2$. By Magma [23], no such graph exists, which is a contradiction. Therefore, we have $d = 1$, and $N = T \trianglelefteq A$ is a nonabelian simple group.

We next prove that $C = 1$. If $C \neq 1$, then C is insoluble, as $C \trianglelefteq A$ and A contain no soluble minimal normal subgroup. In the same argument as for the case N, we have 7 divides $|C_\alpha|$. Because $\langle C, N \rangle = C \times N$ and $C, N \trianglelefteq A$, we have $C_\alpha \times N_\alpha \leq A_\alpha$. Note that 7 divides $|N_\alpha|$; this concludes that $7^2 \mid |A_\alpha|$, which is a contradiction with Lemma 2. Therefore, we have $C = 1$, and thus $A \leq \mathrm{Aut}(T)$ is almost simple. It follows that $T = \mathrm{soc}(A)$ is a nonabelian simple group and satisfies the following condition.

Condition(*): $|T|$ lies in Table 3 such that $28pq \mid |T|$ and $|T| \mid 2^{27} \cdot 3^4 \cdot 5^2 \cdot 7 \cdot p \cdot q$.

Assume first that $T \cong M_{22}$, M_{23}, J_1, A_{11}, $\mathrm{PSL}(2, 2^9)$, $\mathrm{PSL}(3, 16)$, $\mathrm{PSL}(2, 5^3)$, $\mathrm{PSL}(2, 7^2)$, $\mathrm{PSL}(4, 4)$, $\mathrm{PSL}(6, 2)$, $\mathrm{PSp}(4, 8)$, HS, ${}^2D_4(2)$, ${}^3D_4(2)$, or $G_2(4)$. Note that $|T : T_\alpha| = 4pq$ or $8pq$. T has no subgroup of index $4pq$ or $8pq$ by Atlas [35], which is a contradiction.

Assume that $T \cong M_{24}$. Since T has no subgroup of index $4pq$, we show that T is transitive on $V\Gamma$, and thus $|T_\alpha| = 120,960$. In Proposition 1, $\Gamma = \mathrm{Cos}(T, T_\alpha, T_\alpha g T_\alpha)$, where g is a 2-element in T such that $g^2 \in T_\alpha$ and $\langle T_\alpha, g \rangle = T$. In Magma [23], there is no such $g \in T$, which is a contradiction. Similarly, T is not isomorphic to $\mathrm{Sz}(8)$, $\mathrm{PSL}(2, 2^6)$ or $\mathrm{PSL}(5, 2)$.

Assume that $T \cong \mathrm{PSL}(3, 8)$. If T has two orbits on $V\Gamma$, then Γ is bipartite and $|T_\alpha| = 2^7 \cdot 3^2 \cdot 7$. Recall that A is almost simple. Thus, $A \leq \mathrm{Aut}(T)$. Since $\mathrm{Aut}(T) = \mathrm{PSL}(3, 8).\mathbb{Z}_6$, we have $A \cong \mathrm{PSL}(3, 8).\mathbb{Z}_2$, $\mathrm{PSL}(3, 8).\mathbb{Z}_3$ or $\mathrm{PSL}(3, 8).\mathbb{Z}_6$, and thus $|A_\alpha| = 2^7 \cdot 3^2 \cdot 7$, $2^6 \cdot 3^3 \cdot 7$ or $2^7 \cdot 3^3 \cdot 7$, which is impossible according to Lemma 2. Thus, T is transitive on $V\Gamma$. In Proposition 1, $\Gamma = \mathrm{Cos}(T, T_\alpha, T_\alpha g T_\alpha)$, where g is a 2-element in T such that $g^2 \in T_\alpha$ and $\langle T_\alpha, g \rangle = T$. By Magma [23], there is no such $g \in T$, which is a contradiction.

Finally, assume that $T \cong \mathrm{PSL}(2, q)$. Then, $T \leq A \leq \mathrm{Aut}(T) = \mathrm{PGL}(2, q)$ ($\mathrm{PGL}(2, q) = \mathrm{PSL}(2, q).\mathbb{Z}_2$) and $|A : T| \leq 2$. If A_α is insoluble, then T_α is also insoluble as $|A_\alpha : T_\alpha| \leq 2$. $T_\alpha = A_5$ in Lemma 5, contradicting with 7, divides $|T_\alpha|$. Therefore, A_α is soluble, and $|A_\alpha|$ divides by 252 in Lemma 2, and so $|T_\alpha|$ divides 252. This implies that $|T| \mid 2016 \cdot p \cdot q$. Note that $|T| = \dfrac{q(q-1)(q+1)}{2}$ and $(\dfrac{q+1}{2}, \dfrac{q-1}{2}) = 1$. If $p \mid \dfrac{q-1}{2}$, then $q+1 \mid 2016$. It follows that $q = 7, 11, 13, 17, 23, 31, 41, 47, 71, 83, 167, 223, 251$ or 503. If $p \mid \dfrac{q+1}{2}$, then $q-1 \mid 2016$. It follows that $q = 7, 13, 17, 19, 29, 37, 43, 73, 97, 113, 127, 337, 673, 1009$ or 2017. Note that T meets the condition (*) and $5 \leq p < q$. Therefore, T is one of the groups in the following table:

T	Order	T	Order
$\mathrm{PSL}(2, 29)$	$2^2 \cdot 3 \cdot 5 \cdot 7 \cdot 29$	$\mathrm{PSL}(2, 41)$	$2^3 \cdot 3 \cdot 5 \cdot 7 \cdot 41$
$\mathrm{PSL}(2, 43)$	$2^2 \cdot 3 \cdot 7 \cdot 11 \cdot 43$	$\mathrm{PSL}(2, 71)$	$2^3 \cdot 3^2 \cdot 5 \cdot 7 \cdot 71$
$\mathrm{PSL}(2, 83)$	$2^2 \cdot 3 \cdot 7 \cdot 41 \cdot 83$	$\mathrm{PSL}(2, 97)$	$2^5 \cdot 3 \cdot 7^2 \cdot 97$
$\mathrm{PSL}(2, 113)$	$2^4 \cdot 3 \cdot 7 \cdot 19 \cdot 113$	$\mathrm{PSL}(2, 167)$	$2^3 \cdot 3 \cdot 7 \cdot 83 \cdot 167$
$\mathrm{PSL}(2, 223)$	$2^5 \cdot 3 \cdot 7 \cdot 37 \cdot 223$	$\mathrm{PSL}(2, 251)$	$2^2 \cdot 3^2 \cdot 5^3 \cdot 7 \cdot 251$
$\mathrm{PSL}(2, 337)$	$2^4 \cdot 3 \cdot 7 \cdot 13^2 \cdot 337$	$\mathrm{PSL}(2, 503)$	$2^3 \cdot 3^2 \cdot 7 \cdot 251 \cdot 503$
$\mathrm{PSL}(2, 673)$	$2^5 \cdot 3 \cdot 7 \cdot 337 \cdot 673$	$\mathrm{PSL}(2, 1009)$	$2^4 \cdot 3^2 \cdot 5 \cdot 7 \cdot 101 \cdot 1009$
$\mathrm{PSL}(2, 2017)$	$2^5 \cdot 3^2 \cdot 7 \cdot 1009 \cdot 2017$		

Assume that $q = 29, 71, 97, 113, 223, 251, 337$ or 1009. Note that $|T : T_\alpha| = 4pq$ or $8pq$. T has no subgroup of index $4pq$ or $8pq$ in Lemma 5, which is a contradiction.

Assume that $q = 337$. Then, $T = \text{PSL}(2, 337)$, which contradicts with $|T| \mid 2^{27} \cdot 3^4 \cdot 5^2 \cdot 7 \cdot p \cdot q$.

Assume that $q = 43$. Then, $T = \text{PSL}(2, 43)$ and $(p, q) = (11, 43)$, since T has no subgroup of index $8pq$. Then, T is not transitive to $V\Gamma$. If T has two orbits on $V\Gamma$, then $|T_\alpha| = 21$. As A is almost simple, $A = \text{PGL}(2, 43)$, and $A_\alpha = F_{21}$ in Lemma 2. In Proposition 1, $\Gamma = \text{Cos}(A, A_\alpha, A_\alpha g A_\alpha)$, where g is a 2-element in A such that $g^2 \in A_\alpha$ and $\langle A_\alpha, g \rangle = A$. In Magma [23], there is no such $g \in A$, which is a contradiction.

Finally, assume that $q = 41$. Then, $T = \text{PSL}(2, 41)$ and $(p, q) = (5, 11)$. If T has two orbits on $V\Gamma$, then $|T_\alpha| = 42$. As A is almost simple, $A = \text{PGL}(2, 41)$, and $A_\alpha = F_{42}$ in Lemma 2. This is impossible, as $\text{PGL}(2, 41)$ has no subgroup isomorphic to F_{42}. Therefore, T is transitive to $V\Gamma$ and in Lemma 2, $T_\alpha = F_{21}$. In Lemma 5, $\text{PSL}(2, 41)$ has no subgroup isomorphic to F_{21}, which is a contradiction. Similarly, $q \neq 167, 503, 673$ or 2017.

Thus, we complete the proof of Lemma 8. □

By combining Lemma 6, 7 and 8, we have completed the proof of Theorem 1.

4. Conclusions

Through the classification of seven-valent symmetric graphs of the order $8pq$, we obtain many highly symmetric graphs in Table 1. These graphs can be applied to the design of the interconnection network. With induction, we may further classify seven-valent symmetric graphs of the order $8n$, where n is an odd square-free integer. We can even classify p-valent symmetric graphs of the order $2^k n$, where k is a positive integer and n is an odd square-free integer.

Author Contributions: Formal analysis, J.Y. and Y.Z.; Writing—original draft, Y.J.; Writing—review & editing, B.L. All authors have read and agreed to the published version of the manuscript.

Funding: This work was partially supported by the National Natural Science Foundation of China (12061089, 11861076, 11701503, 11761079), and the Natural Science Foundation of Yunnan Province (202201AT070022, 2019FB139).

Data Availability Statement: The data will be made available by the authors on request.

Conflicts of Interest: The authors declare no potential conflicts of interest.

Nomenclature

$G, H, \ldots$	Groups
$a, b, \ldots$	Elements of groups
a^b	$b^{-1}ab$
D_n	Dihedral group of order n
S_n, A_n	Symmetric, alternating groups of degree n
$\mathbb{Z}$	Sets of integers
$\mathbb{Z}_n$	$\mathbb{Z}/n\mathbb{Z}$
M_{22}, M_{23}, M_{24}	Mathieu groups
$\text{ASL}(n, R)$	Affine group over R
$\text{Sz}(2^n)$	Suzuki group
$\text{SL}(n, R)$	Linear groups over R
J_1	Janko group
HS	Higman, Sims group
$\text{PSp}(4, 8)$	Symplectic group
$^2D_4(2)$	Orthogonal group
$^3D_4(2)$	Triality twisted group
$G_2(4)$	Chevalley group
$\text{PGL}(n, R), \text{PSL}(n, R)$	Projective general linear and projective special linear groups
Γ	Graph
$V\Gamma, E\Gamma, A\Gamma$	Vertex set, edge set, arc set of Γ

Γ_N	Quotient graph
α	Element of graph
$\text{Aut}(\Gamma), \text{Aut}(\Gamma_N)$	Automorphism group of Γ and Γ_N
$\mathcal{C}_n$	Symmetric graph of order n
G_α	Stabilizer of α in G
$G \times H, G^n$	Direct product, direct power
$G \text{wr} H$	Wreath product
$G.H$	An extension of G by H
$\lvert G \rvert$	Cardinality of the group G
G/N	Quotient group
F_n	Frobenius group of order n
$H \cong G$	H is isomorphic with G
$\langle N_\alpha, g \rangle$	Group generated by N_α and g
$G \triangleleft A$	G is a normal subgroup of A
$\text{Aut}(T)$	Automorphism group of T
$soc(A)$	Socle of G
$C_A(N)$	Centralizer of N in G
$\lvert A : N \rvert$	Index of the subgroup N in A

References

1. Godsil, C.D.; Royle, G. *Algebraic Graph Theory*; Springer: Berlin, Germany, 2001.
2. Gorenstein, D. *Finite Simple Groups*; Plenum Press: New York, NY, USA, 1982.
3. Abiad, A.; Brimkov, B.; Hayat, S.; Khramova, A.P.; Koolen, J.H. Extending a conjecture of Graham and Lovász on the distance characteristic polynomial. *Linear Algebra Appl.* 2023, in press. [CrossRef]
4. Hayat, S.; Javaid, M.; Koolen, J.H. Graphs with two main and two plain eigenvalues. *Appl. Anal. Discr. Math.* 2017, 11, 244–257. [CrossRef]
5. Hayat, S.; Koolen, J.H.; Liu, F.; Qiao, Z. A note on graphs with exactly two main eigenvalues. *Linear Algebra Appl.* 2016, 511, 318–327. [CrossRef]
6. Hayat, S.; Koolen, J.H.; Riaz, M. A spectral characterization of the s-clique extension of the square grid graphs. *Europ. J. Combin.* 2019, 76, 104–116. [CrossRef]
7. Koolen, J.H.; Hayat, S.; Iqbal, Q. Hypercubes are determined by their distance spectra. *Linear Algebra Appl.* 2016, 505, 97–108. [CrossRef]
8. Xiao, R.; Zhang, X.; Zhang, H. On Edge-Primitive Graphs of Order as a Product of Two Distinct Primes. *Mathematics* 2023, 11, 3896. [CrossRef]
9. Chao, C.Y. On the classification of symmetric graphs with a prime number of vertices. *Trans. Am. Math. Soc.* 1971, 158, 247–256. [CrossRef]
10. Wang, R.J.; Xu, M.Y. A classification of symmetric graphs of order $3p$. *J. Combin. Theory B* 1993, 58, 197–216. [CrossRef]
11. Cheng, Y.; Oxley, J. On the weakly symmetric graphs of order twice a prime, *J. Combin. Theory Ser. B* 1987, 42, 196–211. [CrossRef]
12. Praeger, C.E.; Wang, R.J.; Xu, M.Y. Symmetric graphs of order a product of two distinct primes. *J. Combin. Theory B* 1993, 58, 299–318. [CrossRef]
13. Praeger, C.E.; Xu, M.Y. Vertex-primitive graphs of order a product of two distinct primes. *J. Combin. Theory B* 1993, 59, 245–266. [CrossRef]
14. Conder, M.D.E.; Dobcsańyi, P. Trivalent symmetric graphs on up to 768 vertices. *J. Combin. Math. Combin. Comput.* 2002, 40, 41–63.
15. Feng, Y.Q.; Kwak, J.H. Classifying cubic symmetric graphs of order $10p$ or $10p^2$. *Sci. China A* 2006, 49, 300–319. [CrossRef]
16. Feng, Y.Q.; Kwak, J.H. Cubic symmetric graphs of order a small number times a prime or a prime square. *J. Combin. Theory B* 2007, 97, 627–646. [CrossRef]
17. Feng, Y.Q.; Kwak, J.H.; Wang, K.S. Classifying cubic symmetric graphs of order $8p$ or $8p^2$. *Eur. J. Combin.*, 2005, 26, 1033–1052. [CrossRef]
18. Guo, S.T. 7-valent symmetric graphs of order $12p$. *Ital. J. Pure Appl. Math.* 2019, 42, 161–172.
19. Guo, S.T.; Hou, H.L.; Xu, Y. Heptavalent symmetric graphs of order $8p$. *Ital. J. Pure Appl. Math.* 2020, 43, 37–46.
20. Guo, S.T.; Hou, H.L.; Xu, Y. Heptavalent Symmetric Graphs of Order $16p$. *Algebra Colloq.* 2017, 24, 453–466. [CrossRef]
21. Guo, S.T.; Wu, Y.S. Heptavalent symmetric graphs of order $24p$. *Proc. Indian Acad. Sci.* 2019, 129, 58. [CrossRef]
22. Ling, B.; Lan, T.; Ding, S.Y. On 7-valent symmetric graphs of order $2pq$ and 11-valent symmetric graphs of order $4pq$. *Open Math.* 2022, 20, 1696–1708. [CrossRef]
23. Bosma, W.; Cannon, C.; Playoust, C. The MAGMA algebra system I: The user language. *J. Symbolic Comput.* 1997, 24, 235–265. [CrossRef]
24. Chbili, N.; Dhaheri, S.A.; Tahnon, M.Y.; Abunamous, A.A.E. The Characteristic Polynomials of Symmetric Graphs. *Symetry* 2018, 10, 582. [CrossRef]
25. Lorimer, P. Vertex-transitive graphs: Symmetric graphs of prime valency. *J. Graph Theory* 1984, 8, 55–68. [CrossRef]

26. Li, C.H.; Lu, Z.P.; Wang, G.X. Arc-transitive graphs of square-free order and small valency. *Discret. Math.* **2016**, *339*, 2907–2918. [CrossRef]
27. Guo, S.T.; Li, Y.T.; Hua, X.H. (G,s)-Transitive Graphs of Valency 7. *Algebra Colloq.* **2016**, *23*, 493–500. [CrossRef]
28. Miller, R.C. The trivalent symmetric graphs of girth at most six. *J. Combin. Theory Ser. B* **1971**, *10*, 163–182. [CrossRef]
29. Sabidussi, B.O. Vertex-transitive graphs. *Monatsh Math.* **1964**, *68*, 126–438. [CrossRef]
30. Hua, X.H.; Feng, Y.Q.; Lee, J. Pentavalent symmetric graphs of order $2pq$. *Discrete Math.* **2011**, *311*, 2259–2267. [CrossRef]
31. Dickson, L.E. *Linear Groups and Expositions of the Galois Field Theory*; Dover Publications: Dover, UK, 1958.
32. Gameron, P.J.; Omidi, G.R.; Tayfeh-Rezaie, B. 3-Designs from PGL$(2,p)$. *Electron. J. Combin.* **2006**, *13*, R50. [CrossRef]
33. Pan, J.M.; Ling, B.; Ding, S.Y. On symmetric graphs of order four times an odd square-free integer and valency seven. *Discrete Math.* **2017**, *340*, 2071–2078. [CrossRef]
34. Herzog, M. On finite simple groups of order divisible by three primes only. *J. Algebra.* **1968**, *10*, 383–388. [CrossRef]
35. Conway, J.H.; Curtis, R.T.; Norton, S.P.; Parker, R.A.; Wilson, R.A. *Atlas of Finite Groups*; Oxford University Press: London, UK; New York, NY, USA, 1985.

Disclaimer/Publisher's Note: The statements, opinions and data contained in all publications are solely those of the individual author(s) and contributor(s) and not of MDPI and/or the editor(s). MDPI and/or the editor(s) disclaim responsibility for any injury to people or property resulting from any ideas, methods, instructions or products referred to in the content.

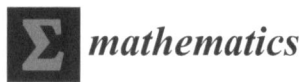

Article

Characterizing Finite Groups through Equitable Graphs: A Graph-Theoretic Approach

Alaa Altassan [1], Anwar Saleh [2,*], Marwa Hamed [1] and Najat Muthana [1,*]

[1] Department of Mathematics, College of Science, King Abdulaziz University, Jeddah 21589, Saudi Arabia; aaltassan@kau.edu.sa (A.A.); mhamed0022@stu.kau.edu.sa (M.H.)
[2] Department of Mathematics and Statistics, Faculty of Science, University of Jeddah, Jeddah 21589, Saudi Arabia
* Correspondence: asaleh1@uj.edu.sa (A.S.); nmuthana@kau.edu.sa (N.M.)

Abstract: This paper introduces equitable graphs of Type I associated with finite groups. We investigate the connectedness and some graph-theoretic properties of these graphs for various groups. Furthermore, we establish the novel concepts of the equitable square-free number and the equitable group. Our study includes an analysis of the equitable graphs for specific equitable groups. Additionally, we determine the first, second and forgotten Zagreb topological indices for the equitable graphs of Type I constructed from certain groups. Finally, we derive the adjacency matrix for this graph type built from cyclic p-groups.

Keywords: equitable graph; equitable group; topological indices

MSC: 05C62; 05C25

1. Introduction

The connection between graphs and groups is an interesting field of research and has wide applications. Research on this subject leads to the investigation of the relationship between the group and the associated graph and explores theoretical properties from one to the other. The graph associated with a group can provide valuable information and offer a combinatorial approach to studying groups. This can give group theorists more tools to work with. Additionally, comparing groups with similar graph-theoretic properties can help classify these groups. The literature is rich with studies on this topic. This concept has been known since 1878, when Cayley graphs were presented [1]. Subsequently, several graphs have been constructed from groups, such as the commuting graph, which was introduced by Brauer and Fowler in 1955 [2]. Then, the prime graphs were defined by Gruenberg and Kegel in 1975 [3]. Later, in 2009, Chackrabarty, Gosh and Sen presented the power graph [4,5]. Many graphs have been introduced in the literature: for instance, the order-divisor graph, intersection graph and cyclic graph. All of these graphs have been thoroughly studied, including their characteristics and their relations with groups. For more details, we refer the reader to [6–11].

In light of the increasing significance of graphs linked to groups and their role in classifying both groups and graphs, as well as the importance of element orders in a finite group, we are inspired to introduce a new type of graph based on the distinctions between element orders within the group. Through this research, we study a graph associated with a finite group called *the equitable graph Type I* and denoted by $\mathcal{E}_1(G)$. The vertex set of this graph is a finite group G, and two distinct vertices x and y are adjacent if and only if $|o(x) - o(y)| \leq \min\{o(x), o(y)\}$.

In our research, we extensively studied important algebraic groups in order to create general formulaic representations of the resulting graphs. These representations were thoroughly analyzed to understand their theoretical properties and topological characteristics.

Citation: Altassan, A.; Saleh, A.; Hamed, M.; Muthana, N. Characterizing Finite Groups through Equitable Graphs: A Graph-Theoretic Approach. *Mathematics* **2024**, *12*, 2126. https://doi.org/10.3390/math12132126

Academic Editors: Irina Cristea and Alessandro Linzi

Received: 2 May 2024
Revised: 3 July 2024
Accepted: 5 July 2024
Published: 6 July 2024

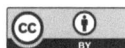

Copyright: © 2024 by the authors. Licensee MDPI, Basel, Switzerland. This article is an open access article distributed under the terms and conditions of the Creative Commons Attribution (CC BY) license (https://creativecommons.org/licenses/by/4.0/).

Moreover, our exploration of this innovative conceptual definition allowed us to establish new specialized terminology: specifically, the concepts of *the equitable square-free number* and *the equitable group*. These new concepts serve as valuable classifications within the respective domains of number theory and graph theory.

In this paper, G denotes a finite group, and e is the identity of G. For any element of G, say g, $o(g)$ is the order of g, and the number of elements of order m in a cyclic group is equal to $\phi(m)$, where ϕ is the *Euler's phi* function. For a real number x, the greatest integer $\leq x$ [or the least integer $\geq x$], called the floor [or ceiling] function and denoted by $\lfloor x \rfloor$ [or $\lceil x \rceil$], respectively.

Let Γ denote a graph with vertex set V and edge set E. Then, $m(\Gamma(V))$ denotes the size of the graph, and the number of edges incident to a single vertex $v \in V$ is called the degree of v, $d(v)$; the maximum and minimum degrees of the graph are denoted by $\Delta(\Gamma(V))$ and $\delta(\Gamma(V))$, respectively. The graph $\Gamma(V)$ is said to be connected if and only if there is a path between any two distinct vertices of V, while the graph is complete if and only if any two vertices are adjacent, and K_m denotes the complete graph on m vertices. The complete subgraph of $\Gamma(V)$ is called a clique, and the clique number, $\omega(\Gamma(V))$, is the cardinality of the maximum clique. The diameter, $\text{diam}(\Gamma(V))$, is defined as the maximum distance between two vertices, and the radius, $r(\Gamma(V))$, is the minimum eccentricity of the graph, where the eccentricity of any vertex v is defined as $e(v) = \max\{d(v,u) : u \in V\}$. The length of the shortest cycle in $\Gamma(V)$ is called the girth of the graph, and it is denoted by $gr(\Gamma(V))$. A set S of vertices is said to be a dominating set if every vertex v belong to $V \setminus S$ is adjacent to at least one vertex in S, and the cardinality of the minimum dominating set, $\gamma - set$, is called the domination number, $\gamma(\Gamma(V))$. The minimum number of colors needed to label the vertices such that no two adjacent vertices have the same color is called the chromatic number of the graph, $\chi(\Gamma(V))$. The adjacency matrix is an $(n \times n)$ matrix, where $|V| = n$, and is denoted by $A(\Gamma(V))$. Almost all of the definitions and notations can be found in [12–14] for group theory and graph theory.

Through this work, we deal with finite groups and simple graphs. We consider the vertex set as the elements of the group and introduce the first type of equitable graph, $\mathcal{E}_1(G)$. In this paper, we study the connectedness of the equitable graph Type I for some groups and investigate some of their theoretical properties in Section 2. In Section 3, we introduce the concepts of the equitable square-free number and the equitable group. Then, the graph of this group is studied. Next, we determine the first, second and forgotten Zagreb indices for the equitable graph Type I of some groups in Section 4. Finally, in Section 5, we obtain the adjacency matrix for $\mathcal{E}_1(G)$, where G is a cyclic p-group, and many examples are included. In this work, since the vertices are the elements of the group G, we use the words "elements" and "vertices" interchangeably. Also, for simplicity, we use $\delta(\mathcal{E}_1)$, for example, rather than $\delta(\mathcal{E}_1(G))$.

2. Equitable Graph Type I

The definition of the first type of an equitable graph from any finite group is introduced in this section. Later, we explore some theoretical properties of this graph from certain groups.

Definition 1. *Let G be a finite group. The equitable graph of Type I of G, denoted by $\mathcal{E}_1(G)$, is a graph with vertex set G in which any two distinct elements of G, x and y are adjacent if and only if*

$$|o(x) - o(y)| \leq \min\{o(x), o(y)\}.$$

Example 1. *Consider the special linear group $G = SL(2,3)$ that is the group of 2×2 matrices with determinant 1 over the field of three elements. Then, the list of the elements is as follows:*

$$v_1 = \begin{pmatrix} 1 & 0 \\ 0 & 1 \end{pmatrix}, v_2 = \begin{pmatrix} 2 & 0 \\ 0 & 2 \end{pmatrix}, v_3 = \begin{pmatrix} 1 & 1 \\ 0 & 1 \end{pmatrix}, v_4 = \begin{pmatrix} 2 & 1 \\ 2 & 0 \end{pmatrix},$$

$$v_5 = \begin{pmatrix} 1 & 0 \\ 2 & 1 \end{pmatrix}, v_6 = \begin{pmatrix} 0 & 1 \\ 2 & 2 \end{pmatrix}, v_7 = \begin{pmatrix} 1 & 2 \\ 0 & 1 \end{pmatrix}, v_8 = \begin{pmatrix} 2 & 2 \\ 1 & 0 \end{pmatrix},$$

$$v_9 = \begin{pmatrix} 1 & 0 \\ 1 & 1 \end{pmatrix}, v_{10} = \begin{pmatrix} 0 & 2 \\ 1 & 2 \end{pmatrix}, v_{11} = \begin{pmatrix} 2 & 1 \\ 0 & 2 \end{pmatrix}, v_{12} = \begin{pmatrix} 1 & 1 \\ 2 & 0 \end{pmatrix},$$

$$v_{13} = \begin{pmatrix} 2 & 0 \\ 2 & 2 \end{pmatrix}, v_{14} = \begin{pmatrix} 0 & 1 \\ 2 & 1 \end{pmatrix}, v_{15} = \begin{pmatrix} 2 & 2 \\ 0 & 2 \end{pmatrix}, v_{16} = \begin{pmatrix} 1 & 2 \\ 1 & 0 \end{pmatrix},$$

$$v_{17} = \begin{pmatrix} 2 & 0 \\ 1 & 2 \end{pmatrix}, v_{18} = \begin{pmatrix} 0 & 2 \\ 1 & 1 \end{pmatrix}, v_{19} = \begin{pmatrix} 0 & 2 \\ 1 & 0 \end{pmatrix}, v_{20} = \begin{pmatrix} 0 & 1 \\ 2 & 0 \end{pmatrix},$$

$$v_{21} = \begin{pmatrix} 1 & 1 \\ 1 & 2 \end{pmatrix}, v_{22} = \begin{pmatrix} 2 & 1 \\ 1 & 1 \end{pmatrix}, v_{23} = \begin{pmatrix} 1 & 2 \\ 2 & 2 \end{pmatrix}, v_{24} = \begin{pmatrix} 2 & 2 \\ 2 & 1 \end{pmatrix},$$

where v_1 has order 1, v_2 has order 2, v_3 to v_{10} have order 3, v_{11} to v_{18} have order 6, and v_{19} to v_{24} have order 4. Then $\mathcal{E}_1(G)$ is depicted in Figure 1.

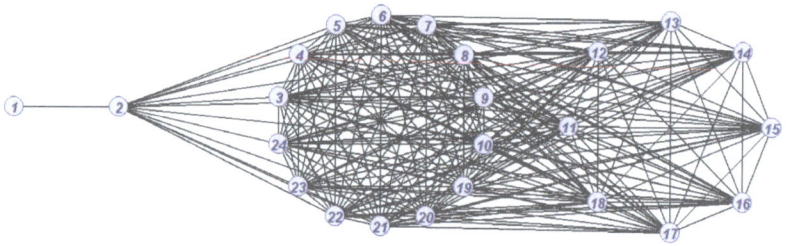

Figure 1. The equitable graph Type I of the group $SL(2,3)$.

- $\delta(\mathcal{E}_1(G)) = 1$, $\Delta(\mathcal{E}_1(G)) = 22$.
- $\chi(\mathcal{E}_1(G)) = \omega(\mathcal{E}_1(G)) = 22$.
- $gr(\mathcal{E}_1(G)) = 3$.
- $\gamma(\mathcal{E}_1(G)) = 2$.
- $diam(\mathcal{E}_1(G)) = 3$.
- $m(\mathcal{E}_1(G)) = 246$.

Lemma 1. $gr(\mathcal{E}_1(G)) = 3$ *for any finite group G with order greater than 3.*

Proof. Let G be a finite group of order n. Then, the result is clear for $n = 1$ or 2, and the only group of order 3 is a cyclic group in which the identity is isolated. Now, assume that $n = 4$; then there are only two possible cases for the group G. Either G is cyclic or G is isomorphic to the Klein four group $V_4 = \langle a, b : a^2 = b^2 = e, ab = ba \rangle$. In the first case, the element of order two is adjacent to the two elements of order four in $\mathcal{E}_1(G)$, forming a cycle with three edges. In the latter case, the graph is complete.

Now, if $n > 4$, it is clear that there exist at least three elements sharing the same order. Hence, $\mathcal{E}_1(G)$ contains K_3 as a subgraph. □

The following lemma has been utilized in numerous proofs throughout this research; therefore, it is prudent to mention it here.

Lemma 2. *Let i be a positive integer. Then*

1. $2^{i-2} + 2^{i-1} + 2^i = (7)2^{i-2}$.

2. $2^{i-2} + 2^{i-1} = (3)2^{i-2}$.

Theorem 1. *Let G be a cyclic group of order 2^k; $k > 1$ is a positive integer. Then $\mathcal{E}_1(G)$ is connected.*

Proof. As G is a cyclic group, the orders of the elements are the divisors of $|G|$. Now, as is well known, $|\ 2^i - 2^{i+1}\ | = 2^i$ for all $0 \leq i \leq k - 1$. Therefore, each element of order 2^i is adjacent to all elements of order 2^{i+1} (as vertices) for all $0 \leq i \leq k - 1$. Thus, we conclude that there is a path between any two vertices, and the graph $\mathcal{E}_1(G)$ can be shown as in Figure 2 such that each circle forms a complete subgraph.

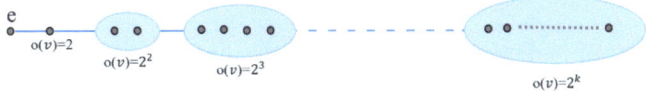

Figure 2. The equitable graph Type I of cyclic groups of order 2^k.
□

Theorem 2. *Let G be a cyclic group of order 2^k; $k > 1$ and is a positive integer. Then $\mathcal{E}_1(G)$ has the following properties:*

1. $\delta(\mathcal{E}_1) = 1$, and $\Delta(\mathcal{E}_1) = (7)2^{k-3} - 1$ unless $k = 2$, in which case $\Delta(\mathcal{E}_1) = 3$.
2. $\omega(\mathcal{E}_1) = (3)2^{k-2}$.
3. $\mathrm{diam}(\mathcal{E}_1) = k$.
4. $\mathcal{E}_1(G)$ is a weakly perfect graph.
5. $\gamma(\mathcal{E}_1) = \left\lceil \dfrac{k+1}{3} \right\rceil$.
6. $r(\mathcal{E}_1) = \begin{cases} \dfrac{k}{2}, & k \equiv 0 \pmod 2; \\ \dfrac{k+1}{2}, & \text{otherwise.} \end{cases}$
7. $m(\mathcal{E}_1) = 1 + \sum\limits_{i=1}^{k-1} 2^{i-1}(2^{i+1} - 1)$.

Proof. Let G be a cyclic group of order 2^k, where $k > 1$ is a positive integer.

1. In this case, the minimum degree and the maximum degree for $k = 2$ are obvious. Now, for $k > 2$, each element of order 2^i is adjacent to each element of order 2^{i-1} and 2^{i+1} for all $1 \leq i \leq k - 1$, and since the number of elements of order 2^m is $\phi(2^m) = 2^{m-1}$ as G is cyclic, for all $1 \leq m \leq k$, we obtain the result.
2. According to the fact that $\phi(2) = 1 < \phi(2^2) < \ldots < \phi(2^k)$ and from the adjacency criteria, the result can be obtained using Lemma 2.
3. This follows from Theorem 1 and the adjacency method of the vertices.
4. Since for any graph Γ, obviously $\chi(\Gamma) \geq \omega(\Gamma)$, we obtain that $\chi(\mathcal{E}_1) \geqslant 3(2^{k-2})$. Then, according to the adjacency order, we can reuse these colors, and hence, $\chi(\mathcal{E}_1) \leqslant 3(2^{k-2})$. Therefore, the equality holds.
5. Through the adjacency method and by Figure 2, we deduce that for each of three consecutive cliques, one vertex of the middle one can be in a dominating set. So the cardinality of $\gamma - \mathrm{set} \geqslant \dfrac{k+1}{3}$, and thus, from the definition of the domination number and the number of sequential cliques, we can obtain $\gamma(\mathcal{E}_1) \leqslant \dfrac{k+3}{3}$.

6. From Figure 2, we obtain that the eccentricity of the vertices ranges between k and $\frac{k}{2}$ (or $\left\lceil\frac{k}{2}\right\rceil$) if k is even (or odd). Therefore, $r(\mathcal{E}_1) = \left\lceil\frac{k}{2}\right\rceil$.

7. This follows from the adjacency method and the fact that the elements of the same order form a complete subgraph. Hence,

$$m(\mathcal{E}_1) = 1 + \sum_{i=2}^{k}\left[\frac{\phi(2^i)(\phi(2^i)-1)}{2} + \phi(2^{i-1})(\phi(2^i))\right]$$

□

Let n be a positive integer. Then the dihedral group of order $2n$ is defined as follows

$$D_{2n} = \langle a, b : a^n = b^2 = e, ab = ba^{-1}\rangle.$$

Example 2. *Consider the dihedral group of order 8, D_8. Then this group has one element of order 1, five elements of order 2, and two elements of order 4. Therefore, the equitable graph of D_8 is shown as in Figure 3, where v_1 denote the identity, $v_2 = a^2$, $v_3 = b$, $v_4 = ab$, $v_5 = a^2b$, $v_6 = a^3b$, $v_7 = a$, and $v_8 = a^3$.*

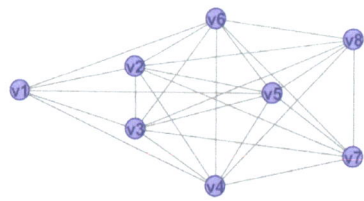

Figure 3. The equitable graph Type I of D_8.

Through the next two results, we explore the theoretical properties of the equitable graph of this group for special cases of n.

Theorem 3. *Consider the dihedral group $G \cong D_{2n}$; $n = 2^k$, $k > 1$. Then*

1. *$\mathcal{E}_1(G)$ is connected.*
2. *$\mathrm{diam}(\mathcal{E}_1(G)) = k$, and $\gamma(\mathcal{E}_1(G)) = \left\lceil\frac{k+1}{3}\right\rceil$.*
3. *$\chi(\mathcal{E}_1(G)) = \omega(\mathcal{E}_1(G)) = 2^k + 3$.*

Proof. Let $G \cong D_{2n}$; $n = 2^k$, $k > 1$. Then

1. The connectedness of this graph is satisfied since the order of the elements of D_{2n} in this case are clearly 2^i for each $1 \leq i \leq k$, which is the same as the cyclic group of order 2^k.
2. From the previous point, we obtain that the equitable graph Type I of this group and any cyclic group of order 2^k share the same *diameter and domination number*. Then by Theorem 2 we obtain the result.
3. The number of elements of order 2 in D_{2n} is equal to $n+1$, and for the remaining divisors of n, there are $\phi(2^m)$ elements for all $1 < m \leq k$. Hence, clearly, the maximum clique consists of the elements of order 2 in addition to the elements of order 2^2 by the connectedness. Therefore, we obtain the outcome.

□

Proposition 1. *Let G be the dihedral group D_{2n}; $n = 2^k$, $k > 1$. Then*

1. $\delta(\mathcal{E}_1(G)) = \begin{cases} 5, & k = 2 \text{ or } 3; \\ 11, & k = 4; \\ 13, & k \geq 5. \end{cases}$

2. $\Delta(\mathcal{E}_1(G)) = \begin{cases} 2^k + 6, & k \geq 3; \\ 7, & k = 2. \end{cases}$

Proof. Let G be the dihedral group D_{2n}; $n = 2^k$, $k > 1$. Then

1. From the adjacency method and according to the number of elements in each order in G, we attain the solution for $k = 2$, 3 or 4. Now, for all $k \geq 5$, we have that the degree of any element of order 2^3 is 13, which is the minimum among all others, and hence, we are done.
2. For the first case, since the elements of order 2^2 are adjacent to all elements of order 2, which include the maximum number of the elements, we obtain that

$$\Delta(\mathcal{E}_1(G)) = 2^k + 1 + \phi(2^2) - 1 + \phi(2^3) = 2^k + 6.$$

Now, when $k = 2$, let $v_{(j)}$ denote a vertex of order j. Then $d(v_{(1)}) = 5$, $d(v_{(2)}) = 7$, and $d(v_{(2^2)}) = 6$. Hence, we can conclude the result. □

Theorem 4. *Let G be a cyclic group of order p^k, where $p > 2$ is a prime number and $k > 1$. Then $\mathcal{E}_1(G)$ is disconnected.*

Proof. Let G be a cyclic group of order p^k, where $p > 2$ is a prime number and $k > 1$. Then the graph $\mathcal{E}_1(G)$ is as shown in Figure 4.

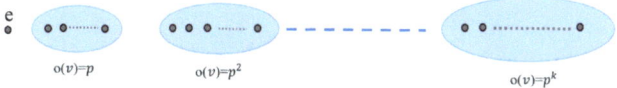

Figure 4. The equitable graph Type I of cyclic groups of order p^k.

Thus, for any $1 \leq i \leq k$, we have $|p^i - p^{i-1}| > \min\{p^i, p^{i-1}\}$. Hence, all elements of order p^i cannot be adjacent to any element of a different order. Therefore, the graph consists of disconnected cliques. □

Theorem 5. *Consider the cyclic group G of order p^k; $p > 2$ is a prime number, and $k > 1$. Then $\mathcal{E}_1(G)$ has the following properties*

1. $\delta(\mathcal{E}_1) = 0$, $\Delta(\mathcal{E}_1) = p^k - p^{k-1} - 1$.
2. *There are $k + 1$ components.*
3. $\gamma(\mathcal{E}_1) = k + 1$.
4. $\omega(\mathcal{E}_1) = p^{k-1}(p - 1)$.
5. $\chi(\mathcal{E}_1) = p^{k-1}(p - 1)$.
6. $m(\mathcal{E}_1) = \sum_{i=1}^{k} \dfrac{(p^i - p^{i-1})[p^i - p^{i-1} - 1]}{2}.$

Proof. Let G be a cyclic group of order p^k; $p > 2$ is a prime number, and $k > 1$. Then

1. The result is clear for the minimum degree. Now, for the maximum degree, the result follows as each element of the same order forms a complete subgraph and since $\phi(p) < \phi(p^2) < \ldots < \phi(p^k)$. Thus, $\Delta(\mathcal{E}_1)$ is equal to the degree of any element of order p^k.
2. Since the elements of the same order form a clique and by Theorem 4, we obtain that the number of the components is the number of the divisors of $|G|$.

3. According to Theorem 4 and the method of the adjacency, one vertex from each clique can be in the dominating set that includes the identity. Thus, the cardinality of the dominating set is at most $k+1$. Therefore, the dominating set, say S, contains the identity and one vertex of order p^i for all $1 \leq i \leq k$, and hence, $|S| = k+1$.
4. The result is direct as the number of vertices in each clique equals $\phi(p^i)$ for all $1 \leq i \leq k$.
5. By the previous point, we obtain that at least $p^{k-1}(p-1)$ colors are needed to label the vertices. Since the components are disjoint, these colors can be reused. Hence, $\chi(\mathcal{E}_1) = \omega(\mathcal{E}_1)$.
6. The result can be obtained through the adjacency method and from the fact that all of the elements of order p^i form a complete subgraph for all $1 \leq i \leq k$.

□

Theorem 6. *Let G be a cyclic group of order $2^k \cdot q$; $q > 2$ is a prime number, and $k > 1$, such that $|2^i - q| \leq \min\{2^i, q\}$ for some $1 \leq i \leq k$. Then $\mathcal{E}_1(G)$ is connected.*

Proof. It is known that the divisors of n consist of 1, 2, 2^2, ..., 2^k, q, $2q$, $2^2 q$, ..., $2^k q$. Then by Theorem 1, we obtain that the vertices of orders 1, 2, ..., 2^k are connected. Consequently, $|2^j q - 2^{j-1} q| = 2^{j-1} q = \min\{2^j q, 2^{j-1} q\}$ for all $1 \leq j \leq k$, and this is achieved by the connectedness of the vertices of orders q, 2q, ..., $2^k q$. Therefore, by the condition $|2^i - q| \leq \min\{2^i, q\}$ for some $1 \leq i \leq k$, the connectedness of this graph holds. □

Proposition 2. *Let G be a cyclic group of order $2^k q$; $q > 2$ is a prime number, and $k > 1$. Then $\mathcal{E}_1(G)$ has the following properties*

1. $\delta(\mathcal{E}_1) = 1$.
2. $\chi(\mathcal{E}_1) = \omega(\mathcal{E}_1) = \phi(n) + \phi(\frac{n}{2})$.
3. $\Delta(\mathcal{E}_1) = \begin{cases} \phi(n) + \phi(\frac{n}{2}) + \phi(\frac{n}{3}) + \phi(\frac{n}{4}) - 1, & \text{if } q = 3; \\ \phi(n) + \phi(\frac{n}{2}) + \phi(\frac{n}{4}) - 1, & \text{if } q > 3. \end{cases}$

Proof. Let G be a cyclic group of order $2^k q$; $q > 2$ is a prime number, and $k > 1$. Then for the first point, the proof is followed, since $deg(e) = 1$, which is the minimum among all vertices. For (2), as the orders n and $\frac{n}{2}$ involve the largest number of elements, and since $|2^k q - 2^{k-1} q| \leq \min\{2^k q, 2^{k-1} q\}$, $|2^k q - 2^k| > \min\{2^k q, 2^k\}$, and $|2^k q - 2^{k-2} q| > \min\{2^k q, 2^{k-2} q\}$, we obtain that the vertices of orders n and $\frac{n}{2}$ form the maximum clique. It is clear that $\chi(\mathcal{E}_1) \geq \omega(\mathcal{E}_1)$. But from the relations above, we deduce that the colors of the vertices of order n can be reused. Thus, $\chi(\mathcal{E}_1) \leq \omega(\mathcal{E}_1)$.

The maximum degree of this graph is the degree of a vertex of order $\frac{n}{2}$; this follows from the previous points and according to the adjacency method. Now, if $q > 3$, we have $|2 - q| > \min\{2, q\}$. Consequently, $|2^k - 2^{k-1} q| > \min\{2^k, 2^{k-1} q\}$. Hence, by the arrangement of the order as in Theorem 6, we obtain the result. Otherwise, if $q = 3$, since $|3 - 2| \leq \min\{3, 2\}$, we obtain that $|2^{k-1} 3 - 2^k| \leq \min\{2^{k-1} 3, 2^k\}$. Also, as $|3 - 1| > \min\{3, 1\}$, then $|2^{k-1} 3 - 2^{k-1}| > \min\{2^{k-1} 3, 2^{k-1}\}$. Then

$$\Delta(\mathcal{E}_1) = \phi(2^k 3) + \phi(2^{k-1} 3) + \phi(2^k) + \phi(2^{k-2} 3) - 1. \tag{1}$$

□

Theorem 7. *Let G be a cyclic group of order $2^k q$; $q > 2$ is a prime number, and $k > 1$. Then $\mathcal{E}_1(G)$ has the following properties:*

1. *If $\mathcal{E}_1(G)$ is connected, then*
   (a) $\begin{cases} \gamma(\mathcal{E}_1) = \lfloor \frac{t-4}{5} \rfloor + 2, & \text{if } q = 3; \\ \lfloor \frac{t-4}{5} \rfloor + 2 \leq \gamma(\mathcal{E}_1) \leq \lceil \frac{t}{3} \rceil, & \text{if } q > 3. \end{cases}$

(b) $\text{diam}(\mathcal{E}_1) = (t-1) - (k-i)$.

where i is a positive integer such that $2^i \leq q \leq 2^{i+1}$, and t denotes the number of divisors of n, which in this case is equal to $2(k+1)$.

2. If $\mathcal{E}_1(G)$ is disconnected, then $\gamma(\mathcal{E}_1) = 2\lceil \frac{k+1}{3} \rceil$.

Proof. Let G be a cyclic group of order $2^k.q$; $q > 2$ is a prime number, and $k > 1$. Then consider the connected case of the graph, and let $q = 3$; then the divisors of n will be in the following order:

$$1, 2, 3, 2^2, 2.3, 2^3, 2^2 3, 2^4, 2^3 3, \ldots, 2^k, 2^{k-1} 3, 2^k 3.$$

Let $v_{(j)}$ denote a single vertex corresponding to an element of order j. Now, as the vertex that is associated with the element of order 2, say $v_{(2)}$, is adjacent to the identity and all vertices that are associated with elements of order 3 and 4, thus $v_{(2)}$ belongs to the dominating set S. For the remaining $t - 4$ divisors, we have the following relation:

It is clear that any vertex associated with an element of order 2^i, say $v_{(2^i)}$, is adjacent to all symmetrical vertices and all $v_{(2^{i-1})}$ and $v_{(2^{i+1})}$ for all $2 \leq i \leq k-1$. This implies that any vertex $v_{(2^i 3)}$ is adjacent to all vertices of orders $2^{i+1} 3$ and $2^{i-1} 3$.

Also, since $|2 - 3| \leq \min\{2, 3\}$, we have $|2^i - 2^{i-1} 3| \leq \min\{2^i, 2^{i-1} 3\}$. And as $|2^2 - 3| \leq \min\{2^2, 3\}$, we obtain $|2^i - 2^{i-2} 3| \leq \min\{2^i, 2^{i-2} 3\}$ for all $2 \leq i \leq k-2$. Therefore, $v_{(2^i 3)}$ is adjacent to all symmetrical vertices and all vertices $v_{(2^{i-1} 3)}, v_{(2^{i+1} 3)}, v_{(2^{i+1})}$ and $v_{(2^{i+2})}$. Also, each vertex $v_{(2^i)}$ is adjacent to all symmetrical vertices and all vertices $v_{(2^{i-1})}, v_{(2^{i+1})}, v_{(2^{i-2} 3)}$ and $v_{(2^{i-1} 3)}$. Thus, according to the order of elements mentioned at the beginning of the proof, we find that the dominating set contains $v_{(2^2 3)}, v_{(2^6)}, v_{(2^7 3)}, v_{(2^{11})}, \ldots, v_{(2^{k-1})}$ or $v_{(2^k)}$; so for every five consecutive divisors, one vertex can be in S, and so $\gamma(\mathcal{E}_1) > \lfloor \frac{t-4}{5} \rfloor + 1$. But since $|2^k 3 - 2^k| > \min\{2^k 3, 2^k\}$, one vertex of $v_{(n)}$ or $v_{(\frac{n}{2})}$ must be in S. Hence, we conclude the result. On the other hand, concerning the case of $q > 3$, $|2 - q| > \min\{2, q\}$, where the minimum value for this occurs at q = 3, so the graph in this case is more interconnected based on the relationships mentioned previously. So $\gamma(\mathcal{E}_1) > \lfloor \frac{t-4}{5} \rfloor + 2$. But the equality is possible given that numerous examples achieve it. For instance, if $n = 2^4 5$, then, according to the order of the divisors, which is as follows:

$$1, 2, 2^2, 5, 2^3, 2(5), 2^4, 2^2(5), 2^3(5), 2^4(5),$$

we obtain that the minimum dominating set contains the vertices $v_{(2)}, v_{(2(5))}$ and $v_{(2^4(5))}$, where $v_{(j)}$ denotes a single vertex associated with an element of order j. Hence, $\gamma(\mathcal{E}_1) = 3 = \lfloor \frac{10-4}{5} \rfloor + 2$, and this yields the desired result. Also, it is clear that $\gamma(\mathcal{E}_1)$ cannot be more than $\lceil \frac{t}{3} \rceil$, whereas the occurrence of the maximum probability arises when for every set of three consecutive divisors (orders), a singular vertex having an order equal to the middle divisor is included in the dominating set.

The diameter of $\mathcal{E}_1(G)$ in this case is clearly equal to the distance between the identity and an element of order $2^k q$ (as each divisor of n corresponds to a clique in $\mathcal{E}_1(G)$). Thus, if $q > 2^k$, then $\text{diam}(\mathcal{E}_1) = t - 1$. Otherwise, if $2^i < q < 2^{i+1}$ for some $1 \leq i \leq k-1$, then

$$2^{i+1} < 2q < 2^{i+2}$$
$$2^{i+2} < 2^2 q < 2^{i+3}$$
$$\vdots$$
$$2^{k-1} < 2^{(k-1)-i} q < 2^k.$$

Then, the path, say P, that joined the identity with $v_{(2^k q)}$ will be as follows: $v_{(1)} - v_{(2)} - \ldots - v_{(2^i)} - v_{(2^{i+1})} - \ldots - v_{(2^k)} - v_{(2^{k-i})q} - \ldots - v_{(2^{k-1} q)} - v_{(2^k q)}$.

Now, as has been shown, all the vertices corresponding to the elements of orders $q, 2q, \ldots,$ and $2^{(k-1)-i} q$ have been excluded from P. This reduces the length by about $(k-1) - i + 1 = k - i$. Therefore, the result is obtained.

Finally, when the graph $\mathcal{E}_1(G)$ is disconnected, meaning $|2^k - q| > \min\{2^k, q\}$ and $q > 2^k$, there are two components by Theorem 6, and each component consists of $k + 1$ cliques that are joined successively as in Theorem 1. Therefore, in this case, the domination number is twice the value of the domination number in Theorem 2. □

Theorem 8. *Let S_n and A_n be the symmetric and alternating groups, respectively, on a set of n elements. Then*

1. *$\mathcal{E}_1(S_n)$, where $n \geq 2$, is connected.*
2. *$\mathcal{E}_1(A_n)$ is connected for all $n > 3$.*

Proof. The proof is straightforward due to the nature of the orders of the elements in these groups. □

The following theorems have been referenced for their applications in verifying the *Eulerian* and planar properties of this graph.

Theorem 9 ([14] (Theorem 6.2.2)). *For nontrivial connected graph Γ, the following statements are equivalent:*

1. *Γ is Eulerian.*
2. *The degree of each vertex of Γ is an even positive integer.*
3. *Γ is an edge-disjoint union of cycles.*

Theorem 10 ([14] (Theorem 8.4.1)). *K_5 is nonplanar.*

Theorem 11. *Let G be a cyclic group of order n; n is a positive integer. Then*

1. *$\mathcal{E}_1(G)$ is not Eulerian for all $n \geq 3$.*
2. *$\mathcal{E}_1(G)$ is not Hamiltonian for all $n \geq 2$.*

Proof. Let G be a cyclic group of order n; n is a positive integer. Then the proof of the first point follows from Theorem 9 since whenever the graph $\mathcal{E}_1(G)$ is connected, the degree of the identity vertex is equal to one, which is an odd integer. Now, for the second point, according to the definition of the graph and since there is exactly one element of order 2 in this group, there is only one edge that is incident to the identity. Hence, it is impossible to have any Hamiltonian cycle in $\mathcal{E}_1(G)$. □

Theorem 12. *Let G be a cyclic group of order n; n is a positive integer. Then $\mathcal{E}_1(G)$ is planar for all $n \leq 6$ and nonplanar otherwise.*

Proof. Let G be a cyclic group of order n; n is a positive integer. Then for each $n > 6$, the graph $\mathcal{E}_1(G)$ contains an induced subgraph K_5, and this implies the nonplanarity of the graph. On the other hand, the proof is obvious for $n = 1, 2, 3$ and 4. Also, if $n = 5$, then $\mathcal{E}_1(G)$ consists of an isolated vertex, which is the identity, and the complete graph k_4, and hence, it is planar. Finally, the planarity of the graph when $n = 6$ is shown in Figure 5.

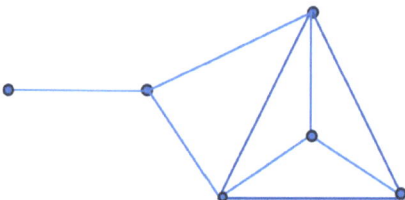

Figure 5. The plane embedding of a cyclic group of order 6.
□

3. Equitable Square-Free Number

This section endeavors to establish the conceptual frameworks of the equitable square-free number and the equitable group. Furthermore, it encompasses a comprehensive study of the connectedness properties inherent to the equitable graph Type I associated with such a group, and we analyze its characteristics in detail.

Definition 2. *Let $p_1 < p_2 < \cdots < p_k$ be distinct prime numbers. The square-free number $n = \prod_{i=1}^{k} p_i$ is called an equitable square-free number if and only if $p_{i+1} - p_i \leq p_i$ for all $i = 1, 2, \cdots, k-1$.*

Theorem 13. *Let n be an equitable square-free number and consider the cyclic group G of order n. Then*

1. *For $p_1 = 2$, $\mathcal{E}_1(G)$ is connected.*
2. *For $p_1 > 2$, $\mathcal{E}_1(G)$ is disconnected.*

Proof. Let G be a cyclic group of order n, where n is an equitable square-free number. Then the divisors of n will be arranged, in general, as follows:

$1, p_1, p_2, \cdots, p_k, p_1p_2, p_1p_3, \cdots, p_1p_k, p_2p_3, \cdots\cdots, p_{k-1}p_k, p_1p_2p_3, p_1p_2p_4, \cdots\cdots, p_{k-2}p_{k-1}p_k, p_1p_2p_3p_4, \cdots\cdots, p_1p_2\cdots p_{k-1}, \cdots, p_2p_3\cdots p_k, p_1p_2\cdots p_k = n$

Since the order of the elements is the divisor of n, we first need to prove that any vertices that have an order equal to the product of the same number of primes form a component; that is, any two vertices of orders with the same number of primes have a path between them. This is clear for order 1 since there is only one vertex that has this order, which is the identity. Also, the vertices with order n clearly form a component.

Now we will prove this for the remaining divisors by using the mathematical induction on the number of primes in the prime factorization of the divisors, say m. The proof is clear for $m = 1$, $n = p_i$; $1 \leq i \leq k$ according to the choice of n.

The base case of $m = 2$:

Let $d_1 = p_i p_j$ and $d_2 = p_t p_s$ be any two divisors such that $j < i, t < s$, and $j \leq t$. By the definition of n, we have

$$|p_{i+1} - p_i| \leq \min\{p_{i+1}, p_i\}; \text{for all } i = 1, 2, \ldots, k-1.$$

Then

$$|p_j p_{i+1} - p_j p_i| \leq \min\{p_j p_{i+1}, p_j p_i\} \qquad (2)$$

So if $t = j$, then this forms a path between the vertices of order d_1 and d_2. If $j < t$, then we have the following:

By inequality (2), we can find a path from the vertices of order $p_j p_i$ to the vertices of order $p_j p_k$. Hence, from the ordering of the divisors, we obtain that:

$$\begin{aligned} p_{j+1}p_{j+2} - p_j p_k &= p_{j+1}p_{j+2} - p_j p_{j+2} + p_j p_{j+2} - p_j p_k & (3) \\ &\leq p_j p_{j+2} + p_j p_{j+2} - p_j p_k & (4) \\ &= p_j(2p_{j+2} - p_k) \leq p_j p_k & (5) \end{aligned}$$

Then

$$|p_{j+1}p_{j+2} - p_j p_k| \leq \min\{p_{j+1}p_{j+2}, p_j p_k\} \qquad (6)$$

This forms an edge between the vertices of these orders. Then by using the same fact as in inequality (2), we obtain that there is a path from the vertices of order $p_j p_i$ to the vertices of order $p_{j+1} p_k$. Continuing the process in the inequalities (2) and (6), we can find a path between vertices of orders d_1 and d_2. Therefore, for all $\alpha \in S_k$ such that $\alpha \neq e$ and $\alpha(j) < \alpha(i)$, there is a path from any vertex of order $p_j p_i$ to any vertex of order $p_{\alpha(j)} p_{\alpha(i)}$, where $1 \leq j < i \leq k$.

The inductive hypothesis: Assume that this is true for all $m < k-1$. That is, for all $\alpha \in S_k$ such that $\alpha \neq 1$ and $\alpha(i_1) < \alpha(i_2) < \cdots < \alpha(i_m)$, there is a path between any two vertices of orders $\prod_{j=1}^{m} p_{i_j}$ and $\prod_{j=1}^{m} p_{\alpha(i_j)}$.

The inductive proof: Let $m = k-1$, and $d_i = \prod_{t=1}^{k-1} p_{i_t}$ and $d_j = \prod_{s=1}^{k-1} p_{j_s}$ are any two divisors such that $p_{i_t} < p_{i_{t+1}}$ and $p_{j_s} < p_{j_{s+1}}$ for all $1 \le t, s \le k-2$. By the inductive hypothesis, we have that there is a path between the vertices of orders $d'_i = \prod_{t=1}^{k-2} p_{i_t}$ and $d'_j = \prod_{s=1}^{k-2} p_{j_s}$. Now if $p_{i_{k-1}} = p_{j_{k-1}}$, we are done. So without loss of generality, let $p_{i_{k-1}} < p_{j_{k-1}}$. Then, similarly to the base case, we can find a path between the vertices of orders $d_i = d'_i p_{i_{k-1}}$ and $d_j = d'_j p_{j_{k-1}}$. Hence, for all $\alpha \in S_k$ such that $\alpha \neq e$ and $\alpha(i_1) < \alpha(i_2) < \cdots < \alpha(i_{k-1})$, there is a path from the vertices of order $\prod_{t=1}^{k-1} p_{i_t}$ to the vertices of order $\prod_{t=1}^{k-1} p_{\alpha(i_t)}$.

Now, assume that $p_1 = 2$. Then by the first part, we need to check the connectedness between the components, and this is clear from the fact that for any integer m,

$$|2m - m| = m = \min\{2m, m\}.$$

Thus, for any divisor $d = p_{i_1} p_{i_2} \ldots p_{i_t}$, where $2 \le t \le k-1$ and $2 < p_{i_1} < p_{i_2} < \cdots < p_{i_t}$, we have

$$|2d - d| = d \le \min\{2d, d\} \qquad (7)$$

Therefore, there is a path from any element of order $\prod_{t=1}^{m} p_{i_t}$ to any element of order $\prod_{j=1}^{m+1} p_{i_j}$, where $1 \le m \le k-1$. Therefore, there is a path between any two vertices in $\mathcal{E}_1(G)$. Otherwise, if $p_1 > 2$, since $|p_i - 1| > \min\{p_i, 1\}$ for all $i = 1, 2, \ldots, k$, we have that for any divisor d of $|G|$,

$$|d - 1| > \min\{d, 1\} \qquad (8)$$

Then, there is no edge between the identity and any other vertex in the graph. Hence, the identity is an isolated vertex. □

For the disconnected case delineated in Theorem 13, the subsequent theorem examines the cardinality of its constituent components.

Theorem 14. *Let G be a cyclic group of order $n = \prod_{i=1}^{k} p_i$, where n is an equitable square-free number, and consider that $p_1 > 2$. Then*

1. *$\mathcal{E}_1(G)$ has 3 or 4 components for $k = 2$ or 3, respectively.*
2. *For $k > 3$, we have*
   - *If $|p_1 p_2 - p_t| \le \min\{p_1 p_2, p_t\}$ for some $3 < t \le k$. Then $\mathcal{E}_1(G)$ has 3 components.*
   - *If $|p_1 p_2 - p_i| > \min\{p_1 p_2, p_i\}$ for all $3 < i \le k$, then the number of the components in $\mathcal{E}_1(G)$ will be as follows:*

$$\begin{cases} 5, & |p_1 p_2 p_3 - p_t p_l| \le \{p_1 p_2 p_3, p_t p_l\} \text{ for some } 1 \le t < l \le k; \\ k+1, & |p_1 p_2 p_3 - p_i p_j| > \{p_1 p_2 p_3, p_i p_j\} \text{ for all } 1 \le i < j \le k. \end{cases}$$

Proof. Let G be a cyclic group of order $n = \prod_{i=1}^{k} p_i$, where n is an equitable square-free number. Now as $p_1 > 2$, we have $|p_i - 1| > \min\{p_i, 1\}$. Then

$$\left| n - \prod_{r=1}^{k-1} p_{i_r} \right| > \prod_{r=1}^{k-1} p_{i_r} = \min\{n, \prod_{r=1}^{k-1} p_{i_r}\} \qquad (9)$$

Thus, there is no edge between the elements of order $\prod_{r=1}^{k-1} p_{i_r}$ and the elements of order equal to n. These two components are depicted in Figure 6.

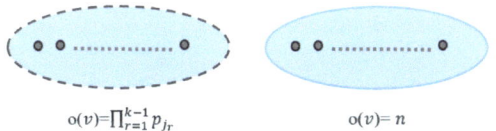

Figure 6. The disconnecting of the last components in $\mathcal{E}_1(G)$.

In the figure, the dotted line circle represents a connected (not complete) subgraph, and $o(v)$ denotes the order of the element v in the group G. Hence, when $k = 2$, $\mathcal{E}_1(G)$ obviously has three components, as is shown in Figure 7.

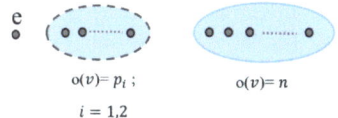

Figure 7. The equitable graph Type I of G with $k = 2$.

Let $k = 3$. Then according to the choice of the prime numbers, we have $|p_1 p_2 - p_3| > \min\{p_1 p_2, p_3\}$. So there is no edge between any element of order p_i and any element of order $p_r p_s$. Thus, the graph has 4 components, as shown in Figure 8.

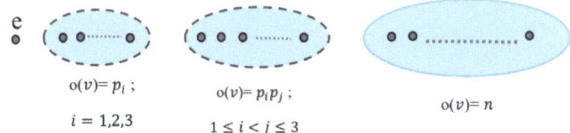

Figure 8. The equitable graph Type I of G with $k = 3$.

Now let $k > 3$ and assume that $|p_1 p_2 - p_t| \leq \min\{p_1 p_2, p_t\}$ for some $3 < t \leq k$. This implies that there is a path between any two elements of order p_i and $p_r p_s$ for all $1 \leq i \leq k$ and $1 \leq r < s \leq k$, respectively. Also, by this assumption, we obtain that

$$|p_1 p_2 \ldots p_{t-1} p_{t+1} \ldots p_k - p_3 \ldots p_{t-1} p_t p_{t+1} \ldots p_k| \leq \min\{p_1 p_2 \ldots p_{t-1} p_{t+1} \ldots p_k, p_3 \ldots p_{t-1} p_t p_{t+1} \ldots p_k\} \quad (10)$$

Hence, there is a path between all elements of order $\prod_{r=1}^{k-1} p_{i_r}$ and $\prod_{s=1}^{k-2} p_{j_s}$. Also, by choosing any $2 < i \leq k$ such that $i \neq t$, we obtain that

$$|p_1 p_2 p_i - p_t p_i| \leq \min\{p_1 p_2 p_i, p_t p_i\} \quad (11)$$

And this forms a path between the elements of order $\prod_{r=1}^{3} p_{i_r}$ and $\prod_{s=1}^{2} p_{j_s}$. Continuing this process, we obtain that there is a path between any two elements of order $\prod_{r=1}^{m} p_{i_r}$ and $\prod_{s=1}^{m-1} p_{j_s}$ for all $3 \leq m \leq k-2$. Therefore, there is a path between any two elements of order $\prod_{r=1}^{m} p_{i_r}$ and $\prod_{s=1}^{t} p_{j_s}$, where $1 \leq m, t \leq k-1$, and hence, these vertices form a component. Thus, the graph in this case is expressed as in Figure 9.

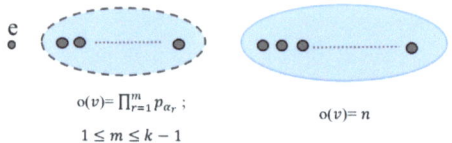

Figure 9. $\mathcal{E}_1(G)$ with 3 components, where $k > 3$.

On the other hand, if $|p_1 p_2 - p_i| > \min\{p_1 p_2, p_i\}$ for all $3 < i \leq k$. By the increasing of the primes, we have that $p_1 p_2 < p_i p_j$ for all $1 \leq i \leq k-1, 2 < j \leq k$ and $i < j$. Then

$$|p_i p_j - p_r| > \min\{p_i p_j, p_r\}; \forall 1 \leq r \leq k \text{ and } 1 \leq i < j \leq k \tag{12}$$

Therefore, there is no path between any two elements of order p_r and $p_i p_j$. Hence, the two components C_1 and C_2 are disjoint, where C_m denotes the components that consist of all elements of order $\prod_{j=1}^{m} p_{i_j}$ for all $1 \leq m \leq k$. Consequently, we have

$$\left|\prod_{r=1}^{k-1} p_{i_r} - \prod_{s=1}^{k-2} p_{j_s}\right| > \min\left\{\prod_{r=1}^{k-1} p_{i_r}, \prod_{s=1}^{k-2} p_{j_s}\right\} \tag{13}$$

Thus, the disjoint components are depicted in Figure 10.

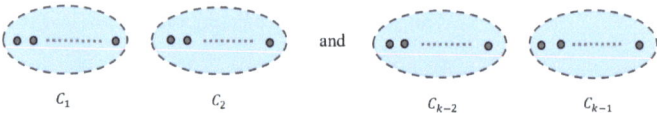

Figure 10. The disconnected components in $\mathcal{E}_1(G)$ with 5 components.

Now consider the case $|p_1 p_2 p_3 - p_t p_l| \leq \min\{p_1 p_2 p_3, p_t p_l\}$ for some $1 \leq t < l \leq k$. Hence, there is a path from any element of order $p_i p_j$ to any element of order $\prod_{r=1}^{3} p_{i_r}$. Then, by choosing any $c \notin \{1, 2, 3, t, l\}$, we obtain that $|p_1 p_2 p_3 p_c - p_t p_l p_c| \leq \min\{p_1 p_2 p_3 p_c, p_t p_l p_c\}$. Thus, this forms a path from any element of order $\prod_{r=1}^{3} p_{i_r}$ to any element of order $\prod_{s=1}^{4} p_{j_s}$. Sustaining this procedure, we obtain that

$$\left|\prod_{r=1}^{m} p_{i_r} - \prod_{s=1}^{m-1} p_{j_s}\right| \leq \min\left\{\prod_{r=1}^{m} p_{i_r}, \prod_{s=1}^{m-1} p_{j_s}\right\}; \forall 4 \leq m \leq k-2 \tag{14}$$

Therefore, there is a path between any two elements of these orders, and hence, it forms a component such as that shown in Figure 11.

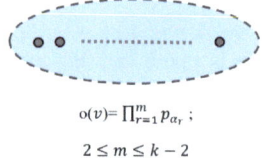

Figure 11. The middle component in $\mathcal{E}_1(G)$ with 5 components.

Otherwise, if $|p_1 p_2 p_3 - p_i p_j| > \min\{p_1 p_2 p_3, p_i p_j\}$ for all $1 \leq i < j \leq k$, then $p_1 p_2 p_3 > p_i p_j$ for all $1 \leq i < j \leq k$. Also, since $p_1 p_2 p_3 < p_i p_j p_r$ for all $1 \leq i < j < r \leq k$, we obtain that

$$|\prod_{r=1}^{3} p_{i_r} - \prod_{s=1}^{2} p_{j_s}| > \min\{\prod_{r=1}^{3} p_{i_r}, \prod_{s=1}^{2} p_{j_s}\} \tag{15}$$

Hence, there is no path between these components, as presented in Figure 12.

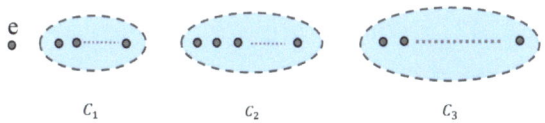

Figure 12. The disconnection of the first four components in $\mathcal{E}_1(G)$ with $k+1$ components.

From inequality (15), we obtain

$$|\prod_{r=1}^{k-2} p_{i_r} - \prod_{s=1}^{k-3} p_{j_s}| > \min\{\prod_{r=1}^{k-2} p_{i_r}, \prod_{s=1}^{k-3} p_{j_s}\} \tag{16}$$

Hence, these components are disjoint, as described in Figure 13.

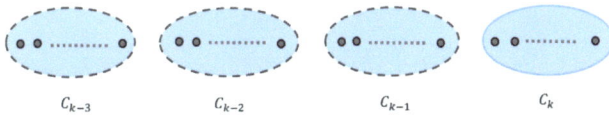

Figure 13. The disconnection of the last four components in $\mathcal{E}_1(G)$ with $k+1$ components.

Then, by the mathematical induction on the number of primes in the prime factorization of the divisors, say m, we will prove that the component containing elements of order $\prod_{r=1}^{m} p_{i_r}$ and the component consisting of elements of order $\prod_{r=1}^{m-1} p_{i_r}$ for all $4 \leq m \leq k-3$ are separated.

The base case, $m = 4$: First, claim $p_1 p_2 p_3 p_4 > p_{k-2} p_{k-1} p_k$. Then

$$p_1 p_2 p_3 p_4 > p_i p_j p_r; \text{ for all } 1 \leq i < j < r \leq k.$$

Now since $p_1 p_2 > p_i$ for all $1 \leq i \leq k$ and $p_1 p_2 p_3 > p_i p_j$ for all $1 \leq i < j \leq k$, then $p_1 p_2 p_3 > p_{k-1} p_k$.

Moreover, as p_4 is greater than every prime on the left side of the inequality and p_{k-2} is smaller than every prime on the other side, according to the choice of the primes, we obtain that

$$p_1 p_2 p_3 p_4 > p_{k-2} p_{k-1} p_k$$

Thus, by the increasing these numbers, we have

$p_1 p_2 p_3 p_4 > p_i p_j p_r$ for all $1 \leq i < j < r \leq k$. From inequality (15) and for any $t \in \{1, 2, \ldots, k\}$, such that $p_t > p_{i_r}$ and $p_t > p_{j_s}$ for all $r = 1, 2, 3$ and $s = 1, 2$, respectively, then

$$|\prod_{r=1}^{3} p_{i_r} p_t - \prod_{s=1}^{2} p_{j_s} p_t| > \min\{\prod_{r=1}^{3} p_{i_r} p_t, \prod_{s=1}^{2} p_{j_s} p_t\} \tag{17}$$

Furthermore, $p_1 p_2 p_3 - p_{k-1} p_k > \min\{p_1 p_2 p_3, p_{k-1} p_k\} = p_{k-1} p_k$

$$p_1 p_2 p_3 p_4 - p_4 p_{k-1} p_k > p_4 p_{k-1} p_k \tag{18}$$

and
$$p_1p_2p_3p_{k-2} - p_{k-2}p_{k-1}p_k > p_{k-2}p_{k-1}p_k \tag{19}$$
Then
$$p_1p_2p_3p_{k-2} - p_4p_{k-1}p_k > p_4p_{k-1}p_k \tag{20}$$
Then, adding the inequalities (18) and (19) gives
$$[p_1p_2p_3p_4 - p_{k-2}p_{k-1}p_k] + [p_1p_2p_3p_{k-2} - p_4p_{k-1}p_k] > p_{k-2}p_{k-1}p_k + p_4p_{k-1}p_k \tag{21}$$
Also, inequality (20) implies that
$$p_1p_2p_3p_4 - p_{k-2}p_{k-1}p_k > p_{k-2}p_{k-1}p_k$$
Then,
$$|\prod_{r=1}^{4} p_{i_r} - \prod_{s=1}^{3} p_{j_s}| > \min\{\prod_{r=1}^{4} p_{i_r}, \prod_{s=1}^{3} p_{j_s}\} \tag{22}$$

Thus, there is no path from any element of order $\prod_{s=1}^{3} p_{j_s}$ to any element of order $\prod_{r=1}^{4} p_{i_r}$.
The inductive hypothesis: Assume that this is true for all $m < k - 3$, that is
$$|\prod_{r=1}^{m} p_{i_r} - \prod_{s=1}^{m-1} p_{j_s}| > \min\{\prod_{r=1}^{m} p_{i_r}, \prod_{s=1}^{m-1} p_{j_s}\} \tag{23}$$

Then the resulting components are depicted in Figure 14.

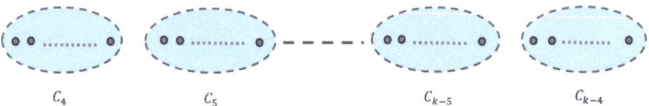

Figure 14. The disconnection of the middle components in $\mathcal{E}_1(G)$ with $k+1$ components.

The inductive proof: Claim that $|\prod_{r=1}^{k-3} p_{i_r} - \prod_{s=1}^{k-4} p_{j_s}| > \min\{\prod_{r=1}^{k-3} p_{i_r}, \prod_{s=1}^{k-4} p_{j_s}\}$. Now from the inductive hypothesis, we have for all $k-4 < s \leq k$ and $p_s > p_{i_j}$ for all $1 \leq j \leq k$,
$$|p_1p_2\ldots p_{k-4}p_s - \prod_{j=1}^{k-5} p_{i_j}p_s| > \min\{p_1p_2\ldots p_{k-4}p_s, \prod_{j=1}^{k-5} p_{i_j}p_s\} \tag{24}$$

Then, similarly to the base case, we obtain
$$p_1p_2\ldots p_{k-3} > p_5p_6\ldots p_k, \text{ and}$$
$$|p_1p_2\ldots p_{k-3} - p_5\ldots p_k| > \min\{p_1p_2\ldots p_{k-3}, p_5\ldots p_k\}$$
Then
$$|p_1p_2\ldots p_{k-3} - \prod_{j=1}^{k-4} p_{i_j}| > \min\{p_1p_2\ldots p_{k-3}, \prod_{j=1}^{k-4} p_{i_j}\} \tag{25}$$

And hence, $p_1p_2\ldots p_{k-3} > \prod_{j=1}^{k-4} p_{i_j}$.
Thus, the increase of the primes implies that
$$|\prod_{r=1}^{k-3} p_{i_r} - \prod_{s=1}^{k-4} p_{j_s}| > \min\{\prod_{r=1}^{k-3} p_{i_r}, \prod_{s=1}^{k-4} p_{j_s}\} \tag{26}$$

Therefore, there is no path between any two elements of orders $\prod_{r=1}^{k-3} p_{i_r}$ and $\prod_{s=1}^{k-4} p_{j_s}$. Hence, there is no path between any element of order $\prod_{r=1}^{m} p_{i_r}$ and any element of order $\prod_{s=1}^{m-1} p_{j_s}$ for all $4 \leq m \leq k-4$, and this complete the proof. □

Definition 3. *Let G be a finite group. Then G is said to be an equitable group if the order of G is an equitable square-free number.*

Example 3. *The symmetric group S_3, the dihedral group D_{30} and the cyclic group of order 1729 are examples of equitable groups.*

Corollary 1. *Let G be a cyclic equitable group of order $n = \prod_{i=1}^{k} p_i$, where p_i are distinct primes for all $1 \leq i \leq k$. Then the only cases in which $\mathcal{E}_1(G)$ is connected to $k = 2, 3$ or 4 are $n = 6, 30$ or 210, respectively.*

Proposition 3. *Let G be a cyclic equitable group of order $n = \prod_{i=1}^{k} p_i$, where $k > 2$ is a positive integer and p_i are distinct primes for all $1 \leq i \leq k$. Consider the disconnected graph $\mathcal{E}_1(G)$. Then $\mathcal{E}_1(G)$ has the following properties:*

1. $\delta(\mathcal{E}_1) = 0$,
2. $\chi(\mathcal{E}_1) = \omega(\mathcal{E}_1) = \phi(n)$,
3. $\Delta(\mathcal{E}_1) = \phi(n) - 1$,
4. $2k - 2 \leq \gamma(\mathcal{E}_1) \leq \lceil \frac{2^k - 2}{3} \rceil + 2$.

Proof. Let G be a cyclic equitable group of order $n = \prod_{i=1}^{k} p_i$, where $k > 2$ is a positive integer and p_i are distinct primes, and consider the disconnected graph $\mathcal{E}_1(G)$. Then, the identity is isolated, and hence, we obtain the result of the minimum degree. Also, since all the vertices that are associated with the elements of order n in G, which occupies the largest number of vertices, form a disjoint clique by Theorem 14, we obtain (2) and (3).

To prove (4), let C_m denote a component that consists of vertices that correspond to the elements of order $d_m = \prod_{j=1}^{m} p_{i_j}$, where $1 \leq m \leq k$ in the group. Then we have $k + 1$ components, including the identity. From Theorem 14, we obtain that the identity and one vertex from C_k belong to the dominating set, say S. The two components C_1 and C_{k-1} consist of $k = \binom{k}{1} = \binom{k}{k-1}$ connected cliques. Hence, taking into view the number of cliques in these components and the difference between the divisors, at least one vertex of each of them can be in S. Each one of the remaining $(k - 3)$ components consists of $\binom{k}{j}$ connected cliques, which is greater than k for all $2 \leq j \leq k - 2$. So again, based on a similar reason, at least two vertices of each component belong to S. Thus, the dominating set S consists of at least $4 + 2(k - 3) = 2k - 2$ components. The highest value that S can attain is $\lceil \frac{2^k - 2}{3} \rceil + 2$ since each divisor of n corresponds to a clique in this graph and, in our case, n has 2^k divisors. As previously explained, the identity and one vertex of C_k are included in the dominating set. Therefore, $2^k - 2$ cliques remain, in which, for each three consecutive cliques, one vertex can be in S, which has an order equal to the middle ones. □

Proposition 4. *Let G be a cyclic equitable group of order $n = \prod_{i=1}^{k} p_i$, where $k > 2$ is a positive integer and p_i are distinct primes. Consider the connected graph $\mathcal{E}_1(G)$. Then $\mathcal{E}_1(G)$ has the following properties:*

1. $\delta(\mathcal{E}_1) = 1$.
2. $\Delta(\mathcal{E}_1) = \phi(n) + \phi(\frac{n}{2}) + \phi(\frac{n}{3}) - 1$.
3. $\chi(\mathcal{E}_1) = \omega(\mathcal{E}_1) = \phi(n) + \phi(\frac{n}{2})$.
4. $\gamma(\mathcal{E}_1) \geq k + 1$ *unless* $k = 2, 3$ or 4, *in which case*, $\gamma(\mathcal{E}_1) = k$.
5. $\text{diam}(\mathcal{E}_1) \geq 2\gamma(\mathcal{E}_1)$ *unless* $k = 2, 3$ or 4, *in which case*, $\text{diam}(\mathcal{E}_1) = 3, 6$ or 10, *respectively.*

Proof. Let G be a cyclic equitable group of order $n = \prod_{i=1}^{k} p_i$, where $k > 2$ is a positive integer and p_i are distinct primes, and consider the connected graph $\mathcal{E}_1(G)$. Then the number of vertices that are associated with the elements of order 2 in G is $\phi(2) = 1$, for which the identity is uniquely adjacent to it, and this yields the result of (1). Now, the two following differences $|n - \frac{n}{2}| \leq \min\{n, \frac{n}{2}\}$ and $|\frac{n}{2} - \frac{n}{3}| \leq \min\{\frac{n}{2}, \frac{n}{3}\}$ lead to any vertex associated with an element of order $\frac{n}{2}$ being adjacent to all symmetrical vertices and all vertices that are associated with elements of order n and $\frac{n}{3}$. Moreover, as $|\frac{n}{2} - \frac{n}{5}| > \min\{\frac{n}{2}, \frac{n}{5}\}$ and $|n - \frac{n}{3}| > \min\{n, \frac{n}{3}\}$, taking into consideration the number of elements in each order, this gives (2) and (3), respectively.

The diameter and the domination number of the graph when $k = 2, 3$ or 4 is obtained obviously. On the other hand, let k be greater than four. Then the first four primes are always 2, 3, 5 and 7, which means that the divisors of n begin as 1, 2, 3, 5, 6, 7, 10, ..., $\frac{n}{2}$, n. Let $v_{(i)}$ denote a single vertex associated with an element of order i in G for all $1 \leq i \leq n$. Then we have $v_{(2)}, v_{(10)}, v_{(42)}, v_{(\frac{n}{2})}$ or $v_{(n)}$ and one vertex from the component C_{k-1}, where C_m is defined as in Proposition 3 are always belonging to S. Now for the residue components (C_3 to C_{k-2}), at least $k - 4$ vertices from these components can be included in the dominating set regarding the connectedness of the graph and the difference between the divisors. Thus, $\gamma(\mathcal{E}_1) \geq k + 1$.

Moreover, the diameter of the graph is clearly the shortest path from the identity to $v_{(n)}$, which, in this case, usually starts as $v_{(1)} \to v_{(2)} \to v_{(3)} \to v_{(6)} \to v_{(10)} \to \cdots \to v_{(n)}$.

So we obtain that each vertex in S gives at least two edges in this path in addition to the edge between $v_{(3)}$ and $v_{(6)}$. Hence, we conclude the result. □

4. Zagreb Indices of the Equitable Graph

Topological indices are crucial for analyzing the physico–chemical characteristics of chemical compounds. They include degree-based and distance-based molecular structures and hybrid formulations. These indices are leading tools for identifying physical properties, chemical reactivity and biological activities of compounds. For any graph Γ with vertex set V and edge set E, the first and second Zagreb indices are defined as $M_1(\Gamma) = \sum_{u \in V} (d(u))^2$ and $M_2(\Gamma) = \sum_{uv \in E} d(u)d(v)$. The forgotten index is similar to the first Zagreb index, which is defined as $F_i(\Gamma) = \sum_{u \in V} (d(u))^3$. For more details, see [15,16]. Through this section, we determine these three indices for the equitable graph Type I from some specific cyclic groups.

Theorem 15. *Let G be a cyclic group of order 2^k; $k > 1$ is a positive integer. Then the first, second and forgotten Zagreb indices of $\mathcal{E}_1(G)$ will be as follows:*

1. $M_1(\mathcal{E}_1(G)) = 10 + 2^{k-1}((3)2^{k-2} - 1)^2 + \sum_{i=1}^{k-2} 2^i((7)2^{i-1} - 1)^2$.

2. $M_2(\mathcal{E}_1(G)) = 3 + \sum_{i=1}^{k-1} 2^{2i-1}[d(v_{2^i})d(v_{2^{i+1}})] + \sum_{i=2}^{k} \left[\frac{s_i(s_i+1)}{2}\right][d(v_{2^i})]^2$
   where $s_i = \phi(2^i) - 1 = 2^{i-1} - 1$.

3. $F(\mathcal{E}_1(G)) = 28 + 2^{k-1}((3)2^{k-2} - 1)^3 + \sum_{i=1}^{k-2} 2^i((7)2^{i-1} - 1)^3$.

Proof. Let G be a cyclic group of order 2^k; $k > 1$ is a positive integer. Then as $\phi(2^i) = 2^{i-1}$ and for any vertex v that associates with an element of order 2^i; $2 \leq i \leq k - 1$, we have $d(v) = \phi(2^{i-1}) + \phi(2^i) - 1 + \phi(2^{i+1})$, and if $i = 1$ or k, $d(v) = 3$ or $[\phi(2^{k-1}) + \phi(2^k)]$, respectively. Then, computing $M_1(\mathcal{E}_1) = \sum_{v \in V(\mathcal{E})} d^2(v)$, we obtain

$M_1(\mathcal{E}_1(G)) = 1 + 9 + \phi(2^2)[1 + \phi(2^2) - 1 + \phi(2^3)]^2 + \phi(2^3)[\phi(2^2) + \phi(2^3) - 1 + \phi(2^4)]^2 + \cdots + \phi(2^{k-1})[\phi(2^{k-2}) + \phi(2^{k-1}) - 1 + \phi(2^k)]^2 + \phi(2^k)[\phi(2^{k-1}) + \phi(2^k) - 1]^2$.

Hence, substituting the value of $\phi(2^i)$ and using Lemma 2, we obtain the result.

Now for the second Zagreb index, let $v_{(2^i)}$ denote the vertex corresponding to an element of order 2^i; then

$$M_2(\mathcal{E}_1(G)) = \sum_{uv\in E(\mathcal{E}_1)} d(u)d(v)$$

$$= (1)(3) + 2[d(v_{(2)})d(v_{(2^2)})] + \left(\sum_{j=1}^{\phi(2^3)-1} j\right)[d(v_{(2^3)})]^2 + (2^2)(2^3)[d(v_{(2^3)})d(v_{(2^4)})]$$

$$+ \left(\sum_{j=1}^{\phi(2^4)-1} j\right)[d(v_{(2^4)})]^2 + \ldots\ldots + (2^{k-2})(2^{k-1})[d(v_{(2^{k-1})})d(v_{(2^k)})] +$$

$$\left(\sum_{j=1}^{\phi(2^k)-1} j\right)[d(v_{(2^k)})]^2.$$

Setting $s_i = \phi(2^i) - 1$, using the fact that $\sum_{j=1}^{n} j = \frac{n(n+1)}{2}$, and since all the vertices that correspond to elements of the same order have the same degree, we obtain what is required. For the forgotten index, we have the following:

$$F(\mathcal{E}_1(G)) = 1 + 27 + \phi(2^2)[1 + \phi(2^2) - 1 + \phi(2^3)]^3 + \phi(2^3)[\phi(2^2) + \phi(2^3) - 1 +$$
$$\phi(2^4)]^3 + \ldots + \phi(2^{k-1})[\phi(2^{k-2}) + \phi(2^{k-1}) - 1 + \phi(2^k)]^3 + \phi(2^k)[\phi(2^{k-1}) + \phi(2^k) - 1]^3.$$

Then, similarly to the first index, we obtain the desired outcome. □

Example 4. *Let G be a cyclic group of order 2^k; $k > 1$. Table 1 shows the value of the topological indices of $\mathcal{E}_1(G)$.*

Table 1. The topological indices of a cyclic group G of order 2^k for some $k > 1$.

	$|G| = 2^2$	$|G| = 2^3$	$|G| = 2^4$	$|G| = 2^5$	$|G| = 2^6$
$M_1(\mathcal{E}_1(G))$	18	182	1726	15,054	125,678
$M_2(\mathcal{E}_1(G))$	19	465	9677	176,325	300,5621
$F(\mathcal{E}_1(G))$	44	960	19,896	361,384	6,151,048

Theorem 16. *Let G be a cyclic group of order p^k; $p > 2$ is a prime number, and $k > 1$ is a positive integer. Then the first, second and forgotten Zagreb indices of $\mathcal{E}_1(G)$ will be as follows:*

1. $M_1(\mathcal{E}_1(G)) = \sum_{i=1}^{k}(p^i - p^{i-1})[p^i - p^{i-1} - 1]^2.$

2. $M_2(\mathcal{E}_1(G)) = \sum_{i=1}^{k}\left[\frac{s_i(s_i+1)}{2}\cdot(s_i)^2\right]$
   where $s_i = \phi(p^i) - 1$; $1 \leq i \leq k$.

3. $F(\mathcal{E}_1(G)) = \sum_{i=1}^{k}(p^i - p^{i-1})[p^i - p^{i-1} - 1]^3.$

Proof. Let G be a cyclic group of order p^k; $p > 2$ is a prime number, and $k > 1$ is a positive integer. Then the result for the first Zagreb and the forgotten indices follows from the fact that each clique in this graph has $\phi(p^i)$ vertices, where p^i is the order of the group elements that correspond to these vertices for all $1 \leq i \leq k$, and hence, the degree of any vertex v in such a clique is $\phi(p^i) - 1$.

Now for the second Zagreb index, since each vertex is adjacent only to the vertices that associate with elements of the same order, consider the clique, say Q, of vertices that correspond to elements of order p^i for some $1 \leq i \leq k$. Let $v_1, v_2, \ldots, v_t$, where $t = \phi(p^i)$.

Then $d(u) = d(v)$, $for\ all\ u \neq v\ in\ Q$, and by computing $\sum d(u).d(v)$, $uv \in E(\mathcal{E}_1)$, we obtain

$d(v_1)d(v_2) + d(v_1)d(v_3) + \ldots + d(v_1)d(v_t)$
$+ d(v_2)d(v_3) + d(v_2)d(v_4) + \ldots + d(v_2)d(v_t)$
$\vdots$
$+ d(v_{t-2})d(v_{t-1}) + d(v_{t-2})d(v_t) + d(v_{t-1})d(v_t)$
$= d(v_1)[(\phi(p^i) - 1)(d(v_1))] + d(v_2)[(\phi(p^i) - 2)(d(v_2))] + \ldots + d(v_{t-2})[2(d(v_{t-2}))]$
$+ d(v_{t-1})[1(d(v_{t-1}))]$
$= \sum_{j=1}^{t-1} j[d(v_j)]^2 = [\frac{t-1(t)}{2}](t-1)^2.$

Therefore, by generalizing this sum to all $1 \leq i \leq k$, we obtain the result. □

Example 5. *Let G be a cyclic group of order p^k; $k > 1$ and $p > 2$. Table 2 shows the value of the topological indices of $\mathcal{E}_1(G)$.*

Table 2. The topological indices of a cyclic group G of order p^k; $p > 2$ for some $k > 1$.

	$|G| = 3^2$	$|G| = 3^3$	$|G| = 5^2$	$|G| = 5^3$	$|G| = 7^2$	$|G| = 7^3$
$M_1(\mathcal{E}_1(G))$	152	157,040	7256	987,356	70,752	1,307,720
$M_2(\mathcal{E}_1(G))$	376	4,064,272	68,644	48,583,594	1,447,716	71,230,240
$F(\mathcal{E}_1(G))$	752	8,128,544	137,288	97,167,188	2,895,432	142,460,480

Theorem 17. *Let G be a cyclic group of order $2^k q$; $q > 2$ a prime number, and $k > 1$. Then the first Zagreb index is given by the following formula:*

- *If $2^t \leq q \leq 2^{t+1}$ for some $1 \leq t < k$, we have*

$M_1(\mathcal{E}_1(G)) = 10 + \sum_{i=1}^{t-1} 2^i[(7)2^{i-1} - 1]^2 + 2^{t-1}[(7)2^{t-2} + q - 2]^2 + (q-1)[(3)2^{t-1} + 2q - 3]^2 + \sum_{i=t+1}^{k-1} 2^{i-1}[(7)2^{i-2} + (3)2^{i-t-2}(q-1) - 1]^2 + \sum_{i=1}^{k-t-1} 2^{i-1}(q-1)[(7)2^{i-2}(q-1) + (3)2^{i+t-1} - 1]^2 + 2^{k-1}[(3)2^{k-2} + (3)2^{k-t-2}(q-1) - 1]^2 + 2^{k-t-1}(q-1)[2^{k-1} + (7)2^{k-t-2}(q-1) - 1]^2 + \sum_{i=k-t+1}^{k-1} 2^{i-1}(q-1)[(7)2^{i-2}(q-1) - 1]^2 + 2^{k-1}(q-1)[(3)2^{k-2}(q-1) - 1]^2.$

- *If $q > 2^k$, and $|q - 2^k| \leq \min\{q, 2^k\}$, we have*

$M_1(\mathcal{E}_1(G)) = 10 + \sum_{i=1}^{k-2} 2^i[(7)2^{i-1} - 1]^2 + 2^{k-1}[(3)2^{k-2} + q - 2]^2 + (q-1)[2^{k-1} + 2q - 3]^2 + \sum_{i=1}^{k-2} 2^i(q-1)[(7)2^{i-1}(q-1) - 1]^2 + 2^{k-1}(q-1)[(3)2^{k-2}(q-1) - 1]^2.$

- *If $q > 2^k$, and $|q - 2^k| > \min\{q, 2^k\}$, we have*

$M_1(\mathcal{E}_1(G)) = 10 + \sum_{i=1}^{k-2} 2^i[(7)2^{i-1} - 1]^2 + 2^{k-1}[(3)2^{k-2} - 1]^2 + (q-1)[2q - 3]^2 + \sum_{i=1}^{k-2} 2^i(q-1)[(7)2^{i-1}(q-1) - 1]^2 + 2^{k-1}(q-1)[(3)2^{k-2}(q-1) - 1]^2.$

Proof. Let G be a cyclic group of order $2^k q$; $q > 2$ a prime number, and $k > 1$. Then consider the arrangement of the divisors according to the position of the prime number q.

Assume the first case; then the divisors will be as follows:
$1, 2, 2^2, \ldots, 2^t, q, 2^{t+1}, 2q, 2^{t+2}, 2^2q, \ldots, 2^k, 2^{k-t}, \ldots, 2^kq$.

For the later cases, the divisors will be as mentioned in the proof of Theorem 6. Hence, applying identical procedures as outlined in Theorem 15 and using Lemma 2, we achieve the desired outcome. □

Theorem 18. *Let G be a cyclic group of order $2^k q$; $q > 2$ is a prime number, and $k > 1$. Then the second Zagreb index is given by the following formula:*

- *If $2^t \leq q \leq 2^{t+1}$ for some $1 \geq t < k$, then*

$$M_2(\mathcal{E}_1(G)) = 3 + \sum_{i=1}^{k-1} 2^{2i-1}[d(v_{(2^i)})d(v_{(2^{i+1})})] + \sum_{i=2^2}^{2^k q} [\frac{s_i(s_i+1)}{2}][d(v_{(i)})]^2$$
$$+ \sum_{i=0}^{k} \phi(2^i q)\phi(2^{i+1} q)[d(v_{(2^i q)})d(v_{(2^{i+1} q)})] + \sum_{i=t}^{k} 2^{2i-t-2}(q-1)[d(v_{(2^i)})d(v_{(2^{i-t} q)})]$$
$$+ \sum_{i=t+1}^{k} 2^{2i-t-3}(q-1)[d(v_{(2^{i-t-1} q)})d(v_{(2^i)})].$$

- *If $q > 2^k$, and $|q - 2^k| \leq \min\{q, 2^k\}$, then*

$$M_2(\mathcal{E}_1(G)) = 3 + \sum_{i=1}^{k-1} 2^{2i-1}[d(v_{(2^i)})d(v_{(2^{i+1})})] + \sum_{i=2^2}^{2^k q} [\frac{s_i(s_i+1)}{2}][d(v_{(i)})]^2 +$$
$$2^{k-1}(q-1)[d(v_{(2^k)})d(v_{(q)})] + \sum_{i=0}^{k-1} \phi(2^i q)\phi(2^{i+1} q)[d(v_{(2^i q)})d(v_{(2^{i+1} q)})].$$

- *If $q > 2^k$, and $|q - 2^k| > \min\{q, 2^k\}$, then*

$$M_2(\mathcal{E}_1(G)) = 3 + \sum_{i=1}^{k-1} 2^{2i-1}[d(v_{(2^i)})d(v_{(2^{i+1})})] + \sum_{i=2^2}^{2^k q} [\frac{s_i(s_i+1)}{2}][d(v_{(i)})]^2$$
$$+ \sum_{i=0}^{k-1} \phi(2^i q)\phi(2^{i+1} q)[d(v_{(2^i q)})d(v_{(2^{i+1} q)})].$$

where $s_i = \phi(i) - 1$ and $d(v_{(j)})$ denote the degree of a vertex that is associated with an element of order j.

Proof. Let G be a cyclic group of order $2^k q$; $q > 2$ a prime number, and $k > 1$. Then applying the same procedure as in Theorems 15 and 17, we obtain the result. □

Theorem 19. *Let G be a cyclic group of order $2^k q$; $q > 2$ is a prime number, and $k > 1$. Then the forgotten index is given by the following formula:*

- *If $2^t \leq q \leq 2^{t+1}$ for some $1 \geq t < k$, we have*

$$F(\mathcal{E}_1(G)) = 28 + \sum_{i=1}^{t-1} 2^i[(7)2^{i-1} - 1]^3 + 2^{t-1}[(7)2^{t-2} + q - 2]^3 + (q-1)[(3)2^{t-1}+$$
$$2q - 3]^3 + \sum_{i=t+1}^{k-1} 2^{i-1}[(7)2^{i-2} + (3)2^{i-t-2}(q-1) - 1]^3 + \sum_{i=1}^{k-t-1} 2^{i-1}(q-1)[(7)2^{i-2}(q-$$
$$1) + (3)2^{i+t-1} - 1]^3 + 2^{k-1}[(3)2^{k-2} + (3)2^{k-t-2}(q-1) - 1]^3 + 2^{k-t-1}(q-1)[2^{k-1}+$$
$$(7)2^{k-t-2}(q-1) - 1]^3 + \sum_{i=k-t+1}^{k-1} 2^{i-1}(q-1)[(7)2^{i-2}(q-1) - 1]^3 + 2^{k-1}(q-1)[(3)2^{k-2}(q-$$
$$1) - 1]^3.$$

- *If $q > 2^k$, and $|q - 2^k| \leq \min\{q, 2^k\}$, we have*

$$F(\mathcal{E}_1(G)) = 28 + \sum_{i=1}^{k-2} 2^i[(7)2^{i-1} - 1]^3 + 2^{k-1}[(3)2^{k-2} + q - 2]^3 + (q-1)[2^{k-1} + 2q -$$
$$3]^3 + \sum_{i=1}^{k-2} 2^i(q-1)[(7)2^{i-1}(q-1) - 1]^3 + 2^{k-1}(q-1)[(3)2^{k-2}(q-1) - 1]^3.$$

- If $q > 2^k$, and $|q - 2^k| > \min\{q, 2^k\}$, we have

$$F(\mathcal{E}_1(G)) = 28 + \sum_{i=1}^{k-2} 2^i[(7)2^{i-1} - 1]^3 + 2^{k-1}[(3)2^{k-2} - 1]^3 + (q-1)[2q - 3]^3 +$$
$$\sum_{i=1}^{k-2} 2^i(q-1)[(7)2^{i-1}(q-1) - 1]^3 + 2^{k-1}(q-1)[(3)2^{k-2}(q-1) - 1]^3.$$

Proof. Let G be a cyclic group of order $2^k q$; $q > 2$ is a prime number, and $k > 1$. Then the proof is similar to Theorems 15 and 17. □

5. The Adjacency Matrix $A(\mathcal{E}_1(G))$

In graph theory, the adjacency matrix of a simple graph Γ is a symmetric matrix $A(\Gamma) = (a_{ij})$ of size $n \times n$, where n represents the number of vertices in the graph. The matrix is defined such that $a_{ij} = 1$ if the vertices v_i and v_j are adjacent and 0 otherwise.

This section deals with obtaining the adjacency matrix of the equitable graph of Type I that arises from cyclic p groups.

Proposition 5. *Let G be a cyclic group of order 2^k; $k > 2$ (or p^k; $k > 1$, and $p > 2$ is a prime number). Then the adjacency matrix of the equitable graph Type I of G will be as follows:*

$$A(\mathcal{E}_1(G)) = \begin{pmatrix} 0 & \cdots & \cdots & \cdots & \cdots & \cdots & \cdots \\ \vdots & J^* & \vdots & J & \vdots & \cdots & \cdots & \vdots & J \\ \cdots & \cdots & \cdots & \cdots & \cdots & \cdots & \cdots \\ \vdots & J & \vdots & J^* & \vdots & \cdots & \cdots & \vdots & J \\ \cdots & \cdots & \cdots & \cdots & \cdots & \cdots & \cdots \\ \vdots & J & \vdots & \cdots & \ddots & \cdots & \vdots & J \\ \cdots & \cdots & \cdots & \cdots & \cdots & \cdots & \cdots \\ \vdots & \vdots & \vdots & \cdots & \ddots & \vdots & \vdots \\ \cdots & \cdots & \cdots & \cdots & \cdots & \cdots & \cdots \\ \vdots & J & \vdots & \cdots & \cdots & \cdots & J^* & \vdots & J \\ \cdots & \cdots & \cdots & \cdots & \cdots & \cdots & \cdots \\ \vdots & J & \vdots & \cdots & \cdots & \cdots & J & \vdots & J^* \end{pmatrix}$$

Proof. Let G be a cyclic group of order n and assume that $n = 2^k$; $k > 2$. Then according to the adjacency method, let J be a 3×3 matrix for which each entry equals one, and J^* is similar to J except that it has zeros in the main diagonal. In $A(\mathcal{E}_1(G))$, the first row consists of zeros except for in the (2^{k-1})th position. The middle row, (2^{k-1}), has one only in the positions $(2^{k-1}, 0)$, $(2^{k-1}, 2^{k-2})$ and $(2^{k-1}, 2^{k-2}3)$. Now for each $(4m)$th row, where $m \geq 1$, if m is odd, then there are zeros in the positions $(4m, i)$, where $i = 0, 4m, 2^{k-1}$, and all odd numbers. On the other hand, if m is even such that $4m \neq 2^{k-1}$, this row has ones in the positions $(4m, 4i)$ for all $i \geq 1$ and $i \neq m$. The corresponding rows and columns are symmetric.

Now suppose that $n = p^k$, where $p > 2$, and $k > 1$. Then by the definition of the graph, in this case, J and J^* are $(p - 1 \times p - 1)$ matrices, and they are as defined as before.

The first row (column) is zeros, and the remaining rows (columns) in $A(\mathcal{E}_1(G))$ have the following explanations

First, if $p = 3$, the $(3m)th$ rows, where $m \geq 1$ and $3m \neq 3^{k-1}$ or $(2)3^{k-1}$, have ones in the positions $(3m, 3i)$, where $i \geq 1$, except for the case when $i = 3^{k-2}$ or $(2)3^{k-2}$ or $i = m$. For the $(3^{k-1})th$ and $((2)3^{k-1})th$ rows (columns), they have one at a unique position where the row and the column intersect mutually. Now if $p > 3$, then the $(pr)th$ rows, where $r \geq 1$, consist of ones only in the positions (pr, pi) for all $i \geq 1$ and $i \neq r$. □

Example 6. *Let $G \cong \mathbb{Z}_8$. Then*

$$A(\mathcal{E}_1(G)) = \begin{pmatrix} 0 & 0 & 0 & 0 & 1 & 0 & 0 & 0 \\ 0 & 0 & 1 & 1 & 0 & 1 & 1 & 1 \\ 0 & 1 & 0 & 1 & 1 & 1 & 1 & 1 \\ 0 & 1 & 1 & 0 & 0 & 1 & 1 & 1 \\ 1 & 0 & 1 & 0 & 0 & 0 & 1 & 0 \\ 0 & 1 & 1 & 1 & 0 & 0 & 1 & 1 \\ 0 & 1 & 1 & 1 & 1 & 1 & 0 & 1 \\ 0 & 1 & 1 & 1 & 0 & 1 & 1 & 0 \end{pmatrix}$$

Example 7. *Let G be a cyclic group of order 2^k; $k = 2$. Then*

$$A(\mathcal{E}_1(G)) = \begin{pmatrix} 0 & 0 & 1 & 0 \\ 0 & 0 & 1 & 1 \\ 1 & 1 & 0 & 1 \\ 0 & 1 & 1 & 0 \end{pmatrix}$$

Example 8. *Let $G \cong \mathbb{Z}_9$. Then*

$$A(\mathcal{E}_1(G)) = \begin{pmatrix} 0 & 0 & 0 & 0 & 0 & 0 & 0 & 0 & 0 \\ 0 & 0 & 1 & 0 & 1 & 1 & 0 & 1 & 1 \\ 0 & 1 & 0 & 0 & 1 & 1 & 0 & 1 & 1 \\ 0 & 0 & 0 & 0 & 0 & 0 & 1 & 0 & 0 \\ 0 & 1 & 1 & 0 & 0 & 1 & 0 & 1 & 1 \\ 0 & 1 & 1 & 0 & 1 & 0 & 0 & 1 & 1 \\ 0 & 0 & 0 & 1 & 0 & 0 & 0 & 0 & 0 \\ 0 & 1 & 1 & 0 & 1 & 1 & 0 & 0 & 1 \\ 0 & 1 & 1 & 0 & 1 & 1 & 0 & 1 & 0 \end{pmatrix}$$

6. Conclusions

In this research, we introduced the equitable graphs Type I on groups. We studied the connectedness of these graphs for some groups and explored some of their theoretical properties. Additionally, the equitable square-free number and the equitable group were established. Furthermore, the connectedness and characteristics of the graph of cyclic equitable groups were investigated. The first, second and forgotten Zagreb indices were determined for the equitable graph Type I of specific groups. Finally, the adjacency matrix for the equitable graph Type I of cyclic p-groups was obtained. The newly introduced graph has significant potential for further investigation into its properties. Promising avenues for future research include analyzing equitable graph Type I, examining its perfectness, computing spectral properties, and elucidating connections with other well-known graph classes associated with finite groups. Addressing these open problems can provide valuable insights into theoretical and practical aspects, advancing our understanding of finite group theory and its interplay with graph theory.

Author Contributions: Conceptualization, A.S.; investigation, M.H.; writing—review and editing, A.A.; supervision, N.M. All authors have read and agreed to the published version of the manuscript.

Funding: This research received no external funding.

Data Availability Statement: The data used to support the findings of this study are available within this article.

Conflicts of Interest: The authors declare no conflicts of interest.

References

1. Chelvam, T.T.; Rani, I. Dominating sets in cayley graphs on Z_n. *Tamkang J. Math.* **2007**, *37*, 341–345. [CrossRef]
2. Dutta, J.; Nath, R.K. Spectrum of commuting graphs of some classes of finite groups. *Mathematika* **2017**, *33*, 87–95.
3. Tong-Viet, H.P. Finite groups whose prime graphs are regular. *J. Algebra* **2014**, *397*, 18–31. [CrossRef]
4. Cameron, P.J. The power graph of a finite group, II. *J. Group Theory* **2010**, *13*, 779–783. [CrossRef]
5. Cameron, P.J.; Gosh, S. The power graph of a finite group. *Discret. Math.* **2011**, *311*, 1220–1222. [CrossRef]
6. Rehman, S.U.; Baig, A.Q.; Imran, M.; Khan, Z.U. Order divisor graphs of finite groups. *Analele Ştiinţifice Univ. Ovidius Constanţa Seria Matematică* **2018**, *26*, 29–40. [CrossRef]
7. Akhbari, S.; Heydari, F.; Maghasedi, M. The intersection graph of a group. *J. Algebra Its Appl.* **2015**, *14*, 1550065. [CrossRef]
8. Ma, X.L.; Wei, H.Q.; Zhong, G. The cyclic graph of a finite group. *Algebra* **2013**, *2013*, 107265 . [CrossRef]
9. Cameron, P.J. Graphs defined on groups. *Int. J. Group Theory* **2022**, *11*, 53–107.
10. Nath, R.K.; Fasfous, W.N.T.; Das, K.C.; Shang, Y. Common neighborhood energy of commuting graphs of finite groups. *Symmetry* **2021**, *13*, 1651. [CrossRef]
11. Sharma, M.; Nath, R.K.; Shang, Y. On g-noncommuting graph of a finite group relative to its subgroups. *Mathematics* **2021**, *9*, 3147. [CrossRef]
12. Hungerford, T.W. *Algebra*; Springer Science and Business Media: New York, NY, USA, 2012; Volume 73.
13. Kumar, A.; Selvaganesh, L.; Cameron, P.J.; Chelvam, T.T. Recent developments on the power graph of finite groups—A survey. *Akce Int. J. Graphs Comb.* **2021**, *18*, 65–94. [CrossRef]
14. Balakrishnan, R.; Ranganathan, K. *A Textbook of Graph Theory*, 2nd ed.; Springer Science and Business Media: New York, NY, USA, 2012.
15. Abdu, A.; Mohammed, A. *Topological Indices Types in Graphs and Their Applications*; Generis Publishing: Chisinau, Moldova, 2021.
16. Ali, F.; Rather, B.A.; Sarfraz, M.; Ullah, A.; Fatima, N.; Mashwani, W.K. Certain topological Indices of non-commuting graphs for finite non-abelian groups. *Molecules* **2022**, *27*, 6053. [CrossRef] [PubMed]

Disclaimer/Publisher's Note: The statements, opinions and data contained in all publications are solely those of the individual author(s) and contributor(s) and not of MDPI and/or the editor(s). MDPI and/or the editor(s) disclaim responsibility for any injury to people or property resulting from any ideas, methods, instructions or products referred to in the content.

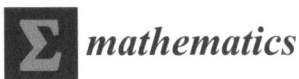

Article

On Non-Commutative Multi-Rings with Involution

Kaique M. A. Roberto [†], Kaique R. P. Santos [†] and Hugo Luiz Mariano [*,†]

Institute of Mathematics and Statistics, University of São Paulo, Rua do Matão, 1010, São Paulo 05508-090, Brazil; kaique.roberto@alumni.usp.br (K.M.A.R.); kaique.rps@ime.usp.br (K.R.P.S.)
* Correspondence: hugomar@ime.usp.br
† The authors contributed equally to this work.

Abstract: The primary motivation for this work is to develop the concept of Marshall's quotient applicable to non-commutative multi-rings endowed with involution, expanding upon the main ideas of the classical case—commutative and without involution—presented in Marshall's seminal paper. We define two multiplicative properties to address the involutive case and characterize their Marshall quotient. Moreover, this article presents various cases demonstrating that the "multi" version of rings with involution offers many examples, applications, and relatives in (multi)algebraic structures. Therefore, we established the first steps toward the development of an expansion of real algebra and real algebraic geometry to a non-commutative and involutive setting.

Keywords: multi-rings; involution; abstract real algebra

MSC: 16Y20; 11E16; 11E81

Citation: Roberto, K.M.A.; Santos, K.R.P.; Mariano, H.L. On Non-Commutative Multi-Rings with Involution. *Mathematics* **2024**, *12*, 2931. https://doi.org/10.3390/math12182931

Academic Editors: Irina Cristea and Alessandro Linzi

Received: 29 July 2024
Revised: 14 September 2024
Accepted: 18 September 2024
Published: 20 September 2024

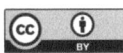

Copyright: © 2024 by the authors. Licensee MDPI, Basel, Switzerland. This article is an open access article distributed under the terms and conditions of the Creative Commons Attribution (CC BY) license (https://creativecommons.org/licenses/by/4.0/).

1. Introduction

Multialgebraic structures are "algebraic-like" structures endowed with multiple valued operations: an n-ary multi-operation on set A is just a function $A^n \to P(A) \setminus \{\emptyset\}$. The definition and study of the concept of multi-group (Definition 1) began in the 1930s by Marty; in the 1950s, the commutative hyperrings were introduced by Krasner (Definition 2). Since then, research on these multi-structures and their broad range of applications has been developed. The concepts of (commutative) multi-ring and superring (Definition 2), are much more recent developments, as discussed in [1,2]. To access advances and results in the theory of multi-ring and hyperring (commutative), we recommend the following: [2–9].

Many instances of multialgebraic structures codify the nature of mathematical objects through operations. Here, we recall some basic examples and provide additional ones, focusing on the non-commutative case.

Moreover, the exploration of this subject remains substantially open compared to the classical case. The natural progression of the subject has led to the development of *polynomials* [2], *linear algebra* [10], and *orderings* [11].

The main purpose of the present work is to outline the fundamental steps necessary to expand Marshall's seminal paper [1] to the context of non-commutative multi-rings with involution. Specifically, we present and analyze the expansion of the notion of the "Marshall's quotient" (see [12]), a crucial construction in abstract concepts of real algebra and real algebraic geometry. This includes applications in the space of signs [13], abstract real spectra [14], real semigroups [15], and real reduced multi-rings [1].

Building on this foundation, future work will focus on developing a real spectrum for non-commutative rings with involution, as a preparation for establishing an abstract theory of Hermitian forms ([16]).

Within this context, we introduce the concept of the Marshall quotient for involutive (non-commutative) multi-rings and discuss some applications to quaternion algebras over formally real fields. The main technical results are presented in Theorems 3–5. To illustrate an application, in Section 5, we provide the following:

Theorem 1 (7). *Let R be a commutative ring and A be an R-algebra with involution σ. We denote*

$$Orth(A) := \{a \in A : a\sigma(a) = \sigma(a)a = 1\}.$$

If $Orth(A) \subseteq Z(A)$, then $A/_m Orth(A)$ is a (non-commutative) hyperring.

Outline

In Section 2, we provide a brief introduction to multi/super-structures relevant to this work. We offer a non-standard example that extends Krasner's hyperfield and the signal hyperfield in Example 2. In Section 3, we introduce the basic objects of the theory of (non-commutative) multi-rings with involution and invite the reader to compare this theory with the classical one. Additionally, we cover various constructions and examples, including multi-groups, products, and matrices.

In Section 4, we define Marshall's quotient on involutive multialgebras and analyze the conditions for their existence using a "coherent" approach. Theorem 3 presents two types of quotients characterized by certain multiplicative subsets. Although many relations can be considered when forming classes in the quotient, we focus on four different possibilities and show how they are similar (Lemma 4). Moreover, in developing particular examples, we verify the independence of the conditions in Theorem 3. Additionally, the available quotient provides a "concrete" framework that encodes several types. In Section 5, we explore some applications and present examples of quotients that generate well-known multi-structures. Finally, in Section 6, we present our final remarks and conclusions.

2. Multi-Structures

In this section, we provide a brief overview of multi-structures and establish the necessary notations for the reader.

Multialgebraic structures are "algebraic-like" structures endowed with multi-valued operations. An n-ary multi-operation on set A is defined as a function $f : A^n \to P(A) \setminus \{\emptyset\}$, where $P(A)$ is the power set of A. Alternatively, the same concept can be described by an $n+1$-ary relation $R_f \subseteq A^{n+1}$, which satisfies the following condition: for all $x_0, x_1, \cdots, x_{n-1} \in A$, there exists $x_n \in A$, such that $R_f(x_0, x_1, \cdots, x_{n-1}, x_n)$.

Definition 1 (Adapted from Definition 1.1 in [1]). *A **multi-group concept** is a first-order structure $(G, \cdot, r, 1)$, where G is a non-empty set, $r : G \to G$ is a function, 1 is an element of G, $\cdot \subseteq G \times G \times G$ is a ternary relation (which will play the role of a binary multi-operation, and we denote $d \in a \cdot b$ for $(a, b, d) \in \cdot$), such that for all $a, b, c, d \in G$, we have the following:*

M1 - *If $c \in a \cdot b$, then $a \in c \cdot (r(b))$ and $b \in (r(a)) \cdot c$. We write $a \cdot b^{-1}$ to simplify $a \cdot (r(b))$.*

M2 - *$b \in a \cdot 1$ iff $a = b$.*

M3 - *If there exists x, such that $x \in a \cdot b$ and $t \in x \cdot c$, then there exists y, such that $y \in b \cdot c$ and $t \in a \cdot y$. Equivalently, if $\exists x(x \in a \cdot b \wedge t \in x \cdot c)$, then $\exists y(y \in b \cdot c \wedge t \in a \cdot y)$.*

The structure $(G, \cdot, r, 1)$ is said to be **commutative (or abelian)** if it satisfies the following condition for all $a, b, c \in G$:

M4 - *$c \in a \cdot b$ iff $c \in b \cdot a$.*

The structure $(G, \cdot, 1)$ is a **commutative multimonoid (with unity)** if it satisfy M3, M4, and condition $a \in 1 \cdot a$ for all $a \in G$.

Definition 2 (Definition 5 in [2]). *A **(commutative) superring** is a tuple $(R, +, \cdot, -, 0, 1)$, satisfying the following:*

1. *$(R, +, -, 0)$ is a commutative multi-group and $(R, \cdot, 1)$ is a (commutative) multimonoid;*
2. *(Null element) $a \cdot 0 = 0$ and $0 \cdot a = 0$ for all $a \in R$;*
3. *(Weak distributive) If $x \in b + c$, then $a \cdot x \in a \cdot b + a \cdot c$ and $x \cdot a \in b \cdot a + c \cdot a$. Equivalently, $(b + c) \cdot a \subseteq b \cdot a + c \cdot a$ and $a \cdot (b + c) \subseteq a \cdot b + a \cdot c$.*

4. The rule of signals holds: $-(ab) = (-a)b = a(-b)$, for all $a, b \in R$.

Note that if $a \in R$, then $0 = 0 \cdot a \in (1 + (-1)) \cdot a \subseteq 1 \cdot a + (-1) \cdot a$, thus $(-1) \cdot a = -a$.

R is said to be a **multi-ring** if $(R, \cdot, 1)$ forms a monoid. A **hyperring** R is a multi-ring such that if for $a, b, c \in R$, $a(b + c) = ab + ac$ and $(b + c)a = ba + ca$. A multi-ring (respectively, a hyperring) R is said to be a **multi-domain (hyperdomain)** if it contains no zero divisors. A commutative multi-ring R will be a **multifield** if every non-zero element of R has a multiplicative inverse.

If $a = 0$, then $a(b + c) = ab + ac$ and $(b + c)a = ba + ca$. **Observe that hyperfields and multifields coincide**. Indeed, by definition, every hyperfield is a multifield, and, for a given multifield, F, if $a \neq 0$, then we have the following:

$$a^{-1}(ab + ac) \subseteq b + c \text{ implies } aa^{-1}(ab + ac) \subseteq a(b + c),$$

whenever $b, c \in F$. Therefore, $a(b + c) = ab + ac$.

Definition 3. *Let A and B be superrings. A map $f : A \to B$ is a morphism if for all $a, b, c \in A$:*
1. *$f(1) = 1$ and $f(0) = 0$;*
2. *$f(-a) = -f(a)$;*
3. *$f(ab) = f(a)f(b)$;*
4. *if $c \in a + b$ then $f(c) \in f(a) + f(b)$.*

*A morphism f is a **full morphism** if for all $a, b \in A$,*

$$f(a + b) = f(a) + f(b) \text{ and } f(a \cdot b) = f(a) \cdot f(b).$$

In this text, we provide some examples and treat (non-commutative) multi-rings. For more details, we recommend the reader to check [2–9] for advances and results in multi-ring/hyperring (commutative) theory.

Example 1.
1. *Suppose that $(G, \cdot, 1)$ is a group. Defining $a * b = \{a \cdot b\}$, and $r(g) = g^{-1}$, we have that $(G, *, r, 1)$ is a multi-group. In this way, every ring, domain, and field is a multi-ring, multi-domain, and hyperfield, respectively.*
2. *Let $K = \{0, 1\}$ with the usual product, and the sum defined by relations $x + 0 = 0 + x = x$, $x \in K$, and $1 + 1 = \{0, 1\}$. This is a hyperfield referred to as **Krasner's hyperfield** [17].*
3. *$Q_2 = \{-1, 0, 1\}$ is the **"signal" hyperfield** with the usual product (in $\mathbb{Z}$) and the multi-valued sum defined by relations*

$$\begin{cases} 0 + x = x + 0 = x, \text{ for every } x \in Q_2 \\ 1 + 1 = 1, (-1) + (-1) = -1 \\ 1 + (-1) = (-1) + 1 = \{-1, 0, 1\} \end{cases}$$

4. *For every multi-ring R, we define the **opposite multi-ring** R^{op}, which has the same structure unless $(R^{op}, \cdot^{op}, 1^{op})$ is the opposite monoid of $(R, \cdot, 1)$, i.e., $\cdot^{op}$ is the reverse multiplication. The null element and the weak distributive properties are satisfied on both sides in R^{op} because they are met on the opposite sides in R.*

The following example codifies the structure of ranks of square matrices:

Example 2 (Superrings of signed ranks). *Consider $n \in \mathbb{N}$ and*

$$K_n^{\pm} = \{0, 1, 2, ..., n - 1, n_-, n_+\}.$$

This set is endowed with a superring structure, which includes the addition $\oplus$ and multiplication $\odot$ operations, defined by the following:

(n = 0,1) $K_0^\pm = K_0 = \{0\}$, $K_1^\pm = Q_2$ and $K_1 = \{0,1\} = K$.

(K1) *0 is the identity with respect to the addition $\oplus$;*

(K2) 1.
$$m \oplus m' = \begin{cases} [|m - m'|, m + m']; m, m' \in \{1, ..., n-1\}, m + m' < n; \\ [|m - m'|, m + m'] \cup \{n_\pm\}; m, m' \in \{1, ..., n-1\}, m + m' \geq n; \end{cases}$$

2. $m \oplus n_\pm = [n - m, n - 1] \cup \{n_\pm\}$ whenever $m \leq n - 1$;
3. (n is even) $n_+ \oplus n_+ = n_- \oplus n_- = K_n^\pm$;
   $n_+ \oplus n_- = K_n^\pm \setminus \{0\}$.
4. (n is odd) $n_+ \oplus n_+ = n_- \oplus n_- = K_n^\pm \setminus \{0\}$;
   $n_+ \oplus n_- = K_n^\pm$.

(K3) n_+ *is the identity with respect to the multiplication $\odot$ and $n_- \odot n_- = n_+$;*

(K4) *For $m, m' < n$,*

$$m \odot m' = \begin{cases} [m + m' - n, \min(m, m')], \text{ whenever } m + m' > n; \\ [0, \min(m, m')], \text{ otherwise.} \end{cases}$$

*We denote the **superrings of ranks** by $K_n = \{0, 1, 2, ..., n-1, n\}$, whose axioms are identical, except for $n_+ = n_- = n$.*

Example 3 (Kaleidoscope, Example 2.7 in [12]). *Let $n \in \mathbb{N}$ and define*

$$X_n = \{-n, ..., 0, ..., n\} \subseteq \mathbb{Z}.$$

*We define the n-**kaleidoscope multi-ring** by $(X_n, +, \cdot, -, 0, 1)$, where $- : X_n \to X_n$ is the restriction of the opposite map in $\mathbb{Z}$, $+ : X_n \times X_n \to \mathcal{P}(X_n) \setminus \{\emptyset\}$ is given by the following rules:*

$$a + b = \begin{cases} \{a\}, \text{ if } b \neq -a \text{ and } |b| \leq |a| \\ \{b\}, \text{ if } b \neq -a \text{ and } |a| \leq |b| \\ \{-a, ..., 0, ..., a\} \text{ if } b = -a \end{cases},$$

and $\cdot : X_n \times X_n \to X_n$ is given by the following rules:

$$a \cdot b = \begin{cases} \text{sgn}(ab) \max\{|a|, |b|\} \text{ if } a, b \neq 0 \\ 0 \text{ if } a = 0 \text{ or } b = 0 \end{cases}.$$

With the above rules we have that $(X_n, +, \cdot, -, 0, 1)$ is a multi-ring, which is not a hyperring for $n \geq 2$ because

$$n(1 - 1) = b \cdot \{-1, 0, 1\} = \{-n, 0, n\}$$

and $n - n = X_n$. Note that $X_0 = \{0\}$ and $X_1 = \{-1, 0, 1\} = Q_2$.

Example 4 (Triangle hyperfield [18]). *Let $\mathbb{R}_+$ be the set of non-negative real numbers endowed with the following (multi)operations:*

$$\begin{cases} a \triangledown b = \{c \in \mathbb{R}_+ \mid |a - b| \leq c \leq |a + b|\}, \text{ for all } a, b \in \mathbb{R}_+, \\ a \cdot b = ab, \text{ the usual multiplication in } \mathbb{R}_+, \\ -a = a. \end{cases}$$

Moreover, this is a hyperfield that does not satisfy the double distributive property (see 5.1 in [18] for more details).

Example 5.

1. The prime ideals of a commutative ring (its Zariski spectrum) are classified by equivalence classes of morphisms into algebraically closed fields; however, they can be uniformly classified by a multi-ring morphism into the Krasner hyperfield $K = \{0, 1\}$.
2. The orderings of a commutative ring (its real spectrum) are classified by classes of equivalence of ring homomorphisms into real closed fields. However, they can be uniformly classified by a multi-ring morphism into the signal hyperfield $Q_2 = \{-1, 0, 1\}$.
3. The Krull valuation on a commutative ring with a group of values $(G, +, -, 0, \leq)$ is just a morphism into the hyperfield $T_G = G \cup \{\infty\}$.

3. Multialgebras with Involution

In this section, we introduce the key concept of this work: multialgebras with involution. For a multi-ring A, we denote

$$Z(A) := \{a \in A : \text{for all } b \in A, \, ab = ba\},$$

the **center** of A. Of course, if A is commutative, $Z(A) = A$. The classical theory of central algebras with involution suggests the development of this subject in a very similar way.

Definition 4.

1. Let R be a commutative multi-ring, A be a (non-necessarily commutative) multi-ring, and $j : R \to A$ a homomorphism of multi-rings, such that $j[R] \subseteq Z(A)$, then (A, j) is an R-**multialgebra**.
2. A **morphism** of R-multialgebras $f : (A, j) \to (A', j')$ is a morphism of multi-rings $f : A \to A'$ such that $f \circ j = j'$.
3. An **involution** σ over the R-multialgebra (A, j) is an (anti)isomorphism of R-multialgebras $\sigma : (A, j) \to (A^{op}, j^{op})$ where A^{op} is the opposite multi-ring, $j^{op} : R^{op} \to A^{op}$ is a homomorphism, and $\sigma^{op} = \sigma^{-1}$. Thus, for all $a, b \in A$, $\sigma(ab) = \sigma(b)\sigma(a)$.
4. A **multialgebra with involution** is just a (R, τ)-multialgebra endowed with an involution, where (R, τ) is a multi-ring with involution. A **morphism of** R-**multialgebras with involution** is a morphism of R-multialgebras $f : (A, j, \sigma) \longrightarrow (A', j', \sigma')$ satisfying $f \circ \sigma = \sigma' \circ f$.
5. For each commutative multi-ring with involution $(\mathcal{R}, \tau)$, there exists the **category of** (R, τ)-**multialgebras with involution**, whose objects are (R, τ)-multialgebras with involution and morphisms are morphisms of R-multialgebras with involution.

Whenever the involution τ is clear, we will omit it and write only $\mathcal{R}$. Note that item 1 implies that (R, τ) is an initial object in $\mathcal{R}$. Item 2 ensures that every morphism $f : (A, j, \sigma) \longrightarrow (A', j', \sigma')$ is represented by a commutative triangle.

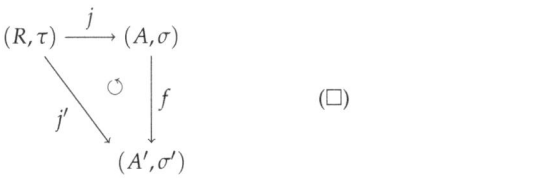

We call (A, σ) a **subalgebra** of (A', σ') if the diagram ($\square$) is satisfied by the restricted identity morphism $f = id_{A'}|_A$. An **ideal** $J \subseteq A$ is a σ-invariant ($\sigma(J) \subseteq J$) non-empty subset satisfying $J \cdot A \subseteq J$ and $x + y \subseteq J$ for all $x, y \in J$. Once J is σ-invariant and σ is an isomorphism, $A \cdot J = \sigma(\sigma(J) \cdot \sigma(A)) \subseteq \sigma(J) \subseteq J$ and, thus, J is a two-sided ideal. A **proper ideal** is an ideal $J \neq A$. We call J a **prime ideal** if J is an ideal such that $ab \in J$ implies $a \in J$ or $b \in J$ for any pair $a, b \in A$. The smallest ideal generated by $a_1, ..., a_k \in A$ is

$$J(a_1,...,a_k) = \sum_{i=1}^{k} Aa_i A + A\sigma(a_i)A.$$

We define the quotient A/J as usual (see, for instance, [2,12,19], or [20]). We have many standard and effusive constructions that raise various examples in category $\mathcal{R}$.

Let I be a non-empty set. For a given family $(A_i, j_i, \sigma_i)_{i \in I}$ of R-multialgebras with involution, the **direct product** $\prod A_i = (\prod_{i \in I}(A_i, \pi_i), \bar{j}, \bar{\sigma})$ is an R-multialgebra with involution such that $\pi_{i_0} : \prod A_i \longrightarrow A_{i_0}$ are projection morphisms for each $i_0 \in I$. Indeed, $\bar{\sigma}(a_i)_{i \in I} = (\sigma_i(a_i))_{i \in I}$ is an involution over $\prod A_i$, and $\bar{j}(r) = (j_i(r))_{i \in I} \in Z(\prod A_i)$ is a well-defined map satisfying the necessary conditions above.

Matrices over a given commutative multi-ring are natural constructions. We denote by $M_n(A)$ the set of square matrices of order n with coefficients in (A, j, σ) and set the sum and product of matrices as follows:

For all matrices $C = (c_{ij})_{n \times n}, B = (b_{ij})_{n \times n} \in M_n(A)$, we define the function $\bar{\sigma} : M_n(A) \longrightarrow M_n(A)$ by $\bar{\sigma}(B) = (\sigma(b_{ji}))_{n \times n}$ and (multi)operations, as follows:

$$C + B := \{(d_{ij}) : d_{ij} \in c_{ij} + b_{ij} \text{ for all } i,j\} \neq \emptyset$$

$$CB := \{(d_{ij}) : d_{ij} \in \sum_{k=1}^{n} c_{ik} b_{kj} = c_{i1} b_{1j} + c_{i2} b_{2j} + ... + c_{in} b_{nj} \text{ for all } i,j\} \neq \emptyset$$

$$\lambda C := (\lambda c_{ij})_{n \times n}, \text{ for all } \lambda \in R.$$

Since σ is an involution and A is a commutative multi-ring, it follows that $\bar{\sigma}$ is also an involution. Finally, let $f : (A, \sigma) \longrightarrow (M_n(A), \bar{\sigma})$ be the diagonal morphism defined by

$$f(a) = \text{diag}(a, a, ..., a) \in M_n(A),$$

which associates each $a \in A$ with a diagonal matrix in $M_n(A)$ and $\bar{j} := f \circ j$ is the injective morphism such that $\bar{j}(R) \subseteq Z(M_n(A))$. We will avoid the verification that $(M_n(A), \bar{j}, \bar{\sigma})$ is an R-multialgebra with involution, but the reader can check Section 2 of [10], Theorem 2.3, and Lemma 2.5. However, we provide an example to illustrate this construction.

Example 6. *Consider the 2-kaleidoscope multi-ring $(X_2, +, \cdot, -, 0, 1)$ as defined in 3 and $(\ )^t$ the matrix transposition. Then, $(M_2(X_2), (\ )^t)$ is an X_2-multialgebra with involution.*

Let $A = \begin{bmatrix} 1 & 2 \\ -1 & 0 \end{bmatrix}$ and $B = \begin{bmatrix} 0 & 1 \\ -1 & 1 \end{bmatrix}$ matrices over X_2. Thus,

$$AB = \begin{bmatrix} 1 \cdot 0 + 2 \cdot (-1) & 1 \cdot 1 + 2 \cdot 1 \\ -1 \cdot 0 + 0 \cdot (-1) & -1 \cdot 1 + 0 \cdot 1 \end{bmatrix}, A^t = \begin{bmatrix} 1 & -1 \\ 2 & 0 \end{bmatrix}, B^t = \begin{bmatrix} 0 & -1 \\ 1 & 1 \end{bmatrix}.$$

Therefore, $(AB)^t = B^t A^t = \begin{bmatrix} -2 & 0 \\ 2 & -1 \end{bmatrix}$.

Example 7. *(Adapted from [21]) Let $G^0 = G \cup \{0\}$ be a group with 0 and define + the multi-operation satisfying the following:*

$$x + 0 = 0 + x = x, \forall x \in G^0;$$

$$x + x = G^0 \setminus \{x\}, \forall x \in G^0;$$

$$x + y = \{x, y\}, \forall x, y \in G^0 \text{ with } x \neq y.$$

We can define an involution σ over this structure by setting $\sigma(x) = x^{-1}$ for all $x \in G$ and $\sigma(0) = 0$. In fact, σ is additive and it is easy to verify that $(G^0, 0, 1, +, \cdot, \sigma)$ is a multi-ring with involution.

4. Marshall's Quotient of Multialgebras with Involution

The notion of Marshall's quotient of a commutative (hyper)ring (resp., multi-ring) by a multiplicative subset always produces a commutative hyperring (resp., a commutative multi-ring), and is the main construction used in the abstract approaches of quadratic forms theory ([1,12]). In this section, we introduce the main technical tool, in the general setting of a (non-commutative) multi-ring with involution, developed in the present work—Marshall's quotient—which will enable us to construct a variety of interesting multialgebras with involution, derived from standard algebraic structures.

Throughout this section, we fix an R-multialgebra with involution (A, j, σ). We are interested in *Marshall-coherent subsets* satisfying at least one of the conditions in Theorem 3, i.e., *normality* or *convexity*. These conditions interact in many ways with the relations below (6) compared to the commutative case. First of all, we explore basic properties due to definitions.

Definition 5. *A subset (without zero divisors) $S \subseteq A$ is called a **Marshall-coherent subset** whenever*

- *S is a multiplicative submonoid of $(A, \cdot, 1)$*
- *$\sigma[S] \subseteq S$ (or, equivalently $\sigma[S] = S$)*

*We call S **standard** if $s\sigma(s) \in Z(A)^\times$, for all $s \in S$. We note that S is **convex** if $xS\sigma(x) \subseteq S$ for all $x \in A_0$ in the subset of nonzero divisors of A. If $x\sigma(x) \in S$ for all $x \in A_0$, we note that S is **1-convex**.*

Immediately, convexity implies 1-convexity. One can check Lemma 5 and Proposition 1 for a reciprocal result. From now on, we fix a Marshall-coherent subset $S \subseteq A$.

The expansion of the theory to this non-commutative and involutive setting, inevitably, leads us to a multitude of definitions that are collapsed to a single one in the traditional commutative setting and where the involution is trivial. Therefore, we present the following:

Definition 6. *Let $a, b \in A$ and $s_1, s_2, t_1, t_2 \in S$. We define the following:*

1. *$a \sim_1 b$ iff $a = s_1 b s_2$ and $b = t_1 a t_2$;*
2. *$a \sim_2 b$ iff $s_1 a s_2 = t_1 b t_2$;*
3. *$a \sim_3 b$ iff $a s_1 = t_1 b$ and $s_2 a = b t_2$;*
4. *$a \sim_4 b$ iff there is $s \in S$ such that $a s \sigma(b) \in S$.*

Despite the diversity of these relations, they are interconnected and, under certain natural conditions, they may coincide. Of course, $a \sim_1 b$ implies $a \sim_2 b$. Further, $\sim_4$ is an equivalence relation when S is 1-convex. Indeed, this relation concurs with $\sim_3$ (see Lemma 4). We start our exploration of these relations and the associated properties of Marshall-coherent subsets.

Lemma 1. *For $\sim \, = \, \sim_1$, as defined above, $\sim$ is an equivalence relation and satisfies the following:*

1. *For all $a \in A$ and all $s \in S$, $\sigma(s)as \sim a$, $sa\sigma(s) \sim a$, and $abs \sim ab$, $sab \sim ab$.*
2. *For all $a, b \in A$ if $a \sim b$ then $\sigma(a) \sim \sigma(b)$.*

Proof. Of course $\sim$ is reflexive (since S has 1) and symmetric. Now, let $a \sim b$ and $b \sim c$, with $a = s_1 b s_2$, $b = t_1 a t_2$ and $b = r_1 c r_2$, $c = w_1 b w_2$, $s_1, s_2, t_1, t_2, r_1, r_2, w_1, w_2 \in S$. Then

$$a = s_1 b s_2 = s_1(r_1 c r_2) s_2 = (s_1 r_1) c (r_2 s_2)$$

and

$$c = w_1 b w_2 = w_1(t_1 a t_2) w_2 = (w_1 t_1) a (t_2 w_2).$$

Since S is multiplicative, we have $s_1r_1, r_2s_2, w_1t_1, t_2w_2 \in S$, which implies $a \sim c$. Hence, $\sim = \sim_1$ is an equivalence relation. Items 1 and 2 are straightforward once S is multiplicative and σ-invariant. □

Lemma 2. *If S is standard, then $\sim = \sim_2$ is an equivalence relation and satisfies the following:*
1. *For all $a \in A$ and all $s \in S$, $\sigma(s)as \sim a$, $sa\sigma(s) \sim a$, and $abs \sim ab$, $sab \sim ab$.*
2. *For all $a, b \in A$ if $a \sim b$ then $\sigma(a) \sim \sigma(b)$.*

Proof. Reflexivity and symmetry follow immediately. Note that $s\sigma(s) \in Z(A)$ enable us to rewrite the definition of $\sim = \sim_2$ as follows:

$$a \sim_2 b \text{ iff } s_1as_2 = t_1bt_2 \text{ iff } \sigma(s_1)s_1as_2\sigma(t_2) = \sigma(s_1)t_1bt_2\sigma(t_2) \text{ iff } as_1' = t_1'b,$$

for $s_1', t_1' \in S$.

Consider $a \sim b$ and $b \sim c$, which means that there exist $s_1, t_1, s_2, t_2 \in S$. such that $as_1 = t_1b$ and $bs_2 = t_2c$. Scaling the previous equation on the right by s_2, and the latter, on the left by t_1, we conclude that $a(s_1s_2) = (t_1t_2)c$. Thus, $\sim$ is transitive; that is, an equivalence relation.

For Item 1, observe that $w(\sigma(s)as)w' = (w\sigma(s))a(sw')$, and $w(abs)w' = w(ab)sw'$ for all $s, w, w' \in S$. Item 2 follows by applying σ to both sides of $as = bt$. □

Back to Example 7, we observe that normal and convex (Marshall-coherent) subgroups coincide in this type of structure. In general, this is not the case, nor is their relationship with the relations above equal. Now, we treat these two cases.

Lemma 3. *Suppose that $x \cdot S = S \cdot x$ for each $x \in A$. Let $a, a' \in A$, and the following statements are equivalent:*
1. *$\exists s, t, s', t' \in S$ such that $sat = s'a't'$*
2. *$\exists u, u' \in S$ such that $ua = u'a'$*
3. *$\exists v, v' \in S$ such that $av = a'v'$*

That is, $a \sim_2 a'$ if, and only if, $a \sim_3 a'$. Furthermore, $\sim_S = \sim_2 = \sim_3$ is an equivalence relation.

Proof. (1) $\iff$ (2) $\iff$ (3) follows immediately from the hypothesis. Thus, $\sim_i = \sim_j$ for each pair (i, j), $i, j \in \{2, 3\}$. For simplicity, denote $\sim_S = \sim_i$, for each $i \in \{2, 3\}$.

The relation $\sim_S$ is an equivalence relation: suppose that $ua = u'a'$ and $r'a' = r''a''$ for $u, u', r', r'' \in S$. Observe the following:

$$ua = u'a' \implies r'ua = r'(u'a') \therefore r'ua = r'(a'v'), \text{ for some } v' \in S.$$

Also

$$(r'u)a = (r'a')v' = (r''a'')v' \implies \exists r'u = v, v'' \in S, \text{ such that } (r'u)a = v''a''.$$

It follows that $a \sim_S a'$, $a' \sim_S a''$ implies $a \sim_S a''$. We already prove that $\sim_S$ is transitive. Reflexivity and symmetry follow from $1 \in S$ and the equivalence of the statements 1, 2, and 3. □

Lemma 3 is a powerful tool to deal with multiplication. It improves efficiency when managing equations, but mainly, it is a sufficient condition for the Marshall's quotient (8) being a multi-ring instead of a superring (Theorem 3).

We observe that, for a given Marshall's coherent subset S, convexity is the reflexivity property of $\sim_4$ by definition. Indeed, there is a suitable relationship between the upward-selected set of relations and Marshall's coherent convex subsets.

Lemma 4. *Suppose that S is convex. Let $a, a' \in A$, and the following statements are equivalent:*

1. $a \sim_2 a'$;
2. $a \sim_3 a'$;
3. $a \sim_4 a'$.

Furthermore, $\sim_S = \sim_2 = \sim_3 = \sim_4$ is an equivalence relation. Additionally, for every 1-convex S', $\sim_4 = \sim_3 \subseteq \sim_2$.

Proof. $1 \implies 2$: There are $s_1, s_2, t_1, t_2 \in S$ such that we have the following:

$$s_1 a s_2 = t_1 a' t_2 \implies \underbrace{s_1 a s_2(\sigma(a)}_{\in S} a) = t_1 a' \underbrace{t_2(\sigma(a) a)}_{\in S} \quad (S \text{ is Marshall convex})$$
$$\therefore \underbrace{(a' \sigma(a')) s_3}_{\in S} a = (a' \underbrace{\sigma(a')) t_1 a' t_2'}_{\in S} \implies sa = a't. \tag{1}$$

$2 \implies 3$: Suppose that $a \sim_3 a'$. Then, there exist $s_1, t_1 \in S$, satisfying the following:

$$a s_1 = t_1 a' \implies a s_1 \sigma(a') = t_1 a' \sigma(a') \in S. \tag{2}$$

$3 \implies 1$: Finally, if $a \sim_4 a'$, then $\exists s, t_1 \in S$ such that we have the following:

$$a \sigma(a') = t_1 \implies a \underbrace{s \sigma(a') a'}_{\in S} = t_1 a' \therefore \quad 1 \cdot a s_2 = t_1 a' \cdot 1. \tag{3}$$

To prove the final assertion, consider $a \sim_S b = a \sim_4 b$, for all $a, b \in A$. Since $1 \in S$ and S is convex, $a\sigma(a) \in S$ for all $a \in A$. Moreover, as long as S is σ-invariant, $a\sigma(b) \in S$ if, and only if, $b\sigma(s)\sigma(a) \in S$. It turns out that $a \sim_S b$ if, and only if, $b \sim_S a$. Thus, $\sim_S$ is reflexive and symmetric.

Finally, we prove the transitivity property. Put $a \sim_S b$ and $b \sim_S c$. Thus, by definition, it follows that

$$\exists r, s, s', s'' \in S; \begin{cases} a\sigma(b) = s' & \mathbf{1} \\ b r \sigma(c) = s'' & \mathbf{2} \end{cases} \overset{1 \cdot 2}{\implies} a \underbrace{s\sigma(b) b r}_{\in S} \sigma(c) = s' s'' \in S.$$

Remember that S is closed under multiplication and 1-convex. We have previously demonstrated that transitivity holds; thus, we conclude that $\sim_S$ is an equivalence relation. The final assertion follows straightforwardly. □

The following lemma summarizes and proves many results concerning the properties of Marshall-coherent subsets and the above relations.

Lemma 5. *Let S be a Marshall-coherent set in (A, σ). The following statements hold:*

1. *If $y \cdot S = S \cdot y$ for all $y \in A$ and S is 1-convex, then S is convex;*
2. *If S is convex and $x\sigma(x) \in Z(A)^\times$ for all non-zero divisors $x \in A$, then $x \cdot S = S \cdot x$ (S is normal);*
3. *If $S \subseteq A^\times$, and S is 1-convex, then $A_0 = A^\times$ denotes the set of non-zero divisors, i.e., every non-zero divisor has an inverse in A;*
4. *If S is standard, then $S \subseteq A^\times$;*
5. *If S is standard then $a \sim_1 a'$ if, and only if, $a \sim_2 a'$ if, and only if, $a \sim_3 a'$;*

Proof. 1. Let $x \in A$ be a non-zero divisor and $s \in S$. Thus, $\sigma(x) s x = z$ for some $z \in A$. Commuting s with x, it follows that $\sigma(x) x s' = y$ for a suitable $s' \in S$. Hence, 1-convexity and the closure of multiplication implies $y \in S$. Therefore, $\sigma(x) S x \subseteq S$.

2. Let $x \in A^*$ be a non-zero divisor. For any $s_1 \in S$, $\sigma(x) s_1 x = s_2$ for some s_2. Therefore $(x\sigma(x)) s_1 x = x s_2$, which implies $s_1 x = x s_2 (x\sigma(x))^{-1}$. Since $x\sigma(x) \in S^\times$ has an

inverse in S, $s_1 x = x s_1'$ for a suitable choice of s_1'. Hence, $S \cdot x \subseteq x \cdot S$. The reverse inclusive follows from symmetry.

3. By definition, $A^\times \subseteq A_0$. For the inverse inclusion, note that A_0 is a Marshall-coherent set and, let $y \in A_0$ and $1 \in S$. Thus, $\sigma(y)y = s' \neq 0$.

$$\sigma(y)y = s' \implies s'^{-1}\sigma(y)y = 1 \therefore y_l^{-1} = s'^{-1}\sigma(y) \text{ is a left inverse for } y. \quad (4)$$

The same argument shows that y has the right inverse y_r^{-1}. Note that $yy_l^{-1} = s_1 \in S$. Thus, $yy_l^{-1}y = s_1 y$ and implies $y = s_1 y$ for some $s_1 \in S$. Scaling by y_r^{-1} on both right sides of the equation, we obtain $1 = s_1$. Hence, $y^{-1} = y_l^{-1} = y_r^{-1}$.

4. By hypothesis, $s\sigma(s) \in Z(A)^\times (\cap S)$. Hence, $\exists x \in A$ such that $(x\sigma(s))s = 1$. Direct calculations confirm that this serves as a unique inverse on both sides.

5. The statement can be straightforwardly proven by scaling and division. □

Item 1 of Lemma 5 provides a sufficient condition for a normal subset to be a convex subset. On the other hand, Item 2 specifies a reciprocal condition; that is, each element, $x \in A_0$, has a norm lying in the center. In the classical theory of rings with involution (see, for instance, [16]), involution with traces $x + \sigma(x)$ and norms $x\sigma(x)$ lying in the center are called *standard*. This justifies the notation above. As we see in Section 5, standard subsets are typical examples.

For each $\sim \in \{\sim_1, \sim_2, \sim_3, \sim_4\}$, we denote an element in $A/\sim$ (whenever it exists) by $[a]$. We have well-defined rules, as follows:

$$[a] + [b] := \{[c] : c = s_1 a s_2 + t_1 b t_2 \text{ for some } s_1, s_2, t_1, t_2 \in S\} \text{ and,}$$
$$[a][b] := \{[c] : c = rasbt \text{ for some } r, s, t \in S\}.$$

Observe that the involutory structure can be defined in the very same way for superrings.

Definition 7. *A **superring with involution** (A, σ) is a superring that satisfies the (mutatis mutandis) axioms for multialgebras with involution.*

Theorem 2. *The structure $(A/\sim_2, +, \cdot, [0], [1])$ is a superring with involution provided by $\sigma([a]) := [\sigma(a)]$. If S is standard, then $(A/\sim_1, +, \cdot, [0], [1])$ is a superring with involution $\sigma([a]) := [\sigma(a)]$.*

Proof. We proceed with a very similar argument to the one used in Theorem 6. □

We define existing quotients for general Marshall-coherent subsets. In the sequel, we deal with normality and convexity.

Definition 8. *We define the superring $(A/\sim, +, \cdot, [0], [1])$ as the **Marshall's quotient** of A by S, and denote it by $A/_m S := A/\sim$.*

Whenever $\sim$ is chosen, we indicate the Marshall subset S by adding it to the index, i.e., writing $\sim_S$.

Theorem 3 has a central result in this section. Since the reverse image of the canonical morphism $j : R \longrightarrow A$ (see Definition 4) lifts Marshall-coherent subsets of A to R, the quotient is a multialgebra (with involution) likewise. The associated Marshall-coherent subset is $S_j = j^{-1}[S] \subseteq R$, where $S \subseteq A$ is Marshall-coherent in A and $[S] = [1]$ is the algebraic class of S under $\sim_S$.

Theorem 3. *Let $S \subseteq A$ be a Marshall-coherent subset of a multi-ring A satisfying one of the additional conditions below:*

1. *(Normal) $xS = Sx$, for all $x \in A$.*

2. (Convex) For all $x \in A$, a nonzero divisor in A, $xS\sigma(x) \subseteq S$.

If (A, σ) is an (R, τ)-multialgebra with involution, the set $S_j := j^{-1}[S] \subseteq R$ is a multiplicative submonoid of $(R, \cdot, 1)$. Moreover, $j_S : R/\sim_{S_j} \to A/\sim_S$, $[r] \mapsto [j(r)]$ defines an $R/\sim_{S_j}$-multialgebra structure over $A/\sim_S$, and $\sigma_S : A/\sim_S \to A/\sim_S$, $[a] \mapsto [\sigma(a)]$ is an involution over the $R/\sim_{S_j}$-multialgebra $(A/\sim_S, j_S)$. In both cases, $A/\sim_S$ is a multi-ring.

Proof. Once $j : (R, \tau) \longrightarrow (A, \sigma)$ is a homomorphism, if $s_1 r s_2 = t_1 r' t_2$ in R, then $j([r]) = [j(r)] = [j(r')] = j([r'])$. It is easy to check that S_j is a multiplicative submonoid of R and, due to S being Marshall-coherent, $\sigma(j(r)) = j(\tau(r)) \in S$ for all $r \in S_j$. Thus, $\tau(r) \in S_j$ whenever $r \in S_j$. We conclude that S_j is Marshall-coherent and, by Theorem 2, $R/\sim_{S_j}$ is a superring endowed with an involution $\tau([r]) := [\tau(r)]$.

For any two elements $[c], [d] \in [a] \cdot [b] \subseteq R/\sim_{S_j}$, $s_1 c = t_1 ab$ and $ds_2 = abt_2$ for some $s_1, t_1, s_2, t_2 \in S_j$, because R is commutative. Scaling these equations, we write $s_1 c t_2 = t_1 d s_2$, i.e., , $[a] \cdot [b] = \{[ab]\}$. Hence, $R/\sim_{S_j}$ is a multi-ring with involution.

Now, consider the following diagram:

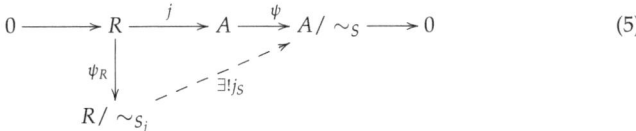 (5)

(1) If $xS = Sx$, then $\sim = \sim_2$ can be read as $a \sim b$ if, and only if, $as = tb$ for some $s, t \in S$. Previous constructions (see Theorem 2) and demonstrations show that $(A/\sim_S)$ is a superring. Let $[c]$ and $[c']$ be elements in $[a] \cdot [b]$; thus, $c = abs$ and $c' = s'ab$ for some $s, s' \in S$. Scaling equations and comparing gives us $s'c = c's = s'abs$, which means that $c \sim c'$. Therefore, $[a] \cdot [b] = \{[ab]\}$ and $A/\sim$ is a multi-ring.

By the universal property of the quotient $R/\sim_{S_j}$, j_S is unique. Since all arrows are homomorphisms, $(A/\sim_S, j_S)$ is $R/\sim_{S_j}$-multialgebra. Furthermore, S is σ-invariant, which means $\sigma(aS) = \sigma(a)S$. Consequently, the induced anti-homomorphism $\sigma_S : A/\sim_S \to A/\sim_S$ such that $\sigma([a]) = [\sigma(a)]$ is well-defined and an involution over $A/\sim_S$.

(2) Let $\sim = \sim_2$. In this case, Lemma 4 and the preceding case show that $A/\sim$ is a multi-ring. The proof is the same as before since Theorem 2 still holds. □

The above theorem provides us with two kinds of quotients lying in the class of multi-rings. One can wonder if the quotient can provide some information about the Marshall-coherent subset.

Proposition 1. *Let $A/\sim_S$ be a multi-ring, and S be a Marshall-coherent subset, such that $1 \in S$ and $\sim = \sim_2$. Then, $[1]$ is 1-convex if, and only if, $[1]$ is convex.*

Proof. (Sketch:) Note that $[S] = [1]$ is Marshall-coherent. The converse is immediate. To prove the reciprocal statement, use $[x] \cdot [s] \cdot [\sigma(x)] = [xs\sigma(x)] = [1]$ (since the quotient is a multi-ring, $\cdot$ is a usual operation) for all $s \in [1]$. We obtain $xs\sigma(x) \in [1]$ and, therefore $[1]$ is convex. □

According to the above results, some immediate examples follow below.

Example 8. *For a given (A, σ), a (R, σ')-multialgebra with involution, the following sets are Marshall-coherent:*

(a) *The set of all non-zero divisors A_0;*
(b) *The set of all invertible elements $A^\times$;*
(c) *The set of all symmetric elements (in A_0) $Sym(A, \sigma) = \{a \in A_0 | a = \sigma(a)\}$;*

(d) If $x\sigma(x) \in Z(A)$ for all $x \in A$, then $A_0\sigma(A_0) = \{a\sigma(a)| \ a \in A_0\}$ is Marshall-coherent and convex.

In the next section, we will provide more examples minutely. For now, we treat another kind of operation in the quotient. For $a, a' \in A$, let $a \sim_S a'$ if, and only if, there exist $s, t, s', t' \in S$ such that $sat = s'a't'$. This can be replaced in terms of the equivalent statements in 3 or 4, whether $x \cdot S = S \cdot x$ or S is convex, respectively. Hence, $\sim_S$ is an equivalence relation. Moreover, each $[a]$ is invariant under S action, $[a] = [sa]$ for all $s \in S$.

In $A/\sim_S$ define $[a] + [b] := \{[c] : \exists r_i, s_i, t_i \in S, r_0 c r_1 \in s_0 a s_1 + t_0 b t_1\}$, $-[a] := [-a]$ and $[a] \cdot [b] := [ab]$.

Theorem 4. *Suppose that $x \cdot S = S \cdot x$. Then, we have the following:*

1. *$A/\sim_S$ is a (non-commutative) multi-ring.*
2. *If A is a hyperring, then $A/\sim_S$ is a hyperring. In particular, if A is a ring, then $A/\sim_S$ is a hyperring.*
3. *It holds the universal property of Marshall's quotient for homomorphisms $f : A \to M$ and anti-homomorphisms (= homomorphism $f : A \to M^{op}$) such that $f[S] = \{1\}$.*

Proof. To demonstrate 1, we note that $+, \cdot,$ and $-$ are well-defined as multi-group operations, and $0 = [0] = \{0\}$ is the null element because A is a multi-ring.

Suppose that $[c] \in [a] + [b]$. Thus, there exists $r, s, t \in S$, satisfying $rc \in sa + tb$ in A. Therefore, $sa \in rc + t(-b)$ (in A). Similarly, $tb \in s(-a) + rc$. Consequently, $[a] \in [c] - [b]$ and $[b] \in -[a] + [c]$.

Let $[b] \in [a] + [0]$. By definition, there exists $r \in S$ such that $rb \in sa + t0$ for some $s, t \in S$. However, it implies $[a] = [b]$. The reciprocal is obvious.

If $[x] \in [a] + [b]$ and $[t] \in [x] + [c]$, then $vt \in wx + zc$ and $r'wx \in s'a + p'b$ for $r', s', p', v, w, z \in S$. Afterward,

$$vt \in wx + zc \implies r'vt \in r'wx + r'zc$$
$$\exists r'wx(r'wx \in s'a + p'b \land r'vt \in r'wx + r'zc) \implies \exists y(y \in p'b + r'zc \land r'vt \in s'a + y)$$

The last implication means $\exists [y]([y] \in [b] + [c] \land [t] \in [a] + [y])$. Once A is a multi-ring, $[c] \in [a] + [b]$ if, and only if, $[c] \in [b] + [a]$ follows.

We already proved that $(A/\sim_S, +, -, 0)$ is a multi-group. Note that there exists $1 = [1] = S \in A/\sim_S$ such that $[a] \cdot [1] = [a]$ for all $[a] \in A/\sim_S$. Thus, $(A/\sim_S, \cdot, 1)$ is a monoid. Moreover, $[a] \cdot 0 = 0$. Finally, let $[c] \in [a] + [b]$ and $pd \in [d] \in A/\sim_S$. By definition, exists $r, s, t \in S$ such that $rc \in sa + tb$. Since A is a multi-ring, $rcpd \in sapd + tbpd$. Using the 'normality property' of S, we rewrite it as follows:

$$r'cd \in s'ad + t'bd \therefore [c][d] \in [a][d] + [b][d].$$

Similarly, $[d][c] \in [d][a] + [d][b]$ holds. It follows that $A/\sim_S$ is a multi-ring. For the second assertion, suppose that A is a hyperring. Let $[e] \in [a][d] + [b][d]$. Thus,

$$\exists s, r, t \in S, se \in rad + tbd \implies se \in (ra + tb)d \quad (A \text{ is hyperring})$$
$$\implies [e] \in ([a] + [b])[d] \quad (\text{by definition of } +).$$

Therefore, $[a][d] + [b][d] = ([a] + [b])[d]$. By symmetry, $[d][a] + [d][b] = [d]([a] + [b])$ also follows.

To demonstrate the third statement, consider $f : A \longrightarrow M$ a homomorphism such that $f([S]) = 1$. Let $a \in A$ and $s \in S$. Thus, $f(sa) = f(s)f(a) = f(a)$. Define the homomorphism $\bar{f} : A/\sim_S \longrightarrow M$ with $\bar{f}([a]) = f(a)$. Hence, $\bar{f}$ is well-defined, and $f = \bar{f} \circ \psi$, with $\psi(a) = [a]$ the canonical projection. It is immediate that another homomorphism $\bar{g} : A/\sim_S \longrightarrow M$ satisfying $f = \bar{g} \circ \psi$ must coincide with $\bar{f}$. $\square$

Remark 1. *Theorem 4 is valid if S is convex. Since both conditions normality and convexity imply $\sim_2 = \sim_3$, we are capable of proving that the distributive laws hold and the entire rest of the proof follows as above.*

The next theorem distinguishes Marshall-coherent subsets that lie in the center $Z(A)$ from an ordinary one.

Theorem 5. *Let A be a multialgebra with involution and $S \subseteq A$ be a Marshall-coherent subset such that $S \subseteq Z(A)$ (thus, in particular, $xS = Sx$, for all $x \in A$). Then, $A/_m S$ is a (non-commutative) hyperring with induced involution.*

Proof. From previous considerations and Theorem 2, we prove that $A/_m S$ is a multi-ring instead of a superring, and the hyperring property still holds.

In fact, if $[c] \in [a][b]$, then $cr = asbt$ for some $r, s, t \in S \subseteq Z(A)$, which means $cr = (ab)(st)$ and $c \sim ab$. Then, $[a][b] = \{[ab]\}$, proving that $A/_m S$ is a multi-ring.

Now, let $[y] \in [c][a] + [c][b]$. Then, $[y] = [d_1] + [d_2]$ for some $[d_1] \in [c][a]$, $[d_2] \in [c][b]$, providing the following equations:

$$y = r_1 d_1 s_1 + r_2 d_2 s_2,$$
$$d_1 = t_1 c v_1 a w_1 \text{ and}$$
$$d_2 = t_2 c v_2 a w_2$$

for some $r_1, r_2, s_1, s_2, t_1, t_2, v_1, v_2, w_1, w_2 \in S$. Then, we have the following:

$$\begin{aligned} y &= r_1 d_1 s_1 + r_2 d_2 s_2 \\ &= r_1 [t_1 c v_1 a w_1] s_1 + r_2 [t_2 c v_2 b w_2] s_2 \\ &= c(r_1 t_1 v_1) a (w_1 s_1) + c(r_2 t_2 v_2) b (w_2 s_2) \\ &= c[(r_1 t_1 v_1) a (w_1 s_1) + (r_2 t_2 v_2) b (w_2 s_2)] \end{aligned}$$

implying that $[y] \in [c]([a] + [b])$. The same reasoning provides $[ac] + [bc] \subseteq ([a] + [b])[c]$. □

5. Applications

This section focuses on results surrounding particular examples. We verify some quotients associated with typical multi-structures, a few of them presented in Section 2. Throughout the subsections below, we deal with technical results and interpret elements in the Marshall quotient as classes of isometric elements.

5.1. Orthogonal

Let R be a commutative ring and A be an R-algebra with involution σ. We denote the following:

$$\text{Orth}(A) := \{a \in A : a\sigma(a) = \sigma(a)a = 1\}.$$

Once we prove that $\text{Orth}(A)$ is a Marshall-coherent subset, then, by definition, the standard property also holds, as follows:

Lemma 6. *The set $\text{Orth}(A)$ is non-empty and if $a, b \in \text{Orth}(A)$ then $\sigma(a), ab \in \text{Orth}(A)$.*

Proof. The set $\text{Orth}(A)$ is non-empty because $1 \in \text{Orth}(A)$. For the rest, note that $\sigma(a)\sigma(\sigma(a)) = \sigma(a)a$ and $(ab)\sigma(ab) = ab[\sigma(b)\sigma(a)]$ for all $a, b \in A$. If $a, b \in \text{Orth}(A)$, these imply $\sigma(a)a = a\sigma(a) = 1$ and

$$(ab)\sigma(ab) = ab[\sigma(b)\sigma(a)] = a[b\sigma(b)]\sigma(a) = a\sigma(a) = 1.$$

□

Now let $a, b \in A$. We define

$$a \sim b \text{ if, and only if, } as = tb \text{ for some } b, t \in \text{Orth}(A).$$

Note that $a \sim b$ if, and only if, $a = sbt$ for some $s, t \in \text{Orth}(A)$, because $S = \text{Orth}(A)$ is a Marshall-coherent standard subset.

Theorem 6. *The structure* $(A/\sim, +, \cdot, [0], [1])$ *is a superring with involution* $\sigma([a]) := [\sigma(a)]$.

Proof. Note that $a \sim 0$ if, and only if, $a = 0$. Moreover, from the very definitions of the sum and the product, we have for all $a, b \in A$,

$$[a] + [0] = [0] + [a] = \{[a]\}, \ [a][1] = [1][a] = \{[a]\},$$
$$[a] + [b] = [b] + [a],$$
$$\sigma([a][b]) = [\sigma(b)][\sigma(a)],$$
$$[0] \in [a] + [b] \iff [b] = -[a].$$

Now, let $a, b, c \in A$ and $[e] \in ([a] + [b]) + [c]$. As a result, $[e]$ also belongs to $[x] + [c]$ for some $[x] \in [a] + [b]$. Consequently, we can express e as $s_1 x s_2 + t_1 c t_2$ and x as $v_1 a v_2 + w_1 b w_2$, where $s_1, s_2, t_1, t_2, v_1, v_2, w_1, w_2 \in \text{Orth}(A)$. Then, we have the following:

$$e = s_1 x s_2 + t_1 c t_2$$
$$= s_1(v_1 a v_2 + w_1 b w_2) s_2 + t_1 c t_2$$
$$= (s_1 v_1) a (v_2 s_2) + (s_1 w_1) b (w_2 s_2) + t_1 c t_2$$
$$= (s_1 v_1) a (v_2 s_2) + [(s_1 w_1) b (w_2 s_2) + t_1 c t_2]$$

Let $y = (s_1 w_1) b (w_2 s_2) + t_1 c t_2$. Then, $[e] \in [a] + [y]$ with $[y] \in [b] + [c]$, implying that $[e] \in [a] + ([b] + [c])$. The same reasoning provides $[a]([b][c]) = ([a][b])[c]$.

Finally, let $[x] \in [c]([a] + [b])$. Therefore, $[x] \in [c][d]$ for some $[d] \in [a] + [b]$. These provide equations $x = rcsdt$ and $d = s_1 a s_2 + t_1 b t_2$. Thus, we have the following:

$$x = rcsdt$$
$$= rcs[s_1 a s_2 + t_1 b t_2]t$$
$$= rcss_1 a s_2 t + rcst_1 b t_2 t$$
$$= rc(ss_1) a (s_2 t) + rc(st_1) b (t_2 t)$$

with $r, ss_1, s_2 t, st_1, t_2 t \in \text{Orth}(A)$, concluding that $[x] \in [c][a] + [c][b]$. Similarly, we conclude that $([a] + [b])[c] \subseteq [a][c] + [b][c]$. □

Observe that S is not necessarily convex, and neither satisfies $xS = Sx$ (see Theorem 2). Thus, $A/\sim$ may not be a multi-ring.

Definition 9. *We define the superring* $(A/\sim, +, \cdot, [0], [1])$ *as the* **orthogonal fragment** *of* A, *and denote by* $A/_m \text{Orth}(A) := A/\sim$.

Theorem 7. *If* $\text{Orth}(A) \subseteq Z(A)$, *then* $A/_m \text{Orth}(A)$ *is a (non-commutative) hyperring.*

Proof. This is a particular case of Theorem 5. □

Theorem 8. *Let F be a field and $A = M_2(F)$. Then $A/_m \text{Orth}(A)$ consists of rotation 2×2 matrices over F.*

Proof. Note that $a \in \text{Orth}(A)$ if, and only if, $aa^t = id_2$, with $\sigma(a) = a^t$ the transpose matrix of $a = (a_{ij})_{2\times 2}$. Applying the definition of matrix product, we have to solve the following system:

$$\begin{cases} a_{11}^2 + a_{12}^2 = 1 \\ a_{21}^2 + a_{22}^2 = 1 \\ a_{11}a_{21} + a_{12}a_{22} = 0 \\ \det(a)^2 = 1 \end{cases}.$$

We conclude the following:

$$\text{Orth}(A) = \left\{ \begin{pmatrix} x & y \\ y & -x \end{pmatrix} \mid x^2 + y^2 = 1,\ x, y \in F \right\} \cup \left\{ \begin{pmatrix} x & -y \\ y & x \end{pmatrix} \mid x^2 + y^2 = 1,\ x, y \in F \right\}. \tag{6}$$

□

If $F = \mathbb{R}$, in (6), the second subset (with the positive determinant equal to 1) is the set of orthonormal matrices or the set of linear transformations in $\mathbb{R}^2$ that are rotations by some angle $\theta \in [0, 2\pi)$ with $x = \cos(\theta)$ and $y = \sin(\theta)$. Moreover, consider the inner product

$$\langle a, b \rangle = \sum_{i,j=1}^{2} a_{ij} b_{ij},\ \text{for } a, b \in A.$$

One may verify that the actions of elements in $\text{Orth}(A)$ function as a set of isometries. By solving a system of equations very similar to the one discussed above, it is possible to demonstrate that these actions form a subset of isometries. The associated matrix, denoted as $T = (t_{ij})$, has a determinant different from $\pm(t_{11} - t_{12})$. Thus, this quotient describes the behavior concerning certain kinds of isometry classes considering the underlined inner product.

5.2. Quaternions over Real Closed Fields

Now, we explore the diversity of quotients in quaternions. Although this includes a lot of calculations, it provides quick verification of independence regarding normal and convex quotients.

Example 9. *Let R be a real closed field and*

$$H = R\{x, y\}/(x^2 + 1, y^2 + 1, xy + yx)$$

the corresponding quaternion algebra $(1,1)_R$; it is an R-division algebra of dimension 4. Put $S = R_{>0} \cdot 1 \subseteq H$. Note that S satisfies the second condition of the Theorem 3 (it is a convex set) in the previous section and $S = \{\sigma(a) \cdot a : a \in H \setminus \{0\}\}$.

Then, $H/_m S \cong \mathbb{S}^3$ is a monoid. And, in this quotient, $\overline{x \cdot \sigma(x) \cdot x} = \overline{x}$, as $\overline{x \cdot \sigma(x)} = 1$.

We observe that, in this case, S is also standard, "normal", and 1-convex (see Lemma 5).

Example 10. *Let $\mathbb{H}$ be the quaternions real algebra endowed with the standard involution $\sigma(a) = \bar{a}$, for all $a \in \mathbb{H}$. Set $S = \mathbb{R} \setminus \{0\}$ and define $a \sim b$ iff $a = \sigma(x)b$ for some $x, y \in S$. Thus, $[0] = \{0\}$, and for a nonzero element a, $[a]$ is the line determined by the origin and the quaternion a (without $\{0\}$), i.e., $\mathbb{H}/_m S \cong \mathbb{RP}^3$.*

Once $S \subseteq Z(\mathbb{H})$ (S has the first "normality" property of the Theorem 3), it is easy to check that $S = [1] = [-1]$, and $[\pm a] = Sa$, and for a, a pure quaternion as well. If $a = a_0 + a_1 i + a_2 j + a_3 k$ and $b = b_0 + b_1 i + b_2 j + b_3 k$ are quaternion numbers, then we have the following:

$$[a] + [b] = \bigcup [x_0 + x_1 i + x_2 j + x_3 k], \tag{7}$$

for $x_i \in \mathbb{R}$, $x_i \in S$, or $x_i = 0$, depending on $a_i, b_i \neq 0$, or $a_i \neq 0$ and $b_i = 0$ (and vice-versa), or both $a_i = b_i = 0$, respectively, for each $i \in \{0,1,2,3\}$. Hence, $[a] + [b]$ is the plane determined by $[a]$ and $[b]$, containing (or not containing) the origin.

Example 11. *Consider the orthogonal fragment* $\mathrm{Orth}(\mathbb{H})$. *Let* $S = \mathbb{S}^3 \subseteq \mathbb{H}$, *representing the sphere of radius with 1 centered at the origin.*

Clearly, $1 \in S$, and S is a multiplicative set, satisfying $x^{-1} \in S$ whenever $x \in S$. Once $|x| = x\sigma(x)$, it is immediate that S is σ-invariant. It remains to verify that the sphere qualifies as "a normal set" in $\mathbb{H}$ (item 1 of Theorem 3) and, thus, the quotient is a multi-ring. In fact, let $a \in \mathbb{H}$ and $x \in S$; given the norm is multiplicative, we have the following:

$$|ax| = |a| \implies a\sigma(a)x\sigma(x) = \sigma(a)a \implies a\sigma(a)x = \sigma(x)^{-1}\sigma(a)a$$
$$\implies \sigma(a)ax = \sigma(x)^{-1}\sigma(a)a \implies ax = (\sigma(a)^{-1}\sigma(x)^{-1}\sigma(a))a. \tag{8}$$

Yet, we have the following: $|\sigma(a)^{-1}\sigma(x)^{-1}\sigma(a)| = |\sigma(a)^{-1}||\sigma(x)^{-1}||\sigma(a)| = |\sigma(a)^{-1}||\sigma(a)| = 1$; therefore,

$$y = \sigma(a)^{-1}\sigma(x)^{-1}\sigma(a) \in S.$$

We conclude that $ax = ya$ for some $y \in S$, i.e., $aS \subseteq Sa$. The reverse inclusion is followed by symmetry. Moreover, in a general division algebra with standard involution, this property holds since $S = \mathrm{Orth}(\mathbb{H})$.

Let $a \sim b$ iff $a = \sigma(x)by$, with $x, y \in S$. Hence, $a \sim b$ iff $|a| = |b|$. It is obvious that $[0] = \{0\}$ and $[1] = \mathbb{S}^3 = S$. The elements $[a]$ are spheres centered at the origin with radius $\sqrt{|a|}$. In fact, $\sqrt{|a|} = a \cdot \frac{\sigma(a)}{\sqrt{|a|}}$, with $x = \frac{\sigma(a)}{\sqrt{|a|}} \in S$. Therefore, $\sqrt{|a|} \sim a$. For $a \in [b]$, $[a] + [b]$ forms a filled sphere with radius $2\sqrt{|a|}$. If $|a| > |b|$, both triangular inequalities $|a+b| \leq |a| + |b|$ and $||a| - |b|| \leq |a - b|$ indicate that $[a] + [b]$ is the 'hollow' surface defined by two spheres with coincident centers at the origin and radii $\sqrt{|a|} + \sqrt{|b|}$ and $\sqrt{|a|} - \sqrt{|b|}$. Moreover, $\mathbb{H}/_m S \cong \mathbb{R}_+$, as a multimonoid with multi-addition, satisfies the following:

$$[a] + [b] = \begin{cases} [a-b, a+b] & \text{if } a \geq b; \\ [b-a, a+b] & \text{if } b \geq a. \end{cases}$$

Thus, this is the triangle hyperfield Example 4. In the last example, S does not satisfy the convexity property. At the same time, Example 9 shows Marshall-coherent sets satisfying many properties simultaneously. These examples illustrate that the definitions provided in the previous section encapsulate elements of different types of structures and demonstrate the independence between the statements outlined in Theorem 3.

6. Conclusions

We have extended the concept of the (commutative) multi-ring, as presented in Marshall's seminal paper [1], to the setting of (non-commutative) and involutive multi-rings (Definition 4). Additionally, we have expanded the concept of Marshall's coherent subset to this new setting (Definition 5) and introduced and studied several equivalence relations related to this notion (Definition 6; Lemmas 4 and 5). Furthermore, we have broadened the concept of Marshall's quotient (Definition 8; Theorems 2 and 3) to accommodate this framework, which serves as a key technical tool for constructing many interesting examples of multialgebras with involution. These examples are derived from standard algebraic structures such as orthogonal groups and quaternion algebras, as thoroughly developed in Section 5.

Thus, we have established the groundwork for extending real algebra and real algebraic geometry into the non-commutative and involutive settings, broadening the abstract methodologies utilized in the space of signs [13], abstract real spectra [14], real semigroups [15], and real reduced multi-rings [1]. Notably, the theory presented here lends itself to model-theoretic methods since every n-multi-operation corresponds to a $n+1$-relation, satisfying an $\forall\exists$ axiom. This is an area we intend to explore in future work. Moreover, the continued development of the theory on non-commutative multialgebras with involution should lay a robust foundation for establishing an abstract theory of Hermitian forms ([16]), similar to how the theory of special groups ([22]) serves as an abstract theory of quadratic forms.

Author Contributions: Writing—original draft, K.M.A.R. and H.L.M.; Writing—review & editing, K.R.P.S. All authors have read and agreed to the published version of the manuscript.

Funding: This research was funded by Coordenação de Aperfeiçoamento de Pessoal de Nível Superior (Capes -Brazil) under the program MATH-AMSUD, project "Abstract theories of quadratic and hermitian forms, and real algebraic geometry", grant number 88881.694471/2022-01.

Data Availability Statement: The original contributions presented in the study are included in the article, further inquiries can be directed to the corresponding author.

Acknowledgments: The authors would like to thank the anonymous referees for their valuable suggestions, which substantially improved our presentation.

Conflicts of Interest: The authors declare no conflict of interest.

References

1. Marshall, M. Real reduced multirings and multifields. *J. Pure Appl. Algebra* **2006**, *205*, 452–468. [CrossRef]
2. Ameri, R.; Eyvazi, M.; Hoskova-Mayerova, S. Superring of Polynomials over a Hyperring. *Mathematics* **2019**, *7*, 902. [CrossRef]
3. Al Tahan, M.; Hoskova-Mayerova, S.; Davvaz, B. Some results on (generalized) fuzzy multi-Hv-ideals of Hv-rings. *Symmetry* **2019**, *11*, 1376. [CrossRef]
4. Ameri, R.; Kordi, A.; Hoskova-Mayerova, S. Multiplicative hyperring of fractions and coprime hyperideals. *Analele Univ. Ovidius-Constanta-Ser. Mat.* **2017**, *25*, 5–23. [CrossRef]
5. Ameri, R.; Eyvazi, M.; Hoskova-Mayerova, S. Advanced results in enumeration of hyperfields. *Aims Math.* **2020**, *5*, 6552–6579. [CrossRef]
6. Massouros, C.G. Theory of hyperrings and hyperfields. *Algebra Log.* **1985**, *24*, 477–485. [CrossRef]
7. Nakassis, A. Recent results in hyperring and hyperfield theory. *Int. J. Math. Math. Sci.* **1988**, *11*, 209–220. [CrossRef]
8. Massouros, G.G.; Massouros, C.G. Homomorphic relation on hyperingoids and join hyperrings. *Ratio Math.* **1999**, *13*, 61–70.
9. Massouros, C.G.; Massouros, G.G. On join hyperrings. In Proceedings of the 10th International Congress on Algebraic Hyperstructures and Applications, Brno, Czech Republic, 3–9 September 2008; pp. 203–215.
10. de Andrade Roberto, K.M.; de Oliveira Ribeiro, H.R.; Mariano, H.L.; Santos, K.R.P. Linear Systems, Matrices and Vector Spaces over Superfields. *arXiv* **2023**, arXiv:2303.14459.
11. Kuhlmann, K.; Linzi, A.; Stojałowska, H. Orderings and valuations in hyperfields. *J. Algebra* **2022**, *611*, 399–421. [CrossRef]
12. de Oliveira Ribeiro, H.R.; de Andrade Roberto, K.M.; Mariano, H.L. Functorial relationship between multirings and the various abstract theories of quadratic forms. *São Paulo J. Math. Sci.* **2022**, *16*, 5–42. [CrossRef]
13. Andradas, C.; Bröcker, L.; Ruiz, J.M. *Constructible Sets in Real Geometry*; Springer Science & Business Media: Berlin/Heidelberg, Germany, 1996; Volume 33.
14. Marshall, M.A. *Spaces of Orderings and Abstract Real Spectra*; Lecture Notes in Mathematics 1636; Springer: Berlin/Heidelberg, Germany, 1996.
15. Dickmann, M.; Petrovich, A. Real semigroups and abstract real spectra. I. *Contemp. Math.* **2004**, *344*, 99–120.
16. Knus, M.A. Quadratic and Hermitian forms over rings. In *Grundlehren der Mathematischen Wissenschaften a Series of Comprehensive Studies in Mathematics*, Springer: Berlin/Heidelberg, Germany, 1991; Volume 294.
17. Jun, J. Algebraic geometry over hyperrings. *Adv. Math.* **2018**, *323*, 142–192. [CrossRef]
18. Viro, O. Hyperfields for Tropical Geometry I. Hyperfields and dequantization. *arXiv* **2010**, arXiv:1006.3034.
19. de Andrade Roberto, K.M. Multirings and the Chamber of Secrets: Relationships between Abstract Theories of Quadratic Forms. Master's Thesis, Universidade de São Paulo, São Paulo, Brazil, 2019.
20. de Andrade Roberto, K.M.; Mariano, H.L. On superrings of polynomials and algebraically closed multifields. *J. Pure Appl. Log.* **2022**, *9*, 419–444.
21. Davvaz, B.; Salasi, A. A Realization of Hyperrings. *Commun. Algebra* **2006**, *34*, 4389–4400. [CrossRef]
22. Dickmann, M.; Miraglia, F. *Special Groups: Boolean-Theoretic Methods in the Theory of Quadratic Forms*; Number 689 in Memoirs AMS; American Mathematical Society: Providence, RI, USA, 2000.

Disclaimer/Publisher's Note: The statements, opinions and data contained in all publications are solely those of the individual author(s) and contributor(s) and not of MDPI and/or the editor(s). MDPI and/or the editor(s) disclaim responsibility for any injury to people or property resulting from any ideas, methods, instructions or products referred to in the content.

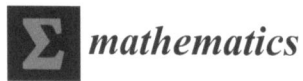 *mathematics*

Article

Optimizing HX-Group Compositions Using C++: A Computational Approach to Dihedral Group Hyperstructures

Andromeda Pătrașcu Sonea [†] and Ciprian Chiruță *,[†]

"Ion Ionescu de la Brad" Iasi University of Life Sciences, 700490 Iași, Romania; andromeda.patrascu@iuls.ro
* Correspondence: ciprian.chiruta@iuls.ro
[†] These authors contributed equally to this work.

Abstract: The HX-groups represent a generalization of the group notion. The Chinese mathematicians Mi Honghai and Li Honxing analyzed this theory. Starting with a group $(G, \cdot)$, they constructed another group $(\mathcal{G}, *) \subset \mathcal{P}^*(G)$, where $\mathcal{P}^*(G)$ is the set of non-empty subsets of G. The hypercomposition "$*$" is thus defined for any A, B from G, $A * B = \{a \cdot b | a \in A, b \in B\}$. In this article, we consider a particular group, G, to be the dihedral group D_n, n is a natural number, greater than 3, and we analyze the HX-groups with the dihedral group D_n as a support. The HX- groups were studied algebraically, but the novelty of this article is that it is a computer analysis of the HX-groups by creating a program in C++. This code aims to improve the calculation time regarding the composition of the HX-groups. In the first part of the paper, we present some results from the hypergroup theory and HX-groups. We create another hyperstructure formed by reuniting all the HX-groups associated with a dihedral group D_n as a support for a natural fixed number n. In the second part, we present the C++ code created in the Microsoft Visual Studio program, and we provide concrete examples of the program's application. We created this program because the code aims to improve the calculation time regarding the composition of HX-groups.

Keywords: HX-group; C++ code; group; hypergroup; dihedral group

MSC: 20N20

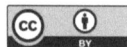

Citation: Sonea, A.P.; Chiruță, C. Optimizing HX-Group Compositions Using C++: A Computational Approach to Dihedral Group Hyperstructures. *Mathematics* **2024**, *12*, 3492. https://doi.org/10.3390/math12223492

Academic Editors: Irina Cristea and Alessandro Linzi

Received: 30 September 2024
Revised: 1 November 2024
Accepted: 2 November 2024
Published: 8 November 2024

Copyright: © 2024 by the authors. Licensee MDPI, Basel, Switzerland. This article is an open access article distributed under the terms and conditions of the Creative Commons Attribution (CC BY) license (https://creativecommons.org/licenses/by/4.0/).

1. Introduction

Hypergroup theory represents a generalization of classical algebraic structures. F. Marty noticed that the quotient group's elements are sets, and he introduced the concept of a hypergroup in 1934 [1]. Over time, the theory of hypergroups has developed greatly from a theoretical point of view. It has applications in numerous fields, such as geometry, topology, cryptography, code theory, graphs, hypergraphs, automata theory, fuzzy degree, probability, etc. [2–8]. Starting with a non-empty set H and the hyperoperation "$\circ$": $H \times H \to \mathcal{P}^*(H)$, where $\mathcal{P}^*(H)$ represents the collection of all non-empty subsets of H, we obtained a semihypergroup if and only if the hyperoperation satisfies the associativity relation, i.e., $(a \circ b) \circ c = a \circ (b \circ c)$, for any $a, b, c \in H^3$. Also, $(H, \circ)$ is a quasihypergroup if and only if the hyperoperation satisfies the reproducibility relation, i.e., $H \circ a = a \circ H = H$, for any $a \in H$. We say that $(H, \circ)$ is a hypergroup if and only if "$\circ$" satisfies the associativity and reproducibility relation. In hypergroup theory, we can compute two sets in the following way: for any A, B sets from H, $A \circ B = A \circ B = \cup \{a \circ b / a \in A, b \in B\}$. In 1985, three Chinese mathematicians, HongXing Li, QinZhi Duan, and PeizHuang, used the term "hypergroup" [9]. Later, Li renamed the concept with the term HX-groups [10]. Zhenliang studied the properties of HX-groups [11], and, recently, the interest in this concept has increased. Corsini studied the hypergroups associated with $\mathbb{Z}/n\mathbb{Z}$, the Chinese hypergroupoid of an HX-group, and found conditions such that the Chinese hypergroupoid becomes a hypergroup; see [12–14]. Cristea established a link between HX-groups and hypergroups [15]. Sonea determined the HX-groups with dihedral group D_n as a support [16], created a new commutative hyperstructure that considered the union of all the HX-groups [17], and studied the NeutroHX-groups [18]. Also, Mousavi, Jafarpour, and Cristea studied the HX-Polygroups [19]. This article is divided into three sections. The first section refers to the introductory notions from the theory of HX-groups and the theory of hypergroups. Also, a new hyperstructure $\mathcal{G}_n$ formed by the union of all the HX-groups associated with the dihedral group D_n for a fixed natural number n is presented [17]. Until now, HX-groups have been analyzed only from an algebraic point of view. In the second part of the article, a computational approach to HX-groups is presented using code in the C++ programming language. This code facilitates the calculation time regarding the composition of HX-groups, and the third section refers to the connection between HX-groups and graph theory.

2. The Construction of the Hyperstructure $\mathcal{G}_n$

In this section, we will present the construction of the hyperstructure $\mathcal{G}_n$. We consider a new hyperstructure formed by the union of all HX-groups with the dihedral group D_n as support for a fixed natural number $n > 3$ [17]. In what follows, we recall the basic notions of HX-groups.

Definition 1 ([10]). *Let $(G, \cdot)$ be a group and $\mathcal{G} \subset \mathcal{P}^*(G)$, where $\mathcal{P}^*(G)$ is the set of non-empty subsets of G. An HX-group is a non-empty subset H of $\mathcal{P}^*(G)$, which is a group with respect to the operation "$*$" defined by*

$$\forall A, B \in \mathcal{G}, A * B = \{a \cdot b \mid a \in A, b \in B\}. \tag{1}$$

We say that $\mathcal{G}$ has group G as support.

The HX-groups with the dihedral group D_n as support denoted by $\mathcal{G}_{p_1}^{q_1}$ are determined [16].

Theorem 1 ([16]). *For $n = p_1 q_1$, $p_1, q_1 \in \mathbb{N}^*$, the $(\mathcal{G}_{p_1}^{q_1}, *)$ is an HX-group associated with the dihedral group D_n with elements*

$$\begin{aligned} A_i &= \{\rho^i, \rho^{q_1+i}, \rho^{2q_1+i}, \ldots, \rho^{(p_1-1)q_1+i}\}; \\ A_{q_1+i} &= \{\rho^i \sigma, \rho^{q_1+i} \sigma, \rho^{2q_1+i} \sigma, \ldots, \rho^{(p_1-1)q_1+i} \sigma\}; \end{aligned}$$

where $i \in \{0, 1, \ldots, q_1 - 1\}$.

Proposition 1. *The $<\rho^q>$ is a normal subgroup in D_n, where $n = pq$, p, q are natural numbers.*

Proof. In what follows, we will recall the definition of a normal subgroup, which we will apply [20] in the demonstration. Let $(G, \cdot)$ be a group and H a subgroup of G. For any x in G, H is a normal subgroup in G if and only if $xH = Hx$. In this case,

$$H = <\rho^q> = \{e, \rho^q, q^{2q}, \ldots, q^{(p-1)q}\}.$$

Therefore, the elements in H are of the form ρ^{kq}, $k \in \{0, 1, \ldots, p-1\}$. We have to show that $x \rho^{kq} x^{-1} \in H$ for any $x \in D_n$ and $k \in \{0, 1, \ldots, p-1\}$. For $x = \rho^t$, $t \in \{0, 1, \ldots, n-1\}$, we obtain

$$xhx^{-1} = \rho^t \rho^{kq} (\rho^t)^{-1} = \rho^{t+kq+n-t} = \rho^{n+kq} = \rho^n \rho^{kq} = e \rho^{kq} = \rho^{kq} \in H.$$

For $x = \rho^t \sigma$,

$$\begin{aligned} xhx^{-1} &= \rho^t \sigma \rho^{kq} (\rho^t \sigma)^{-1} = \rho^t \sigma \rho^{kq} \rho^t \sigma = \rho^t \sigma \rho^{kq+t} \sigma \\ &= \rho^t \sigma \sigma \rho^{n-(kq+t)} = \rho^t e \rho^{n-(kq+t)} = \rho^{t+n-(kq+t)} \\ &= \rho^{n-kq} = \rho^{(p-k)q} \in H. \end{aligned}$$

In conclusion, $<\rho^q>$ is a normal subgroup in the dihedral group D_n. □

Proposition 2. *The HX-group obtained previously represents the quotien group $G_p^q = \frac{D_n}{<\rho^q>}$ for $n = pq$.*

Proof. We proved before that $<\rho^q>$ is a normal subgroup in D_n, so

$$\frac{D_n}{<\rho^q>} = \{x <\rho^q> / x \in D_n\}.$$

For $x = \rho^t$, $t \in \{0, 1, \ldots, n-1\}$, we obtain

$$\rho^t <\rho^q> = \rho^t \cdot \{e, \rho^q, q^{2q}, \ldots, q^{(p-1)q}\} = \{\rho^t, \rho^{t+q}, \ldots, \rho^{t+(p-1)q}\} = A_t,$$

where A_t is defined by Theorem 1.

For $x = \rho^t \sigma$, $t \in \{0, 1, \ldots, n-1\}$, we have

$$\begin{aligned} \rho^t \sigma <\rho^q> &= \rho^t \sigma \cdot \{e, \rho^q, q^{2q}, \ldots, q^{(p-1)q}\} = \{\rho^t \sigma, \rho^t \sigma \rho^q, \rho^t \sigma q^{2q}, \ldots, \rho^t \sigma q^{(p-1)q}\} \\ &= \{\rho^t \sigma, \rho^t \rho^{n-q} \sigma, \rho^t \rho^{n-2q} \sigma, \ldots, \rho^t \rho^{n-(p-1)q} \sigma\} \\ &= \{\rho^t \sigma, \rho^{t+(p-1)q} \sigma, \rho^{t+(p-2)q} \sigma, \ldots, \rho^{t+q} \sigma\} \\ &= \{\rho^t \sigma, \rho^{t+q} \sigma, \ldots, \rho^{t+(p-2)q} \sigma, \rho^{t+(p-1)q} \sigma\} = A_{q+t}, \end{aligned}$$

where A_{q+t}, is defined by Theorem 1. Therefore, we can conclude that $\frac{D_n}{<\rho^q>} = G_p^q$. □

After that, we took into consideration the union of all HX-groups associated with a dihedral group D_n as support, and we obtained a new hyperstructure defined in [17].

$$\mathcal{G}_n = \left\{ \mathcal{G}_{p_1}^{q_1} \mid HX - \text{groups for any } p_1, q_1 \in \mathbb{N}^* \text{ such that } n = p_1 q_1 \right\}$$

is the set of all HX-groups. We define the hyperoperation "$\circ$": $\mathcal{G}_n \times \mathcal{G}_n \to P^*(\mathcal{G}_n)$; thus,

$$\begin{aligned} \mathcal{G}_{p_1}^{q_1} \circ \mathcal{G}_{p_2}^{q_2} &= \bigcup_{0 \leq s \leq 2p_1 - 1} \left(\bigcup_{0 \leq t \leq 2p_2 - 1} C_{s,t} \right), \\ C_{s,t} &= X_s^{q_1} * Y_t^{q_2}; \; X_s^{q_1} \in \mathcal{G}_{p_1}^{q_1}, Y_t^{q_2} \in \mathcal{G}_{p_2}^{q_2} \\ n &= p_1 q_1 = p_2 q_2, \; p_1, q_1, \; p_2, q_2 \in \mathbb{N}^*. \end{aligned}$$

We analyzed the hyperstructure $(\mathcal{G}_4, \circ)$ and obtained some results; see [17].

Proposition 3. *The hyperstructure $(\mathcal{G}_4, \circ)$ is a commutative structure where*

$$\mathcal{G}_4 = \left\{ \mathcal{G}_{p_1}^{q_1} \mid HX - \text{groups, for any } p_1, q_1 \in \mathbb{N}^* \text{ such that } 4 = p_1 q_1 \right\}.$$

Remark 1. *The elements of the hyperstructure $(\mathcal{G}_4, \circ)$ satisfy the following equality*

$$\mathcal{G}_{p_1}^{q_1} \circ \mathcal{G}_{p_2}^{q_2} = \mathcal{G}_{p_2}^{q_2} \circ \mathcal{G}_{p_1}^{q_1} = \mathcal{G}_{\text{GCD}\{p_1, p_2\}}^{\text{LCM}\{q_1, q_2\}}, \qquad (2)$$

for any $p_1, q_1, q_2, p_2 \in \mathbb{N}^*$ such that $4 = p_1 q_1 = p_2 q_2$.

LCM$\{q_1, q_2\}$ represents the least common multiple of numbers q_1, q_2, and GCD $\{p_1, p_2\}$ represent the greatest common divisors of p_1, p_2.

Proposition 4. *The hyperstructure $(\mathcal{G}_4, \circ)$ is a semihypergroup, but not a quasihypergroup.*

Now, we present the connection between the number of cyclic subgroups and the cardinality of $\mathcal{G}_n$.

Remark 2. *The cyclic subgroups of the dihedral group D_n are $<\sigma>$, $<\rho\sigma>$,...,$<\rho^{n-1}\sigma>$, and $<\rho^d>$, where d is a divisor of n. So, the number of all cyclic subgroups is $n + \tau(n)$, where $\tau(n) = (\alpha_1 + 1)(\alpha_2 + 1)\ldots(\alpha_k + 1)$, $n = p_1^{\alpha_1} p_2^{\alpha_2} \ldots p_k^{\alpha_k}$.*

Proposition 5. *The cardinality of the hyperstructure $\mathcal{G}_n$ is equal to the number of normal subgroups of a dihedral group D_n.*

Proof. According to Proposition 1 and Remark 2, we can state that the normal subgroups of the dihedral group D_n are $<\rho^d>$, where d is a divisor of n. Also, the construction of the hyperstructure $\mathcal{G}_n$ implies that the $|\mathcal{G}_n| = \tau(n)$, where $\tau(n) = (\alpha_1 + 1)(\alpha_2 + 1)\ldots(\alpha_k + 1)$, $n = p_1^{\alpha_1} p_2^{\alpha_2} \ldots p_k^{\alpha_k}$. The conclusion is immediate. □

Example 1. *We determine the composition between the HX-groups $\mathcal{G}_1^4$ and $\mathcal{G}_2^2$, where*

$$\mathcal{G}_2^2 = \{\{e, \rho^2\}, \{\rho, \rho^3\}, \{\sigma, \rho^2\sigma\}, \{\rho\sigma, \rho^3\sigma\}\};$$
$$\mathcal{G}_1^4 = \{\{e, \rho, \rho^2, \rho^3\}, \{\sigma, \rho\sigma, \rho^2\sigma, \rho^3\sigma\}\}.$$

Therefore,

$$\mathcal{G}_1^4 * \mathcal{G}_2^2 = \{C_{0,0}, C_{0,1}, C_{0,2}, C_{0,3}, C_{1,0}, C_{1,1}, C_{1,2}, C_{1,3}\},$$

and the sets $X_s^{q_1}, Y_t^{q_2}$, where $s \in \{0,1\}$, $t \in \{0,1,2,3\}$, $q_1 = 4, q_2 = 2$, are

$$X_0^4 = \{e, \rho, \rho^2, \rho^3\}, \ X_1^4 = \{\sigma, \rho\sigma, \rho^2\sigma, \rho^3\sigma\},$$
$$Y_0^2 = \{e, \rho^2\}, \ Y_1^2 = \{\rho, \rho^3\}, \ Y_2^2 = \{\sigma, \rho^2\sigma\}, Y_3^2 = \{\rho\sigma, \rho^3\sigma\}.$$

In the following, we calculate the elements $C_{i,j}, i \in \{0,1\}, j \in \{0,1,2,3\}$.

$$\begin{aligned}
C_{0,0} &= X_0^4 * Y_0^2 = \{e, \rho, \rho^2, \rho^3\} * \{e, \rho^2\} = e \cdot e \cup e \cdot \rho^2 \cup \rho \cdot e \cup \\
&\cup \rho \cdot \rho^2 \cup \rho^2 \cdot e \cup \rho^2 \cdot \rho^2 \cup \rho^3 \cdot e \cup \rho^3 \cdot \rho^3 \\
&= \{e, \rho, \rho^2, \rho^3\} = X_0^4; \\
C_{0,1} &= X_0^4 * Y_1^2 = \{e, \rho, \rho^2, \rho^3\} * \{\rho, \rho^3\} = \\
&= e \cdot \rho \cup e \cdot \rho^3 \cup \rho \cdot \rho \cup \rho \cdot \rho^3 \cup \\
&\cup \rho^2 \cdot \rho \cup \rho^2 \cdot \rho^3 \cup \rho^3 \cdot \rho \cup \rho^3 \cdot \rho^3. \\
&= \{e, \rho, \rho^2, \rho^3\} = X_0^4 \\
C_{0,2} &= X_0^4 * Y_2^2 = \{e, \rho, \rho^2, \rho^3\} * \{\sigma, \rho^2\sigma\} = \\
&= \{\sigma, \rho\sigma, \rho^2\sigma, \rho^3\sigma\} = X_1^4. \\
C_{0,3} &= X_0^4 * Y_3^2 = \{e, \rho, \rho^2, \rho^3\} * \{\rho\sigma, \rho^3\sigma\} = X_1^4.
\end{aligned}$$

Similarly, we obtain

$C_{1,0} = X_1^4 * Y_0^2 = X_1^4$, $C_{1,1} = X_1^4 * Y_1^2 = X_1^4$, $C_{1,2} = X_1^4 * Y_2^2 = X_0^4$, $C_{1,3} = X_1^4 * Y_3^2 = X_0^4$.

So, we have

$$\mathcal{G}_1^4 \circ \mathcal{G}_2^2 = \mathcal{G}_1^4.$$

Remark 3. *The calculation time for composing two HX-groups can be quite high. This represents the starting point of the idea of creating code in the C++ programming language because we can improve the calculation time and analyze higher-order HX-groups.*

3. Materials and Methods

Implementing C++ Code into Microsoft Visual Studio 2022

This section will present the code in the C++ programming language, created in *Microsoft Visual Studio* 2022. The code describes the HX-groups associated with the dihedral group D_n and their composition. Creating such a program was needed to improve the calculation time for composing the HX-groups. The composition problem can become quite complex, as observed in the works [17,18]. The input data will be n (the order of the dihedral group D_n), and the divisors p_1, q_1, p_2, q_2 so that $n = p_1 q_1 = p_2 q_2$. In the program, we identify the HX-group $\mathcal{G}_{p_1}^{q_1}$ with $G(p_1, q_1)$; the elements of $\mathcal{G}_{p_1}^{q_1}$ formed a matrix and are noted with $a[i][j]$, and similarly the elements of $\mathcal{G}_{p_2}^{q_2}$ are noted through $b[i][j]$. We identify the elements of the dihedral group with natural numbers. So, we consider the function $f : (D_n, \cdot) \to (\mathbb{N}, +)$ as follows:

$$f\left(\rho^k\right) = k, \tag{3}$$
$$f(\rho^k \sigma) = n + k,$$

where $k \in \{0, 1, \ldots, n-1\}$. For a fixed natural number n, we consider the restriction of function f, so $f : (D_n, \cdot) \to (\{0, 1, \ldots, 2n-1\}, +)$. In these conditions, we can state the following:

Proposition 6. *For a fixed natural number n, the function $f : (D_n, \cdot) \to (\{0, 1, \ldots, 2n-1\}, +)$*

$$f\left(\rho^k\right) = k, \tag{4}$$
$$f(\rho^k \sigma) = n + k,$$

is a bijective function.

Proof. The injectivity results immediately because, for any $x, y \in D_n$ such that $f(x) = f(y)$, it implies $x = y$. The elements from D_n have the form ρ^k or $\rho^k \sigma$. As we can see, $f(\rho^k) \neq f(\rho^k \sigma)$ for any $k \in \{0, 1, \ldots, n-1\}$. So, to have the equality $f(x) = f(y)$ means that $x = \rho^k$, $y = \rho^p$, $k, p \in \{0, 1, \ldots, n-1\}$, or $x = \rho^k \sigma$, $y = \rho^p \sigma$. In both cases, it results that $p = k$; this means that $x = y$. To study the surjectivity, we have to prove that, for any element k from $\{0, 1, \ldots, 2n-1\}$, there is $x \in D_n$ such that $f(x) = k$. For $k \in \{0, 1, \ldots, n-1\}$, we consider $x = \rho^k$, and, for $k \geq n$, we consider $x = \rho^{k-n} \sigma$. In conclusion, f is a bijective function. □

To determine the composition of groups $\mathcal{G}_{p_1}^{q_1} \circ \mathcal{G}_{p_2}^{q_2}$, where $n = p_1 q_1 = p_2 q_2$, we have four cases. We denote by $\oplus$ the composition law created in the program mentioned above, and we provide the composition rules in each case.

Case 1. We compute the elements that have the form ρ^k with ρ^p, for any $k, p \in \{0, 1, \ldots, n-1\}$ in the following way

$$k \oplus p = f(\rho^k) \circ f(\rho^p) = k + p \pmod{n} \tag{5}$$

Case 2. We compute the elements that have the form ρ^k with $\rho^p \sigma$

$$k \oplus (n+p) = f(\rho^k) \circ f(\rho^p \sigma) = \begin{cases} n+k+p, & k+p < n \\ k+p, & k+p \geq n \end{cases} \tag{6}$$

Case 3. The composition of the elements that has the form $\rho^p \sigma$ with ρ^k is

$$(n+p) \oplus k = f(\rho^p \sigma) \circ f(\rho^k) = \begin{cases} 2n + p - k, & p < k \\ n + p - k, & p \geq k \end{cases} \qquad (7)$$

Case 4. The composition of the elements that has the form $\rho^p \sigma$ with $\rho^k \sigma$ is

$$(n+p) \oplus (n+k) = f(\rho^p \sigma) \circ f(\rho^k \sigma) = \begin{cases} p - k, & p \geq k \\ p + n - k, & p < k \end{cases}. \qquad (8)$$

In the following, we present the code in the C++ programming language.

```
#include<iostream>
#include<stdio.h>
#include<algorithm>
using namespace std;
int main()
{
int n, i, j, p1, q1, p2, q2, k, l, s, t, a[100][100],
b[100][100],c[200],p,d,e,aux,v[200][200],x, m;
cout << "n=";
cin >> n; cout << "p1=";
cin >> p1;cout << "q1=";
cin >> q1;
if (n == p1 * q1)
{
cout << "The HX Group G(" << p1 << ", " << q1 << ")" << endl;
for (i = 0; i < 2 * p1; i++)
{
for (j = 0; j < q1; j++)
{
if (i < p1)
   a[i][j] = i + j * p1;
   else
   a[i][j] = i + n - p1 + j * p1;
   cout << a[i][j] << " ";
}
cout << endl;
}
}
cout << endl;

cout << "p2="; cin >> p2;
cout << "q2="; cin >> q2;
if (n == p2 * q2)
{
cout << "The HX Group G (" << p2 << ", " << q2 << ")" << endl;
d = 2 * p2;
for (i = 0; i < 2 * p2; i++)
{
for (j = 0; j < q2; j++)
{
if (i < p2)
   b[i][j] = i + j * p2;
   else
   b[i][j] = i + n - p2 + j * p2;
```

```
            cout << b[i][j] << " ";
        }
        cout << endl;
    }
    cout << endl;
}

if ((n == p1 * q1)&&(n == p2 * q2))
    {
cout << "Composition between the HX group G(" << p1<<
", " << q1 << ") and HX group G(" << p2 << ", " << q2 <<
") is " << endl;

m = p1 * p2;

for (p = 0; p < p1 * p2; p++)
{
for (j = 0; j < q1; j++)
{
for (t = 0; t < q2; t++)
{
c[p] = (a[p / p2][j] + b[p % p2][t]) % n;
cout << c[p] << " ";
}
}
cout << endl;
}
cout << endl;
cout << endl;

for (p = p1 * p2; p < 2 * p1 * p2; p++)
{
for (j = 0; j < q1; j++)
{
for (t = 0; t < q2; t++)
{
c[p] = (a[p / p2][j] + b[p % p2][t]) % n + n;
cout << c[p] << " ";
}
}
cout << endl;
}
cout << endl;

for (p = 2 * p1 * p2; p < 3 * p1 * p2; p++)
{
for (j = 0; j < q1; j++)
{
for (t = 0; t < q2; t++)
{
c[p] = ((a[p1 + p % p1][j] - b[p % p2][t]) % n) + n;
cout << c[p] << " ";
}
}
```

```
cout << endl;
}
cout << endl;

for (p = 3 * p1 * p2; p < 4 * p1 * p2; p++)
{
for (j = 0; j < q1; j++)
{
for (t = 0; t < q2; t++)
{
c[p] = ((a[p1 + p % p1][j] - b[p2 + p % p2][t]) + n) % n;
cout << c[p] << " ";
}
}
cout << endl;
}
cout << endl;
cout << " Composition between the HX group G(" <<
p2 << ", " << q2 <<") and HX group G(" << p1 << ", "
<< q1 << ") is " << endl;

e = 2 * p1;

for (p = 0; p < p1 * p2; p++)
{
for (j = 0; j < q2; j++)
{
for (t = 0; t < q1; t++)
{
c[p] = (b[p / p1][j] + a[p % p1][t]) % n;
cout << c[p] << " ";
}
}
cout << endl;
}
cout << endl;

for (p = p1 * p2; p < 2 * p1 * p2; p++)
{
for (j = 0; j < q2; j++)
{
for (t = 0; t < q1; t++)
{
c[p] = (b[p / p1][j] + a[p % p1][t]) % n + n;
cout << c[p] << " ";
}
}
cout << endl;
}
cout << endl;

for (p = 2 * p1 * p2; p < 3 * p1 * p2; p++)
{
for (j = 0; j < q2; j++)
```

```
{
for (t = 0; t < q1; t++)
{
c[p] = (b[p / e][j] - a[p % p1][t]) % n + n;
cout << c[p] << " ";
}
}
cout << endl;
}
cout << endl;

for (p = 3 * p1 * p2; p < 4 * p1 * p2; p++)
{
for (j = 0; j < q2; j++)
{
for (t = 0; t < q1; t++)
{
c[p] = ((b[p2 + p % p2][j] - a[p1 + p % p1][t]) + n) % n;
cout << c[p] << " ";
}
}
cout << endl;
}
cout << endl;
}
}
```

4. Results

4.1. The Results Are Provided by the C++ Code Implemented for N = 4

The following will present the results obtained using the C++ code realized in Microsoft Visual Studio 2022. To better understand the above program, we will explain how it works. For $n = 4$, we have the hyperstructure

$$\mathcal{G}_4 = \left\{ \mathcal{G}_2^2, \mathcal{G}_1^4, \mathcal{G}_4^1 \right\}$$

Moreover, we apply the program presented in the previous section in each situation.

First situation: We consider $p_1 = 2$, $q_1 = 2$, $p_2 = 1$, $q_2 = 4$, respectively. In [16], we presented the composition of HX-groups $\mathcal{G}_2^2$ and $\mathcal{G}_1^4$. In the presented cod, these HX-groups are equivalent to the following HX-groups

$$
\begin{aligned}
\mathcal{G}_2^2 &= \{\{0,2\}, \{1,3\}, \{4,6\}, \{5,7\}\}, \text{where} \\
\{0,2\} &= \left\{ f(\rho^0), f(\rho^2) \right\}, \{1,3\} = \left\{ f(\rho^1), f(\rho^3) \right\}, \\
\{4,6\} &= \left\{ f(\sigma), f\left(\rho^2 \sigma\right) \right\}, \{5,7\} = \left\{ f(\rho\sigma), f\left(\rho^3 \sigma\right) \right\}; \\
\mathcal{G}_1^4 &= \{\{0,1,2,3\}, \{4,5,6,7\}\}, \text{where} \\
\{0,1,2,3\} &= \left\{ f(\rho^0), f(\rho^1), f(\rho^2), f(\rho^3) \right\}, \\
\{4,5,6,7\} &= \left\{ f(\sigma), f(\rho\sigma), f\left(\rho^2 \sigma\right), f\left(\rho^3 \sigma\right) \right\}.
\end{aligned}
$$

(1) We compute the elements from case 1, where

$$k \oplus p = f(\rho^k) \cdot f(\rho^p) = (k+p)(mod\ n)$$

$$\begin{aligned}
\{0,2\} \oplus \{0,1,2,3\} &= \left(\bigcup_{k\in\{0,2\}} f(\rho^k)\right) \circ \left(\bigcup_{p=0}^{3} f(\rho^p)\right) = \\
&= 0\oplus 0 \cup 0\oplus 1 \cup 0\oplus 2 \cup 0\oplus 3 \cup 2\oplus 0 \cup 2\oplus 1 \cup 2\oplus 2 \cup 2\oplus 3 \\
&= \{0,1,2,3,2,3,0,1\} = \{0,1,2,3\}, \\
\{1,3\} \oplus \{0,1,2,3\} &= \left(\bigcup_{k\in\{1,3\}} f(\rho^k)\right) \circ \left(\bigcup_{p=0}^{3} f(\rho^p)\right) = \\
&= 1\oplus 0 \cup 1\oplus 1 \cup 1\oplus 2 \cup 1\oplus 3 \cup 3\oplus 0 \cup 3\oplus 1 \cup 3\oplus 2 \cup 3\oplus 3 \\
&= \{1,2,3,0,3,0,1,2\} = \{0,1,2,3\}.
\end{aligned}$$

(2) We applied the formulas from case (2), where

$$k \oplus (n+p) = f(\rho^k) \circ f(\rho^p \sigma) = \begin{cases} n+k+p, & k+p < n \\ k+p, & k+p \geq n \end{cases}.$$

$$\begin{aligned}
\{0,2\} \oplus \{4,5,6,7\} &= \left(\bigcup_{k\in\{0,2\}} f(\rho^k)\right) \circ \left(\bigcup_{p=0}^{3} f(\rho^p \sigma)\right) = \\
&= 0\oplus 4 \cup 0\oplus 5 \cup 0\oplus 6 \cup 0\oplus 7 \cup 2\oplus 4 \cup 2\oplus 5 \cup 2\oplus 6 \cup 2\oplus 7 \\
&= \{4,5,6,7,6,6,4,5\} = \{4,5,6,7\}.
\end{aligned}$$

We explain the second rule in this situation:

$$\begin{aligned}
0\oplus 4 &= 4+0+0 = 4 : (k=0, p=0, k+p<4), \\
0\oplus 5 &= 4+0+1 = 5 : (k=0, p=1, k+p<4), \\
0\oplus 6 &= 4+0+2 = 6 : (k=0, p=2, k+p<4), \\
0\oplus 7 &= 4+0+3 = 7 : (k=0, p=3, k+p<4), \\
2\oplus 4 &= 4+2+0 = 6 : (k=2, p=0, k+p<4), \\
2\oplus 5 &= 4+2+1 = 6 : (k=2, p=1, k+p<4), \\
2\oplus 6 &= 2+2 = 4 : (k=2, p=2, k+p\geq 4), \\
2\oplus 7 &= 2+3 = 5 : (k=2, p=3, k+p\geq 4).
\end{aligned}$$

Similarly, we calculate

$$\begin{aligned}
\{1,3\} \oplus \{4,5,6,7\} &= \left(\bigcup_{k\in\{1,3\}} f(\rho^k)\right) \circ \left(\bigcup_{p=0}^{3} f(\rho^p \sigma)\right) = \\
&= 1\oplus 4 \cup 1\oplus 5 \cup 1\oplus 6 \cup 1\oplus 7 \cup 3\oplus 4 \cup 3\oplus 5 \cup 3\oplus 6 \cup 3\oplus 7 \\
&= \{5,6,7,4,7,4,5,6\} = \{4,5,6,7\}.
\end{aligned}$$

(3) We applied the formulas from case (3), where

$$(n+p) \oplus k = f(\rho^p \sigma) \circ f(\rho^k) = \begin{cases} 2n+p-k, & p < k \\ n+p-k, & p \geq k \end{cases}.$$

$$\begin{aligned}
\{4,6\} \oplus \{0,1,2,3\} &= \left(\bigcup_{p\in\{0,2\}} f(\rho^p \sigma)\right) \circ \left(\bigcup_{k=0}^{3} f(\rho^k)\right) = \\
&= 4\oplus 0 \cup 4\oplus 1 \cup 4\oplus 2 \cup 4\oplus 3 \cup 6\oplus 0 \cup 6\oplus 1 \cup 6\oplus 2 \cup 6\oplus 3 \\
&= \{4,7,6,5,6,5,4,3\} = \{4,5,6,7\},
\end{aligned}$$

where

$$\begin{aligned}
4 \oplus 0 &= 4+0-0 = 4 : (p=0, k=0, p \geq k), \\
4 \oplus 1 &= 2*4+0-1 = 7 : (p=0, k=1, p < k), \\
4 \oplus 2 &= 2*4+0-2 = 6 : (p=0, k=2, p < k), \\
4 \oplus 3 &= 2*4+0-3 = 5 : (p=0, k=3, p < k), \\
6 \oplus 0 &= 4+2-0 = 6 : (p=2, k=0, p \geq k), \\
6 \oplus 1 &= 4+2-1 = 5 : (p=2, k=1, p \geq k), \\
6 \oplus 2 &= 4+2-2 = 4 : (p=2, k=2, p \geq k), \\
6 \oplus 3 &= 2*4+2-3 = 7 : (p=2, k=3, p < k).
\end{aligned}$$

Analogously, we have

$$\begin{aligned}
\{5,7\} \oplus \{0,1,2,3\} &= \left(\bigcup_{p \in \{1,3\}} f(\rho^p \sigma)\right) \circ \left(\bigcup_{k=0}^{3} f(\rho^k)\right) = \\
&= 5 \oplus 0 \cup 5 \oplus 1 \cup 5 \oplus 2 \cup 5 \oplus 3 \cup 7 \oplus 0 \cup 7 \oplus 1 \cup 7 \oplus 2 \cup 7 \oplus 3 \\
&= \{5,4,7,6,7,6,5,4\} = \{4,5,6,7\}.
\end{aligned}$$

(4) The fourth case refers to computing the elements that are greater than n. We have the relation

$$(n+p) \oplus (n+k) = f(\rho^p \sigma) \circ f(\rho^k \sigma) = \begin{cases} p-k, & p \geq k \\ p+n-k, & p < k \end{cases}.$$

$$\begin{aligned}
\{4,6\} \oplus \{4,5,6,7\} &= \left(\bigcup_{p \in \{0,2\}} f(\rho^p \sigma)\right) \circ \left(\bigcup_{k=0}^{3} f(\rho^k \sigma)\right) = \\
&= 4 \oplus 4 \cup 4 \oplus 5 \cup 4 \oplus 6 \cup 4 \oplus 7 \cup 6 \oplus 4 \cup 6 \oplus 5 \cup 6 \oplus 6 \cup 6 \oplus 7 \\
&= \{0,3,2,1,2,1,0,3\} = \{0,1,2,3\}
\end{aligned}$$

because

$$\begin{aligned}
4 \oplus 4 &= 0-0 = 0 : (p=0, k=0, p \geq k); \\
4 \oplus 5 &= 0+4-1 = 3 : (p=0, k=1, p < k); \\
4 \oplus 6 &= 0+4-2 = 2 : (p=0, k=2, p < k); \\
4 \oplus 7 &= 0+4-3 = 1 : (p=0, k=3, p < k); \\
6 \oplus 4 &= 2-0 = 2 : (p=2, k=0, p \geq k); \\
6 \oplus 5 &= 2-1 = 1 : (p=2, k=1, p \geq k); \\
6 \oplus 6 &= 2-2 = 0 : (p=2, k=2, p \geq k); \\
6 \oplus 7 &= 2+4-3 = 3 : (p=2, k=3, p < k).
\end{aligned}$$

Therefore, $\mathcal{G}_2^2 \circ \mathcal{G}_1^4 = \{\{0,1,2,3\}, \{4,5,6,7\}\} = \mathcal{G}_1^4$.

The composition $\mathcal{G}_1^4 \circ \mathcal{G}_2^2$ is analyzed analogously and will be described in Table 1:

Table 1. The composition between HX-groups $\mathcal{G}_1^4$ and $\mathcal{G}_2^2$.

$\mathcal{G}_1^4 \circ \mathcal{G}_2^2$	$\{0,2\}$	$\{1,3\}$	$\{4,6\}$	$\{5,7\}$
$\{0,1,2,3\}$	$\{0,1,2,3\}$	$\{0,1,2,3\}$	$\{4,5,6,7\}$	$\{4,5,6,7\}$
$\{4,5,6,7\}$	$\{4,5,6,7\}$	$\{4,5,6,7\}$	$\{0,1,2,3\}$	$\{0,1,2,3\}$

We have $\mathcal{G}_1^4 \circ \mathcal{G}_2^2 = \{\{0,1,2,3\}, \{4,5,6,7\}\} = \mathcal{G}_1^4$. In conclusion,

$$\mathcal{G}_2^2 \circ \mathcal{G}_1^4 = \mathcal{G}_1^4 \circ \mathcal{G}_2^2 = \mathcal{G}_1^4.$$

Second situation: We consider $p_1 = 2$, $q_1 = 2$, and $p_2 = 4$, $q_2 = 1$ so that the composition $\mathcal{G}_2^2 \circ \mathcal{G}_4^1$ is illustrated in the following table according to the rules presented above for each case.

We can state that $\mathcal{G}_2^2 \circ \mathcal{G}_4^1 = \{\{0,2\}, \{1,3\}, \{4,6\}, \{5,7\}\} = \mathcal{G}_2^2$, and, proceeding similarly, we obtain $\mathcal{G}_4^1 \circ \mathcal{G}_2^2 = \{\{0,2\}, \{1,3\}, \{4,6\}, \{5,7\}\} = \mathcal{G}_2^2$.

Third situation: We have to compute $\mathcal{G}_4^1 \circ \mathcal{G}_1^4$ and $\mathcal{G}_1^4 \circ \mathcal{G}_4^1$, where

$$\mathcal{G}_4^1 = \{\{0\}, \{1\}, \{2\}, \{3\}, \{4\}, \{5\}, \{6\}, \{7\}\}.$$

4.2. A Graph Representation of the HX-Groups with Dihedral Group D_n as Support

Graph theory is applied in many fields, such as computer science, physics, biology [4,21,22], and social and information systems. A graph represents connected points along with their connections. Lines or curves can represent these connections. The points are called nodes or vertices; the lines between points are edges. The sets of nodes are denoted by V, and the sets of edges are denoted by E; therefore, a graph is represented by $G = (V, E)$. In this section, we construct the graph associated with the hyperstructures $(\mathcal{G}_4, \circ)$ and $(\mathcal{G}_6, \circ)$. The vertices represent the elements of the set $\mathcal{G}_n$, and we say that x, y formed an edge if and only if

$$[x, y] = x \circ y \cap \{x, y\} \neq \emptyset. \tag{9}$$

So, let $G_4 = (V_4, E_4)$ be the graph associated with the hyperstructures $(\mathcal{G}_4, \circ)$, where $V_4 = \{\mathcal{G}_1^4, \mathcal{G}_2^2, \mathcal{G}_4^1\}$. In relation (2), we established the connection between the composition of two HX-groups. So, according to them, we can draw the following graphs G_4, and, similarly, we obtained the graph G_6. For graph G_4, the node i is represented by the HX-group $\mathcal{G}_i^{\frac{4}{i}}$, where i is a divisor of 4, and, for the graph G_6, the node j is represented by the HX-group $\mathcal{G}_j^{\frac{6}{j}}$, where j is a divisior of 6. In graph theory, it is important to determine the degree of a vertex. The degree of a vertex v is denoted by $deg(v)$ and represents the number of edges that are incident to the vertex. In our situation, we can say that $\deg(1) = \deg(2) = \deg(4) = 2$ for G_4, and $\deg(1) = 3$, $\deg(2) = 2$, $\deg(3) = 2$, and $\deg(6) = 3$ for G_6.

5. Discussion

The main objective of the study was to analyze the HX-groups associated with the dihedral group D_n through the IT theory. A code in the C++ programming language, created in the Microsoft Visual Studio 2022 program, was presented in detail. This code represents a novelty in the field of HX-groups. In the first part of the paper, we discussed the HX-groups associated with the dihedral group from an algebraic point of view. In the second part of the work, the innovative part of the article was revealed. In Proposition 6, we established a connection between the elements of the dihedral group and natural numbers to implement the HX-groups in the C++ code programming language. The compositions between $\mathcal{G}_4^1$ and $\mathcal{G}_2^2$ and $\mathcal{G}_2^2$ and $\mathcal{G}_4^1$, respectively, are described in Tables 1 and 2. This code is necessary to improve the calculation time for the composition of two HX-groups. In Figures 1 and 2, we can notice how the program works for $n = 4$. Finally, a connection between the HX-groups $\mathcal{G}_4$, $\mathcal{G}_6$ and graph theory was presented in Figure 3.

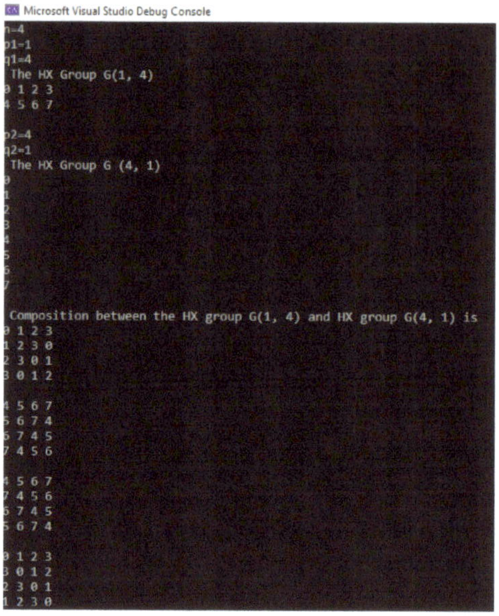

Figure 1. The groups $\mathcal{G}_4^1$, $\mathcal{G}_1^4$, and $\mathcal{G}_1^4 \circ \mathcal{G}_4^1$.

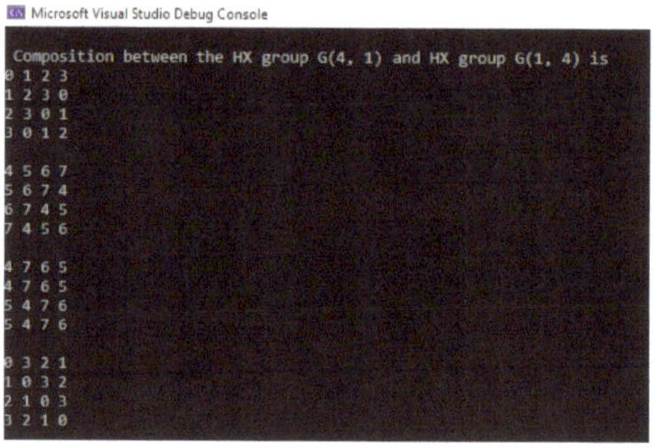

Figure 2. The composition $\mathcal{G}_4^1 \circ \mathcal{G}_1^4$.

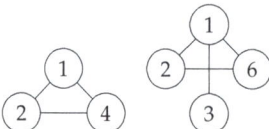

Figure 3. Graph G_4 and graph G_6.

Table 2. Composition of HX-groups $\mathcal{G}_2^2$ and $\mathcal{G}_4^1$.

$\mathcal{G}_2^2 \circ \mathcal{G}_4^1$	{0}	{1}	{2}	{3}	{4}	{5}	{6}	{7}
{0,2}	{0,2}	{1,3}	{0,2}	{1,3}	{4,6}	{5,7}	{4,6}	{5,7}
{1,3}	{1,3}	{0,2}	{1,3}	{0,2}	{5,7}	{4,6}	{5,7}	{4,6}
{4,6}	{4,6}	{5,7}	{4,6}	{5,7}	{0,2}	{1,3}	{0,2}	{1,3}
{5,7}	{5,7}	{4,6}	{5,7}	{4,6}	{1,3}	{0,2}	{5,7}	{0,2}

Author Contributions: Conceptualization, A.P.S. and C.C.; Methodology, A.P.S. and C.C.; Code created in Microsoft Visual Studio 2022 program, A.P.S. and C.C.; Writing—original draft, A.P.S. All authors have read and agreed to the published version of the manuscript.

Funding: This research received no external funding.

Data Availability Statement: The original contributions presented in the study are included in the article; further inquiries can be directed to the corresponding author.

Acknowledgments: The authors would like to thank the referees for the advice provided as they significantly contributed to the improvement of the article.

Conflicts of Interest: The authors declare no conflicts of interest.

References

1. Marty, F. Sur une generalization de la notion de group. In Proceedings of the Congress of Scandinavian Mathematicians, Stockholm, Sweden, 14–18 August 1934; pp. 45–49.
2. Corsini, P.; Leoreanu, V. *Applications of Hyperstructures Theory*; Kluwer Academic Publishers: Boston, MA, USA; Dordrecht, The Netherlands; London, UK, 2003.
3. Davvaz, B.; Cristea, I. *Fuzzy Algebraic Hyperstructures—An Introduction*; Studies in Fuzziness and Soft Computing; Springer: Cham, Switzerland, 2015; Volume 321.
4. Kalampakas, A.; Spartalis, S.; Tsigkas, A. The Path Hyperoperation. *An. Şt. Univ. Ovidius Constanţa* **2014**, *22*, 141–153. [CrossRef]
5. Linzi, A.; Cristea, I. Dependence Relations and Grade Fuzzy Set. *Symmetry* **2023**, *15*, 311. [CrossRef]
6. Massourous, C.; Mittas, J. Languages-automata and hypercompositional structure. In *Algebraic Hyperstructures and Applications, Proceeding of the 4th International Congress, Xanthi, Greece, 27–30 June 1990*; World Scientific: Singapore, 1991; pp. 137–147.
7. Vougiouklis, T. On some representations of hypergroups. *Ann. Sci. L'Univ. Clermont Mathématiques* **1990**, *95*, 21–29.
8. Tofan, I.; Volf, A.C. On some conections between; hyperstructures and fuzzy sets. *Ital. J. Pure Appl. Math.* **2000**, *7*, 63–68.
9. Li, H.X.; Duan, Q.Z.; Wang, P.Z.; Wang, P.Z. Hypergroup(I). *BUSEFAL* **1985**, *23*, 22–29.
10. Li, H.X. HX-groups. *BUSEFAL* **1987**, *33*, 31–37.
11. Zhenliang, Z. The properties of HX-groups. *Italian J. Pure Appl. Math.* **1997**, *2*, 97–106.
12. Corsini, P. HX-groups and Hypergroups. *An. Şt. Univ. Ovidius Constanţa* **2016**, *24*, 101–121. [CrossRef]
13. Corsini, P. HX-Hypergroups associated with the direct product of some Z/nZ. *J. Algebr. Struct. Their Appl.* **2016**, *3*, 1–15.
14. Corsini, P. Hypergroups associated with HX-groups. *An. Şt. Univ. Ovidius Constanţa* **2017**, *25*, 49–64. [CrossRef]
15. Cristea, I.; Novák, M.; Onasanya, B.O. Links Between HX-Groups and Hypergroups. *Algebra Coll.* **2021**, *28*, 441–452. [CrossRef]
16. Sonea, A. HX-groups associated to the dihedral group D_n. *J. Mult. Valued Log. Soft Comput.* **2019**, *33*, 11–26.
17. Sonea, A. A Way to Construct Commutative Hyperstructures. *Comput. Sci. Math. Forum.* **2023**, *7*, 22. [CrossRef]
18. Sonea, A.; Al-Kaseasbeh, S. An introduction to NeutroHX-Groups. In *Theory and Applications of NeutroAlgebras as Generalizations of Classical Algebras*; IGI Global Publishing Tomorrow's Research Today: Hershey, PA, USA, 2022. [CrossRef]
19. Mousavi, S.S.; Jafarpour, M.; Cristea, I. From HX-Groups to HX-Polygroups. *Axioms* **2024**, *13*, 7. [CrossRef]
20. Rotman, J.J. *An Introduction to the Theory of Groups*; Springer: New York, NY, USA, 1995.
21. Cristea, I.; Kocijan, J.; Novák, M. Introduction to Dependence Relations and Their Links to Algebraic Hyperstructures. *Mathematics* **2019**, *7*, 885. [CrossRef]
22. Kalampakas, A.; Spartalis, S. Hyperoperations on directed graphs. *J. Discret. Math. Sci. Cryptogr.* **2023**, *27*, 1011–1025. [CrossRef]

Disclaimer/Publisher's Note: The statements, opinions and data contained in all publications are solely those of the individual author(s) and contributor(s) and not of MDPI and/or the editor(s). MDPI and/or the editor(s) disclaim responsibility for any injury to people or property resulting from any ideas, methods, instructions or products referred to in the content.

Review

Feynman Diagrams beyond Physics: From Biology to Economy

Nicolò Cangiotti

Department of Mathematics, Politecnico di Milano, Via Bonardi 9, Edificio 14 "Nave", Campus Leonardo, 20133 Milan, Italy; nicolo.cangiotti@polimi.it

Abstract: Feynman diagrams represent one of the most powerful and fascinating tools developed in theoretical physics in the last century. Introduced within the framework of quantum electrodynamics as a suitable method for computing the amplitude of a physical process, they rapidly became a fundamental mathematical object in quantum field theory. However, their abstract nature seems to suggest a wider usage, which actually exceeds the physical context. Indeed, as mathematical objects, they could simply be considered graphs that depict not only physical quantities but also biological or economic entities. We survey the analytical and algebraic properties of such diagrams to understand their utility in several areas of science, eventually providing some examples of recent applications.

Keywords: Feynman diagrams; quantum field theory; graph theory; combinatorics; RNA folding; quantum finance; mathematical physics

MSC: 81T18; 81Q30; 81Q65; 91B80; 92-10

Citation: Cangiotti, N. Feynman Diagrams beyond Physics: From Biology to Economy. *Mathematics* **2024**, *12*, 1295. https://doi.org/10.3390/math12091295

Academic Editor: Bo Zhou

Received: 18 March 2024
Revised: 18 April 2024
Accepted: 23 April 2024
Published: 25 April 2024

Copyright: © 2024 by the author. Licensee MDPI, Basel, Switzerland. This article is an open access article distributed under the terms and conditions of the Creative Commons Attribution (CC BY) license (https://creativecommons.org/licenses/by/4.0/).

1. Introduction

In the late 1940s, Richard Feynman published a renowned paper [1], in which he proposed a pictorial formulation of the quantum field theory (QFT) by introducing the so-called *Feynman diagrams* for describing particle interaction as field propagation (see Figure 1). His original attempt was to simplify the tricky computations coming from quantum electrodynamics theory (QED), namely the quantum description of electromagnetic phenomena. As highlighted by David Kaiser [2], the contribution to quantum physics was enormous and, at least, twofold. On the one hand, Feynman diagrams provide a powerful tool to simplify the critical calculations emerging from the perturbative approach in QFT. From this point of view, the diagrams become a topological way to treat enumeration and combinatorical issues. On the other hand, the pedagogical influence that this diagrams had in the second half of the 20th century cannot be overlooked.

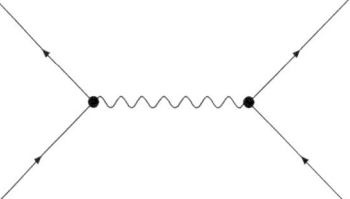

Figure 1. Standard representation of a second-order Feynman diagram in QED. The usual interpretation is the following: fix a time direction; consider the external lines physical particles and the internal lines virtual particles.

The usage of analogous instruments has, not so surprisingly, spread in many other physical field theories. For instance, their application in quantum chromodynamics

(QCD) [3–5], or even in quantum gravity (QG) [6,7], effective field theory (EFT) [8], and condensed matter physics [9], is quite common nowadays.

There also exists a third philosophical interpretation that considers Feynman diagrams not only merely computational tools, but something that actually provides an in-depth depiction of physical processes [10–12]. However, most quantum field theorists actually lean in favour of Feynman diagrams as merely book-keeping devices (namely, they are conveniently employed for calculations) [13–15]. In some sense, this work actually shows that, at least as powerful organizational tools, Feynman-type diagrams can be used in different domains not directly linked with quantum phenomena. Indeed, inspired by this intriguing formulation of fundamental physics, namely the graphical description, with its intrinsic topological and algebraic nature, the diagrams began to be used in different domains, such as mathematical biology and economic science. In this manuscript, we survey different applications of Feynman-type diagrams in order to aim at a broad audience, in the hope that these techniques can provide an inspiring starting point for future developments in many scientific areas. We remark that this work fits into the context of a renewed interest in Feynman diagrams, as evidenced by the recent experimentation of their use in a high school setting [16] or the more technical reformulation in categorical semantics [17].

This paper is organized as follows: In Section 2, we briefly introduce the diagrams, stressing their mathematical significance. Section 3 is devoted to the first application of these kinds of graphs in a biological context. A completely different example is given in Section 4, where we review the usage of diagrams in the field of the so-called quantum economy. Finally, in Section 5, we conclude by taking stock of the overview by proposing some other fascinating applications of these particular mathematical tools.

2. From Matrix Integrals to Diagrams

In this section, we propose a brief summary of how diagrams can be generated from a classical mathematical apparatus. There are many authors who discuss the construction of Feynman diagrams and the contextual *Feynman rules* in QFT [3,5]. In this section, we plan to point out the most important steps in the creation of such graphs, in terms of mathematical operators. Naturally, once you have fixed the graphical apparatus, one can skip the evaluation of the generating functional and the associated Green functions for obtaining amplitudes, as presented in this section. Indeed, the Feynman rules allow us to easily compute the amplitude just by using a list of several formal steps. However, for our purpose, it is important to explain the mathematical formulation behind the diagrams, in order to understand how the same techniques can be used in different scientific domains. Now, we are going to work in a finite-dimensional setting to provide a better explanation of the various passes. Analogous arguments can be found, for instance, in [3,5,18–21].

As is often the case in mathematics, we start by considering an integral, that is,

$$Z_0 = \int_{\mathbb{R}^n} d\mathbf{x}\, \exp\left(-\frac{1}{2}\mathbf{x}^T A \mathbf{x}\right) = (2\pi)^{\frac{n}{2}} (\det A)^{-\frac{1}{2}}, \tag{1}$$

where $\mathbf{x} = (x_1, \ldots, x_n) \in \mathbb{R}^n$ and $A \in \mathcal{M}_n$ is a symmetric matrix. After some straightforward computation, it is also possible to prove that, given a generic vector $\mathbf{b} \in \mathbb{R}^n$, we can write the following integral:

$$Z_b = \int_{\mathbb{R}^n} d\mathbf{x}\, \exp\left(-\frac{1}{2}\mathbf{x}^T A \mathbf{x} + \mathbf{b}^T \mathbf{x}\right), \tag{2}$$

as

$$Z_b = Z_0 \exp\left(\frac{1}{2}\mathbf{b}^T A^{-1} \mathbf{b}\right). \tag{3}$$

We can now fix a set of k indices as $i_1, \ldots, i_k$ in $\{1, 2, \ldots, n\}$, so that we can define the so-called *k-point function* as follows:

$$\langle x_{i_1}, \ldots, x_{i_k} \rangle = \frac{1}{Z_0} \int_{\mathbb{R}^n} d\mathbf{x} \exp\left(\frac{1}{2} \mathbf{x}^T A \mathbf{x}\right) x_{i_1} \cdots x_{i_k}. \tag{4}$$

This kind of function plays a central role in the development of the theory. Indeed, it is possible to compute Equation (4) by differentiating $Z_\mathbf{b}$:

$$\begin{aligned} \frac{\partial Z_\mathbf{b}}{\partial b_i} &= \frac{\partial}{\partial b_i} \int_{\mathbb{R}^n} d\mathbf{x} \exp\left(\frac{1}{2} \mathbf{x}^T A \mathbf{x} + \mathbf{b}^T \mathbf{x}\right) \\ &= \int_{\mathbb{R}^n} d\mathbf{x} \frac{\partial}{\partial b_i} \exp\left(\frac{1}{2} \mathbf{x}^T A \mathbf{x} + \mathbf{b}^T \mathbf{x}\right) \\ &= \int_{\mathbb{R}^n} d\mathbf{x} \exp\left(\frac{1}{2} \mathbf{x}^T A \mathbf{x} + \mathbf{b}^T \mathbf{x}\right) x_i. \end{aligned} \tag{5}$$

Thus, we immediately obtain the following expression for the one-point function:

$$\langle x_i \rangle = \frac{1}{Z_0} \left. \frac{\partial Z_\mathbf{b}}{\partial b_i} \right|_{\mathbf{b}=0}, \tag{6}$$

and then the generic formulation for the k-points function:

$$\langle x_{i_1}, \ldots, x_{i_k} \rangle = \frac{1}{Z_0} \left. \left(\frac{\partial}{\partial b_{i_1}} \cdots \frac{\partial}{\partial b_{i_k}} Z_\mathbf{b} \right) \right|_{\mathbf{b}=0} = \left. \frac{\partial}{\partial b_{i_1}} \cdots \frac{\partial}{\partial b_{i_k}} \exp\left(\frac{1}{2} \mathbf{b}^T A^{-1} \mathbf{b}\right) \right|_{\mathbf{b}=0}. \tag{7}$$

Thanks to these computational steps, we have actually translated the original problem into another one: now, we simply need to compute the derivatives of the exponential function in Equation (3). To reduce this intricate operation to a combinatoric affair, we make use of the well-known *Wick's theorem* (which is stated and proved in every book concerning QFT; see, for instance, [5]). In our framework, this theorem immediately leads to a combinatorical expression of the form

$$\left. \frac{\partial}{\partial b_{i_1}} \cdots \frac{\partial}{\partial b_{i_k}} \exp\left(\frac{1}{2} \mathbf{b}^T A \mathbf{b}\right) \right|_{\mathbf{b}=0} = \sum_{\text{all pairings}} A^{-1}_{i_{i_1}, i_{i_2}} \cdots A^{-1}_{i_{i_{k-1}}, i_{i_k}}. \tag{8}$$

With "all parings", here we denote all possible pairings of the indices $i_1, \ldots, i_k$. Now, it seems to be clear that the sum of Equation (8) can be split in different contributions by using the N-order series expansion of the exponential function as follows:

$$\exp\left(\frac{1}{2} \mathbf{b}^T A^{-1} \mathbf{b}\right) = \left(\frac{1}{N!}\right)\left(\frac{1}{2^N}\right)\left(\sum_{i,j=1}^n A^{-1}_{i,j} b^i b^j\right)^N, \tag{9}$$

In particular, if we use a lighter notation for the derivative, namely

$$\frac{\partial}{\partial b_i} \equiv \partial_i, \tag{10}$$

by fixing $N = 1$, we immediately obtain the following from Equation (9):

$$\begin{aligned} \partial_2 \partial_1 \left(\frac{1}{2} \sum_{i,j=1}^n A^{-1}_{i,j} b^i b^j\right) &= A^{-1}_{1,2} = \langle x_1, x_2 \rangle, \\ \partial_1 \partial_1 \left(\frac{1}{2} \sum_{i,j=1}^n A^{-1}_{i,j} b^i b^j\right) &= A^{-1}_{1,1} = \langle x_1, x_1 \rangle, \end{aligned} \tag{11}$$

Let us remark that the paring (∂_1, ∂_2) is equivalent to the paring (∂_2, ∂_1), because of the symmetry of the matrix A^{-1}. Similarly, for $N = 2$, expressions involve other combinations of indices, for instance,

$$\partial_4 \partial_3 \partial_2 \partial_1 \left(\frac{1}{2!}\right)\left(\frac{1}{2}\right)^2 \left(\frac{1}{2}\sum_{i,j=1}^n A_{i,j}^{-1} b^i b^j\right)^2 = A_{2,3}^{-1} A_{1,4}^{-1} + A_{2,4}^{-1} A_{1,3}^{-1} + A_{3,4}^{-1} A_{1,2}^{-1}, \qquad (12)$$

$$= \langle x_1, x_2, x_3, x_4 \rangle$$

$$\partial_4 \partial_3 \partial_1 \partial_1 \left(\frac{1}{2!}\right)\left(\frac{1}{2}\right)^2 \left(\frac{1}{2}\sum_{i,j=1}^n A_{i,j}^{-1} b^i b^j\right)^2 = 2 \cdot A_{1,4}^{-1} A_{1,3}^{-1} + A_{3,4}^{-1} A_{1,1}^{-1} \qquad (13)$$

$$= \langle x_1, x_1, x_3, x_4 \rangle.$$

Thus, Wick's theorem provides a practical way to compute n-points functions as we show in the latter formulas for the two-points and four-points functions (the generalization is quite obvious). Now, the combinatorial computations arising from Wick's argument can actually be graphically represented. In particular, let us consider the right-hand side of Equations (12) and (13). They can be depicted as graphs, where the indices of the points x_i in the m-point function become the vertices and and each term $A_{i,j}^{-1}$ becomes an edge from vertex x_i to vertex x_j. Practically speaking, it turns out that it is possible to visualize such an expression by means of graphs, as we propose in Figures 2 and 3.

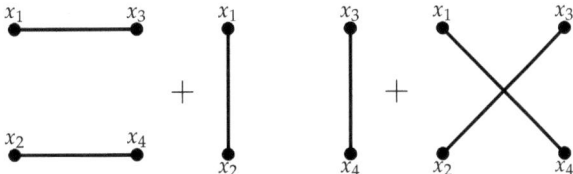

Figure 2. The three graphs representing the 4-points function $\langle x_1, x_2, x_3, x_4 \rangle$, which is explicitly given by Equation (12).

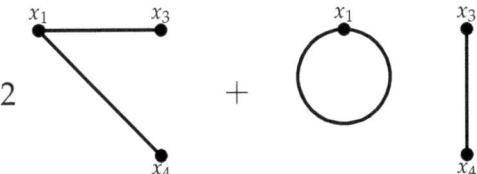

Figure 3. The two graphs representing the 4-points function $\langle x_1, x_1, x_3, x_4 \rangle$. The first graph is multiplied by the same factor, 2, appearing even in the explicit formula of Equation (13).

Remark 1. *The previous paragraphs have explored in depth the link between the mathematical framework and the graphical structures. As mentioned above, the construction of these diagrams can be formulated in a pure formal context by the list of Feynman rules. The latter formulation really provides an easier way to construct the diagrams. However, as we are going to see in the next sections, the mathematical background represents one of the cores of this work, which one needs in order to have a better understanding of the translation of these techniques in other studies.*

Physically speaking, the structure of Feynman diagrams arises directly from the integrals (namely the generating function) due to the path integral approach to QFT [5]. In fact, in the quantum field theory realm the studied integrals assume (by adapting the previous notations) the following form, which involves some potential function $U(\mathbf{x})$ and the *reduced Planck constant* $\hbar$:

$$Z_U = \int d\mathbf{x} \exp\left(-\frac{1}{2}\mathbf{x}^T A \mathbf{x} + \hbar U(\mathbf{x})\right). \tag{14}$$

Equation (14) is trivially linked with the above discussion (we remark that the construction in QFT is actually more complicated, as it involves infinite quantities. However, for the purpose of this illustrative section, the most important thing is to capture the spirit of the mathematical formulation linked to Feynman diagrams). Now, as one can deduce from the proposed construction, it is possible to fix some formal rules in order to connect this abstract mathematical formulation to the corresponding physical significance. This procedure imposes the classical QED interpretation first provided by Feynman (and formally developed by Dyson [22]), in which objects as *virtual particles* are introduced in order to explain the physical phenomena underlying the diagrams (the ontological nature of virtual particles is still an open debate in the philosophical community [23,24]). However, for the purpose of this work, we just consider the mathematical formulation of such diagrams and how their generality can be translated to other scientific domains. Indeed, in this section, we show how it is possible to construct a graph theory starting from a specific class of integrals.

In the next two sections, we apply this impressive trick coming from QFT to develop a graph theory for approaching the problem of RNA folding and for modelling the bond prices in quantum finance.

Remark 2. *It is important to underline that the application of diagrams in the biological and economical contexts actually comes from two different perspectives. In fact, in the first case, the analogy inspiring the construction comes, as we are going to see, directly from the similarity between the pictures in the QFT and RNA framework. Instead, in the second case, the analogy is mediated by the path integral formulation. It is now quite clear that the formal mathematical construction can be based directly on the path integral formulation instead of its diagrammatic version. However, we consider the choice of Feynman-type diagrams for developing and studying the most suitable theories in order to disseminate such an approach to different scientific communities. For the role of the analogy in the mathematical reasoning and discovery, we refer interested readers to [25,26].*

3. RNA Folding Problem

In the previous section, we formally show the connection between matrices and diagrams. This deep link can be exploited to study many kinds of problems once one has reformulated the link in terms of matrix field theory. In this spirit, in 2002 Orland and Zee [27] proposed a method for predicting the tertiary structure of RNA based on such a matrix theory. Indeed, the usage of diagrams to describe secondary and tertiary RNA structures is actually a common practice, as testified by a large number of representations, which one can find in the literature [27–35].

We briefly recall that RNA is usually defined as a single-filament polymer, made of ribonucleosides with four main nucleobases: adenine (A), cytosine (C), guanine (G), and uracil (U). Despite being single-filament, RNA bases can form bonds (similarly to DNA) with bases from other molecules, or even within the same molecule, thus creating more complicated 2D and 3D structures. In standard *Watson–Crick base-pairings*, A binds U with two hydrogen bonds, and G binds C with three hydrogen bonds. Moreover, RNA structural motifs are made up of two components: the first one consists of free bases, like in bulges, loops, or junctions, and the second one is made up of stems of paired bases. While the secondary structure could be assimilated to RNA's planar conformation (i.e., planar graphs), the tertiary structure is its 3D conformation, which determines its specific function (see [36]). The main role in the passage between 2D and 3D models is played by the so-called *pseudoknots*. Roughly speaking, a pseudoknot is composed of at least two helices with both internal bonds and free bases interacting across the two motifs and separated by an additional stretch of free bases (see [37]). In the next paragraphs, we explore in-depth the contribution of pseudoknots in this framework and their graph representation.

Returning to the main topic, Orland and Zee noticed a profound analogy between the model obtained by stretching the manipulation of RNA secondary structures (see Figure 4) and the classical Feynman diagrams defined above.

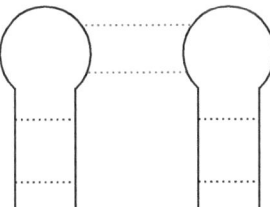

Figure 4. Classical diagram of a *kissing hairpin* pseudoknot.

It turns out that such an approach is strictly related to the topology of such diagrams, as it was already proved by t'Hooft [38]. Thanks to this topological perspective, we can introduce the fundamental notion of *genus*, which can be used to topologically classify RNA structures [30,32,33,39]. It is important to underline that the formal construction, which we are going to explain in the following, is none other than a particular case of a the so-called *maps enumeration problem* belonging to the theory of *dessin d'enfant*, whose contemporary formulation in terms of graph embedding into manifolds is due to Grothendieck [40]. Readers interested in the latter topic may also consult the manuscript published by Zvonkin [41]. The matrix formalism introduced in [27] and then developed in [32] is based on the standard energy models for RNA studied in recent years. These energetic models are based on the following partition function:

$$\mathcal{Z} = \int \prod_{k=1}^{L} d^3 \mathbf{r}_k f(\mathbf{r}) Z_L(\mathbf{r}), \tag{15}$$

where $\mathbf{r}_k$ is the 3D position vector k-th base, L is the length of the sequence, and $f(\mathbf{r})$ is a function, which takes into account the properties of the RNA chain. A fundamental role is played by the function $Z_L(\mathbf{r})$, which provides the description of base interactions; it is given by

$$Z_L = 1 + \sum_{\langle i,j \rangle} V_{ij}(\mathbf{r}_{ij}) + \sum_{\langle i,j,k,l \rangle} V_{ij}(\mathbf{r}_{ij}) V_{kl}(\mathbf{r}_{kl}) + \cdots, \tag{16}$$

where $\langle i,j \rangle$ denotes the pair relation $j > i$, $\langle i,j,k,l \rangle$ the quadruplets relation $l > k > j > i$, and so on. In this formalism, the function $V_{ij}(\mathbf{r})$ represents the Boltzmann factor with energy ϵ_{ij} that relates the i-th and the j-th bases at the distance induced by the vector $\mathbf{r}_{ij}$:

$$V_{ij}(\mathbf{r}_{ij}) = \exp(-\beta \epsilon_{ij} s_{ij}(\mathbf{r}_{ij})), \tag{17}$$

where $\beta = 1/k_B T$ is the usual symbol for the inverse temperature multiplied to the Boltzmann constant, and $s_{ij}(\mathbf{r}_{ij})$ is the space-dependent part of the interaction. And, precisely in this context, Orland and Zee noticed the analogy with QCD that induced them to rewrite the above problem in terms of integrals over the space of $N \times N$ dimensional Hermitian matrices:

$$Z_n(a, N) = \frac{1}{A(N)} \int d^{N \times N} \phi \exp\left(-\frac{N}{2a}\right) \operatorname{Tr} \phi^2 \times \frac{1}{N} \operatorname{Tr}(\mathbb{I} + \phi)^n, \tag{18}$$

where ϕ is a Hermitian matrix, $\operatorname{Tr}(\cdot)$ represents the trace operator, and $A(N)$ is a computable normalization factor.

These latter integrals can be represented by means of diagrams inspired by the Feynman diagrams that we introduced in the previous section. Let us consider for the sake of simplicity the one-dimensional case ($\mathbb{R}$), with $n = 2$. By basic computations, we obtain $Z_2(a) = 1 + a$, namely, if one depicts a circle with two points, the addendum 1 is the no-chord diagram, and the term a is the diagram with chords joining the two points. Now, it is also possible to represent $Z_4(a) = 1 + 6a + 3a^2$, where, in addition to the no-chord diagram, there are also six one-chord diagrams (all the possible combinations) that provide the term $6a$. Finally, $3a^2$ are intuitively the three possible combinations of two-chord diagrams (see Figure 5 for some examples).

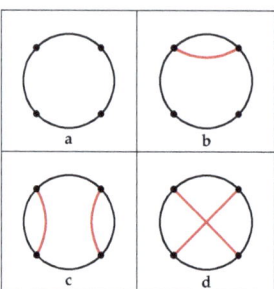

Figure 5. Four examples of diagrams representing terms of the integral $Z_4(a) = 1 + 6a + 3a^2$. We represent here the no-chord diagram (**a**), that is, the addendum 1, a one-chord diagram (**b**) contributing to the first-order term $6a$, and two of the three second-order two-diagrams in $3a^2$: one planar (**c**) and one non-planar (**d**).

Remark 3. *As we are going to explain in the next paragraphs, the power of this approach becomes relevant for large N and large −N expansion. In particular, one can notice that the computation of $Z_2(a, N) = 1 + a$ does not depend on N; instead, by computing $Z_4(a, N) = 1 + 6a + 2a^2 + a^2/N^2$, one explicitly obtains the dependence on N. We remark that, in this example, the term involving $1/N^2$ actually represents the non-planar diagram.*

Once the matrix framework is recovered, it is possible to evaluate such integrals in terms of diagrams, by using the already mentioned Wick's theorem. Moreover, thanks to this graphical approach we can also describe pseudoknots in terms of topological quantities, namely the *genus*. Figure 4 depicts the standard way to represent a well-known pseudoknot, called *kissing hairpin* [42]. This picture can be used to derive (by stretching the backbone) two other useful graphs, namely the *stretching* (or *arc*) *diagram* (Figure 6a) and the *circle* (or *disk*) *diagram* (Figure 6b).

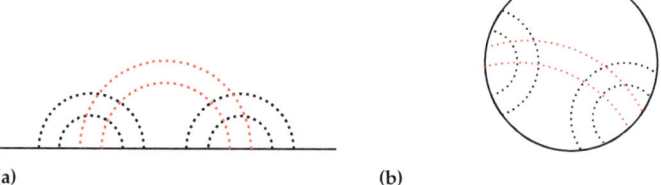

Figure 6. Stretching (or arc) diagram of a *kissing hairpin* pseudoknot (**a**). Circle diagram of *kissing hairpin* pseudoknot (**b**).

Now, in terms of crossing diagrams, pseudoknots can be computed by using the genus of a surface. Topologically speaking, the genus of a surface is the number of *holes* or *handles* of a (orientable) surface. In this framework, the genus of a diagram can be defined as the genus of the surface with the lowest genus, in which our diagram can be drawn with no intersections. In particular, if we consider the case of the kissing hairpin, we obtain the representation in Figure 7, in which the diagram appears embedded in a surface with genus $g = 1$, namely a torus.

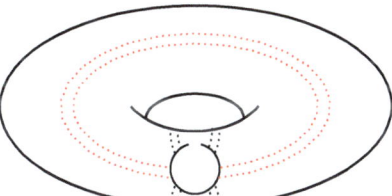

Figure 7. *Kissing hairpin* pseudoknot embedded on a torus. Notice that the circle diagram can be actually drawn without any crossings. This corresponds to the topological genus of the torus, namely $g = 1$ (adapted from [43]).

It is clear now how the topology allows us to classify pseudoknots, which have a central role in the theory. We remark, indeed, that the genus g is included explicitly in the original formulation of the theory [27,32,43], in which the authors consider power series of Equation (18) with respect to terms of the form N^{-2g} (where N is the dimension of the matrix), so that Equation (16) can be rewritten by also including the topological contribution due to pseudoknots (we can assume that the chains are infinitely flexible, so that all spatial degrees of freedom are gotten rid of when simplifying the notation):

$$Z_L(N) = 1 + \sum_{\langle i,j \rangle} V_{ij} + \sum_{\langle i,j,k,l \rangle} V_{ij}V_{kl} + \frac{1}{N^2} \sum_{\langle i,j,k,l \rangle} V_{ik}V_{jk} + \cdots. \tag{19}$$

Remark 4. *We point out that Equation (19) explicitly provides the link between secondary and pseudoknot structures from a topological perspective. In particular, the topological considerations that lead to Equation (19) are based on the N expansion used in the already mentioned matrix field theories. Indeed, this approach predicts that non-planar Feynman diagrams have amplitudes proportional to the negative power of N, and then we can get rid of them when N is large. The same technique has been applied to the problem of RNA folding, leading to the same sort of cancellation of non-planar configurations [27].*

The standard way to compute the genus of a diagram is the well-known *Euler characteristic* that, in the case of diagrams, is provided by the celebrated formula $\chi = V - E + F$, where V, E, and F are the numbers of vertices, edges, and faces, respectively. We remark that, in this view, a vertex is a nucleotide, an edge is any line connecting two nucleotides, and a face is a part of the surface within a closed loop of edges. In the case of n arcs, one trivially obtains $E = V + n$. There is also a famous theorem due to Euler stating that any polyhedron homeomorphic to a sphere with a boundary has an Euler characteristic $\chi = 1$. As a corollary, all RNA secondary structures with no pseudoknots can be represented by disk diagrams with $\chi = 1$. Let us suppose that the RNA secondary structure admits pseudoknots; as in the case of kissing hairpin, the computation of the Euler characteristic leads to the value $\chi = -1$. The geometrical significance of such a value is strictly related to the number of holes on a surface. In particular, we recall that for any orientable surface, we have $\chi = 2 - 2g - p$, where p is the number of punctures. In conclusion, the kissing hairpin pseudoknot induces a genus $g = 1$, and can be drawn without crossing on a surface with one *hole*, that is exactly a *torus* (Figure 7).

Now, we want to stress two more properties about pseudoknots that turn out to be very important for computational reasons. The genus of a diagram is an additive quantity, and so it is possible to provide two notions to characterize the intrinsic complexity of a pseudoknot, namely the concepts of *irreducibility* and *nested* pseudoknots [42]. A diagram is said to be irreducible if it cannot be split into two disconnected parts by cutting a single line, as in Figure 8b. In parallel, a diagram is said to be nested in another one if it can be removed by cutting two lines and keeping the rest of the diagram connected in a single component, as in Figure 8d. These two definitions can be combined as follows: if a diagram is both irreducible and non-nested, it is called a *primitive* diagram. Other interesting details about genuses and pseudoknots can be found in [32,33,39,42,44].

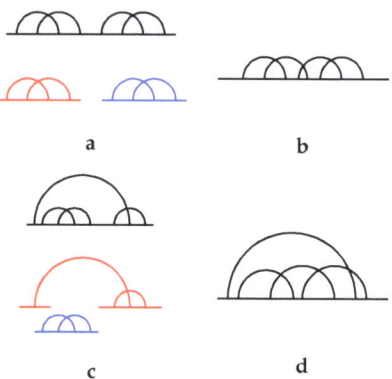

Figure 8. Four example of pseudoknots (reproduced from [42]). A reducible (**a**) and an irreducible (**b**) pseudoknot. (**a**) can be split in two disconnected pieces with a single cut. A nested (**c**) and a non-nested (**d**) pseudoknot. Two disconnected components can be obtained in (**c**) by making two cuts.

Remark 5. *This section is devoted to the explanation of how the matrix theory can be applied in the context of RNA folding prediction problems and the way to connect pseudoknots with genuses by using graphs and their embedding into manifolds. The interests for this method assume a greater significance when such an approach is used to developed specific software for modelling and predicting RNA structures. In particular, we want to mention McGenus* [45] *and its precursor TT2NE* [46]. *Indeed, the notion of pseudoknots and the graphical apparatus outlined above allow us to consider, in producing a suitable predictive software, having both the perspectives: the global one (provided by genuses and pseudoknots) and the local one (provided by the energy function due to the coupling rules of the biological theory). A useful overview about these topics and the most recent applications of McGenus is eventually proposed in* [47].

For the sake of completeness, finally, we want to mention some other recent works that describe a topological approach based on graphs to RNA folding problems. A similar outlook to the one described above is given in [28], where the authors studied a Hermitian matrix model with a given potential that enumerates the number of chord diagrams by using the formalism of the topological recursion, and in [29], where the authors provided a classification and an enumeration of RNA structures by genus. Moreover, two interesting generalizations of the concept of genuses were introduced [31,35]. The first one is the *genus trace*, a function $g(i) : \mathbb{N} \to \mathbb{N}$ providing the genus of a segment of the chain between the first and the i-th residue. The second one is the *fingerprint matrix*, which gives a useful mathematical visualization of all the genuses computed between two elements of a chain; namely, if one fixes the notation $\mathbf{G} = (g_{ij})$ for the matrix, the generic element g_{ij} represents the genus of the sub-chain between the i-th and the j-th residue. Another computational approach based on pseudoknot prediction is given in [34], where the authors proposed a quantitative analysis of the topological constraints on RNA three-dimensional conformational space, with specific attention to the distribution of helix orientations, for pseudoknots and loop–loop kissing structures. The results showed a strong topological coupling between helices and loops in RNA tertiary motifs.

4. Quantum Finance Experience

In this fourth section, we describe a completely different application of Feynman-type diagrams in the interdisciplinary field of econophysics [48–50]. In general, this field of study exploit methods and approaches developed in the domain of physics to solve economical and financial problems.

In the following paragraphs, we focus on an intriguing topic, which is based on quantum theories, and therefore it is called *quantum econophysics*. Although there are several doubts about the ontological foundation of the analogy between quantum mechanics and finance [51], it is still interesting to describe the framework proposed by several authors in the last two decades based on the path integral formulation, which can even be reformulated with the graphical techniques introduced by Feynman and discussed in Section 2. The first attempt to merge quantum and economic theory dates back to the end of the 1970s with the first works of Qadir [52] and Samuelson [53]. Specifically, the first one proposed, under suitable assumptions, the use of quantum formalism to model micro-economics (in analogy with micro-physics). A renewed interest in these ideas started to emerge between the end of the 1990s and the beginning of the 2000s, thanks to researchers coming from the social sciences such as Shubik [54] and Haven [55].

However, at the same time, the two most important approaches to quantum econophysics came onto the stage, that is, the works of Ilinski [56] and Baaquie [57]. In the following years, Baaquie has considerably developed his own approach with several manuscripts [58–62] and books [63,64], which represent the core of this section. Interested readers can find further materials on quantum methods for economics and finance in [65–69]. In the following paragraphs, we explore the formalism developed by Baaquie [57,59,70] for modelling European options on coupon bonds.

Remark 6. *European options represent the most used* path-independent options. *An option is said to be path-independent if the payoff function is independent of how the security arrives at its final price. On the contrary,* path-dependent options *(such as American or Asian options) are ones in which payoff functions depend on the whole path that the security takes before the option expires. For further details, see [57,71]. Moreover, we recall that a* bond *is a primary negotiable financial instrument that at the pre-established maturity gives its owner the right to repayment of the capital lent to the issuer plus a fixed or variable interest rate, the* coupon *(basically, it is a special type of investment). A derivative financial instrument is instead the* option, *which gives to the owner the possibility to buy or sell the underlying bond at a certain price on or before the option expiry date.*

The formalism introduced by Baaquie is inspired by QFT and it naturally leads to Feynman representation of a perturbative series, which, in this case, models a financial instrument, namely the *forward interest rate* (the forward interest rate is just the future yield on a coupon bond). More formally [70], we can denote by $f(x,t)$ the function representing the forward interest rates for a fixed time t and a loan at some future times $x > t$. With this notation, it is possible to define the forward price of a bond (maturing at time T_i) in terms of the interest rate:

$$F_i = \exp\left(-\int_{t^*}^{T_i} dx f(t_0, x)\right), \quad t^* > t_0, \tag{20}$$

where t^* is the future time (with respect to the initial time t_0) for which a zero coupon bond is going to be issued. The development of a rigorous mathematical formulation of the forward interest rates starts from the following equation that describes the time evolution of such rates $f(t,x)$:

$$\frac{\partial}{\partial t} f(t,x) = \alpha(t,x) + \sigma(t,x) \cdot \mathcal{A}(t,x), \tag{21}$$

where $\mathcal{A}(t,x)$ denotes the two-dimensional quantum field (a stochastic random field) associated with the forward interest rates, $\alpha(t,x)$ is the drift fixed by a choice of numeraire, and $\sigma(t,x)$ is the volatility given by the market itself. In this context, one can consider $f(t,x)$ and $\mathcal{A}(t,x)$ as two-dimensional quantum fields [70]. In this framework, it is possible to express the quantum field theory of the forward interest rates thanks to the following generating function [57]:

$$Z(h) = \frac{1}{Z} \int D\mathcal{A} e^{S + \int_{t_0}^{\infty} dt \int_0^{\infty} dz h(t,z)\mathcal{A}(t,z)}, \qquad (22)$$

where the stiff action S and the partition function Z are, respectively,

$$S := S(\mathcal{A}) = \int_0^{\infty} dt \int_t^{\infty} dx \, \mathcal{L} \quad \text{and} \quad Z = \int D\mathcal{A} e^S. \qquad (23)$$

Here, $\mathcal{L}$ denotes a suitable Lagrangian describing the evolution of instantaneous forward rates depending on the three parameters, as explained in [57].

Now, following the argument in [59], in the case of (European) options for coupon bonds, the price of the call option has a partition function of the form

$$Z(\eta) = \frac{1}{Z} \int D\mathcal{A} e^S e^{i\eta V}, \qquad (24)$$

where Z was already defined in Equation (23), and V is the so-called *notional principal amount*. Mathematically speaking, the price at time t of a Treasury Bond maturing at some future time $T > t$ can be defined by using the forward interest rates $f(t, x)$ as

$$B(t, T) = \exp\left(-\int_t^T dx f(t, x)\right).$$

As explained in [59], it is also possible to rewrite the price of the coupon bond in terms of a zero coupon bond $B(t^*, T)$ and the interest rate F_i, defined in Equation (20) as

$$\sum_{i=1}^N k_i B(t^*, T_i) = \sum_{i=1}^N k_i F_i + \sum_{i=1}^N k_i (B(t^*, T) - F_i) = F + V, \quad \text{with } V = \sum_{i=1}^N k_i (B(t^*, T) - F_i).$$

Here, k_i denotes (fixed) dividends payed at time T_i, for $i = 1, \ldots, N$. Moreover, in these settings, one can prove (see [70]) that V is actually a small perturbation of F.

As highlighted by Baaquie [57], the volatility of the forward interest rates is actually a little quantity, namely it is approximately 10^{-2}/year. Thus, the volatility function $\sigma(x, t)$ can be used as a perturbation, that is, an expansion parameter, and the approximation of the partition function can be systematically improved by expanding to higher orders. In other words, the goal now becomes the construction of an analytical expression that yields the price of the coupon bond option in terms of the power series (in σ) of the partition function $Z(\eta)$ given in Equation (24). The analogy with QFT is exploited to develop the rigorous perturbation expansion for the partition function, whose terms can be computed in terms of Feynman diagrams. In particular, we have the following cumulant expansion:

$$Z(\eta) = \exp\left(i\eta a_1 - (1/2)\eta^2 a_2 - i(1/3!)\eta^3 a_3 + (1/4!)\eta^4 a_3 + \cdots\right), \qquad (25)$$

where the parameters a_i are computed thanks to the Feynman diagram representations. There is now a technical–financial hypothesis to add on our argument, namely the *put–call parity* constraint. Roughly speaking, put-call parity is a relationship between the price of a call option and a put option, which mathematically leads to the following conditions:

$$Z(0) = 1 \quad \text{and} \quad \partial_\eta Z(\eta)|_{\eta=0} = 0.$$

This imposes $a_1 = 0$, and it leads to the simplified version of Equation (25):

$$Z(\eta) = \exp\left(-(1/2)\eta^2 a_2 - i(1/3!)\eta^3 a_3 + (1/4!)\eta^4 a_3 + \cdots\right). \qquad (26)$$

It is possible to expand the partition function even in a power series in η. Such an expansion yields to

$$Z(\eta) = \frac{1}{Z}\int D\mathcal{A} e^{i\eta V}\left(1 + i\eta V + \frac{1}{2!}(i\eta)^2 V^2 + \frac{1}{3!}(i\eta)^3 V^3 + \frac{1}{4!}(i\eta)^4 V^4 + \cdots\right). \quad (27)$$

By comparing Equations (26) and (27), it is possible to find the relation between the coefficients a_2, a_3, a_4 and V (see also Remarks 7 and 8). Remarkably, one can see that the martingale condition implies that $a_1 = 0$, so that put–call parity is satisfied. Moreover, these coefficients can be described more specifically by introducing a suitable correlation function G_{ij} (a real symmetric matrix) for expressing the correlation in the fluctuations of the forward bond prices F_i and F_j. If we denote the magnitude of the matrix elements G_{ij} as G and use the relation $G \simeq \sigma^2$, we can rewrite partition function as

$$Z(\eta) \simeq \exp\left(-c_2\zeta^2 - c_3\zeta^3\sigma - c_4\zeta^4\sigma^2 + \cdots\right), \quad \text{with } \zeta = \sigma\eta, \quad (28)$$

where the coefficients c_i are $O(1)$. Here, the quadratic term in the exponential for Z fixes the magnitude of the perturbations as $O(1)$. As a consequence, the remaining terms are of order σ, σ^2, and so on. This argument allows us to compute the partition function to any order of accuracy with respect to the parameter G (or, equivalently, σ).

Remark 7. *In the previous paragraphs, we described the construction of the series expansion of the partition function $Z(\eta)$. It is now clear that the next step involves the computation of the following coefficients emerging from the comparisons of Equations (26) and (27), namely the following (we recall that the coefficient $a_1 = \langle V \rangle$ has to be 0 because of the put–call parity condition):*

$$a_2 = \langle V^2 \rangle; \quad (29)$$
$$a_3 = \langle V^3 \rangle; \quad (30)$$
$$a_4 = \langle V^4 \rangle - 3A^2. \quad (31)$$

The analytic computation of these values is given in full in Appendix of [59].

Once we fix this formalism, it appears quite natural to connect the perturbative expansion of the partition function Z with the Feynman diagrams. Specifically, the forward bond propagator G_{ij} that denotes the correlation between the forward bond price F_i and F_j can be depicted with a wavy line as in Figure 9.

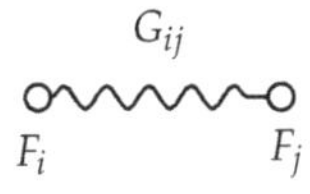

Figure 9. The wavy line is the correlator G_{ij} between the two forward bond prices, F_i and F_j, represented by the small circles. Adapted from [59].

This graph formalism can be used to compute the coefficients a_2, a_3, and a_4 of Equation (27) as represented in Figure 10.

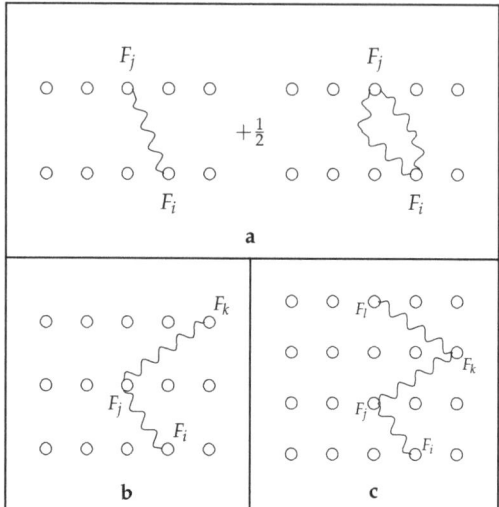

Figure 10. Diagrams representing the evaluation of parameters a_2 (**a**), a_3 (**b**), and a_4 (**c**). Adapted from [59].

We remark that all the diagrams contributing in the series of the partition function Z are connected, namely none of the forward bond prices are decoupled from the forward bond propagator G_{ij}. However, it is also possible to produce disconnected Feynman diagrams (that do not contribute to any of the coefficients), as one can see in Figure 11.

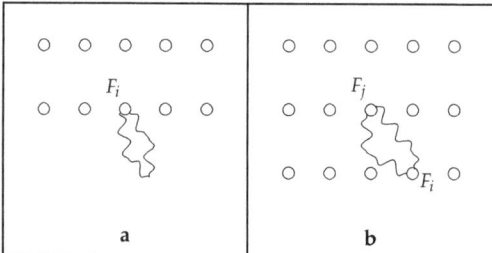

Figure 11. Disconnected diagrams of the second (**a**) and third (**b**) order. As one can notice, the forward bond prices, namely the dots on the top line, have no link with the other forward bond prices. Adapted from [59].

The application of Feynman pictorialism in modelling financial objects represents an intriguing possibility for using such a formalism in a practical framework. In particular, it is interesting to underline that such a theoretical construction has a corresponding empirical study, which can be found in [62]. Apart from the interpretive aspects that surely represent a non trivial issue, the visualization of the terms arising from the series expansion (28) by means of Feynman-type diagrams provides a powerful tool, in order to compute the price of the option for a coupon bond in the framework of quantum finance. However, the works mentioned above can be considered the first technical step in a wider study in this fascinating field.

Remark 8. *The computations of Remark 7 are summarized by the graphs represented in Figure 10. In particular, by some intricate calculations (see Appendix of [59]), it is possible to obtain the following expression for the coefficient a_1 depending on the propagator G_{ij}:*

$$a_2 = \sum_{i,j=1}^{N} J_i J_j (\exp(G_{ij}) - 1), \tag{32}$$

where $J_i = k_i F_i$ and $J_j = k_j F_j$, with $k_i, k_j \in \mathbb{R}$. Thus, by expanding the exponential functions, we obtain

$$a_2 = \sum_{i,j=1}^{N} J_i J_j \left(G_{ij} + \frac{1}{2} G_{ij}^2 \right) + O(G_{ij}^3), \tag{33}$$

which is equivalent to the Feynman-type representation in Figure 10a. Analogous expressions can be found also for coefficients a_3 and a_4, which are equivalent to the graphs in Figure 10b and Figure 10c, respectively.

5. Conclusions

In this work, we have presented two different applications of the Feynman diagrammatic formalism belonging to two completely different domains. On the one hand, RNA secondary and tertiary structures can be modelled intuitively in terms of graphs by involving the matrix theory as theoretical support. On the other hand, the field of econophysics, based on the path integral formulation of the theory, finds a strong ally for studying nonlocal and nonlinear problems.

The abstract nature of the mathematics behind Feynman diagrams suggest the wider use of these tools, which actually transcends the original physical domain. Indeed, we remark that the mathematical significance of Feynman diagrams is well studied in terms of algebraic lattice structures in the framework of Hopf algebras [72,73] and tensor models [74].

In this concluding section, we want to propose a few more attempts to use Feynman diagrams in unusual scientific areas of study. One of the most natural applications of Feynman diagrams has arisen in geophysics for modelling different scenarios involving wave propagation. In this field, we indicate, by way of example, two interesting works. The first one regards wave propagation in a laterally heterogeneous medium [75]. Here, the authors used diagrams to find a solution for random media elastic wave problems involving Dyson's equation and the Bethe–Salpeter equation. The second study exploits the closer link between the perturbation graphs and collision diagrams for modelling scattering processes in oceanic wave guides involving surface and internal gravity waves [76].

Other stimulating employments of Feynman-type graphs come from the field of chemistry, where this kind of representation is used to derive a more accurate reaction–diffusion equation starting from a path integral formulation [77], or even for the so-called 2D-Raman-THz spectroscopy of liquid water [78].

A fascinating arrangement of Feynman diagrams is given in information theory for distributed quantities, which actually provides a Bayesian statistical field theory named *information field theory*. In this framework, interacting information field theories can be diagrammatically expanded in terms of Feynman diagrams [79,80].

Finally, we mention three different applications in the medical area. In the first case, the authors proposed a method for studying some neuronal function signal propagations based on the cable equation [81]. The benefit of this approach is the possibility of working with Green's function, corresponding to the propagator of the system that may be handled with techniques employed in the many body systems theory and then represented by Feynman diagrams. The second case aimed to investigate brain function by using electroencephalogram (EEG) combined with a set of Feynman rules inspired by quantum particle interactions [82]. In particular, the author introduces the brain state matrix, which is composed of several EEG indicators, for predicting several brain reactions that are analyzed as sensory-evoked and event-related potentials. The last medical example regards cardiac arrhythmia. In [83], the authors introduced three *quasiparticles* (heads, tails, and pivots) in order to capture the rich dynamics in excitable systems (which are a large class of chemical and biological systems). Specifically, they used Feynman-like diagrams to represent the dynamical creation, annihilation, and recombination of the identified quasiparticles.

As we have seen in this paper, the usage of Feynman diagrams, as powerful computational tools, seems to go beyond the original physical setting. The graphical approach that many satisfactions gave to QED has an intrinsic capacity to reproduce complicated abstract concepts (such as matrix integrals) in a more suitable and intuitive way. We hope that such a work could be good inspiration for researchers coming from different scientific areas who want to look at things from a different and fascinating angle.

Funding: This research received no external funding.

Acknowledgments: The author would like to express his gratitude to Gianni Arioli and Giovanni Valente for the numerous discussions on the interpretation of Feynman diagrams. Many thanks also to Jacopo Cangiotti, Marco Capolli, Stefano Grasso, and Mattia Sensi for their precious support and important suggestions to improve this work. The author is a member and acknowledges the support of *Gruppo Nazionale per l'Analisi Matematica, la Probabilità e le loro Applicazioni* (GNAMPA) of *Istituto Nazionale di Alta Matematica* (INdAM), and, moreover, acknowledges the support of the MIUR—PRIN 2022 project "Nonlinear dispersive equations in presence of singularities" (Prot. N. 20225ATSTP). Finally, the author thanks the anonymous reviewers for their careful reading of the manuscript and their many insightful comments and suggestions.

Conflicts of Interest: The author declares no conflicts of interest.

References

1. Feynman, R.P. Space-Time Approach to Quantum Electrodynamics. *Phys. Rev.* **1949**, *76*, 769–789. [CrossRef]
2. Kaiser, D. *Drawing Theories Apart: The Dispersion of Feynman Diagrams in Postwar Physics*; University of Chicago Press: Chicago, IL, USA, 2005.
3. Griffiths, D. *Introduction to Elementary Particles*; Harper & Row: New York, NY, USA, 1987.
4. Mangano, M.L. Introduction to QCD. In Proceedings of the 1998 European School of High-Energy Physics, St. Andrews, UK, 23 August–5 September 1998; pp. 53–97.
5. Peskin, M.E.; Schroeder, D.V. *An Introduction to Quantum Field Theory*; Westview Press: New York, NY, USA, 1995.
6. Barrett, J.W. Feynman diagrams coupled to three-dimensional quantum gravity. *Class. Quantum Gravity* **2006**, *23*, 137–141. [CrossRef]
7. Reisenberger M.P.; Rovelli, C. Spacetime as a Feynman diagram: The connection formulation. *Class. Quantum Gravity* **2001**, *18*, 121–140. [CrossRef]
8. Goldberger, W.D.; Rothstein, I.Z. Effective field theory of gravity for extended objects. *Phys. Rev. D* **2006**, *73*, 104029. [CrossRef]
9. Jishi R.A. *Feynman Diagram Techniques in Condensed Matter Physics*; Cambridge University Press: Cambridge, UK, 2013.
10. Meynell, L. Why Feynman diagrams represent. *Int. Stud. Philos. Sci.* **2008**, *22*, 39–59. [CrossRef]
11. Stöltzner, M. Feynman Diagrams as Models. *Math. Intell.* **2017**, *39*, 46–54. [CrossRef]
12. Stöltzner, M. Feynman Diagrams: Modelling between Physics and Mathematics. *Perspect. Sci.* **2018**, *26*, 482–500. [CrossRef]
13. Dorato, M.; Rossanese, E. The Nature of Representation in Feynman Diagrams. *Perspect. Sci.* **2018**, *26*, 443–458. [CrossRef]
14. Passon, O. On the interpretation of Feynman diagrams, or, did the LHC experiments observe $H \to \gamma\gamma$? *Eur. J. Philos.* **2019**, *9*, 20. [CrossRef]
15. Redhead, M. Models in physics. *Br. J. Philos. Sci.* **1980**, *31*, 145–163. [CrossRef]
16. Dahlkemper, M.N.; Klein, P.; Müller, A.; Schmeling, S.M.; Wiener, J. Opportunities and Challenges of Using Feynman Diagrams with Upper Secondary Students. *Physics* **2022**, *4*, 1331–1347. [CrossRef]
17. Shaikh, R.A.; Gogioso, S. Categorical Semantics for Feynman Diagrams. *arXiv* **2022**, arXiv:2205.00466.
18. Polyak, M. Feynman diagrams for pedestrians and mathematicians. *Graphs Patterns Math. Theor. Phys.* **2005**, *73*, 15–42.
19. Srednicki, M. *Quantum Field Theory*; Cambridge University Press: Cambridge, UK, 2007.
20. Ticciati, R. *Quantum Field Theory for Mathematicians*; Cambridge University Press: Cambridge UK, 1999.
21. Wüthrich, A. *The Genesis of Feynman Diagrams*; Springer: Berlin/Heidelberg, Germany, 2016.
22. Dyson, F.J. Divergence of perturbation theory in quantum electrodynamics. *Phys. Rev.* **1952**, *85*, 631–632. [CrossRef]
23. Fox, T. Haunted by the Spectre of Virtual Particles: A Philosophical Reconsideration. *J. Gen. Philos. Sci.* **2008**, *39*, 35–51. [CrossRef]
24. Jaeger, G. Are Virtual Particles Less Real? *Entropy* **2019**, *21*, 141. [CrossRef] [PubMed]
25. Cangiotti, N.; Nappo, F. Reasoning by Analogy in Mathematical Practice. *Philos. Math.* **2023**, *31*, 176–215. [CrossRef]
26. Nappo, F.; Cangiotti, N.; Sisti, C. Confirming Mathematical Conjectures by Analogy. *Erkenntnis* 2023, *Online First Articles*.
27. Orland, H.; Zee, A. RNA folding and large N matrix theory. *Nucl. Phys. B* **2002**, *620*, 456–476. [CrossRef]

28. Andersen, J.E.; Chekhov, L.O.; Penner, R.C.; Reidys, C.M.; Sułkowski, P. Topological recursion for chord diagrams, RNA complexes, and cells in moduli spaces. *Nucl. Phys. B* **2013**, *866*, 414–443. [CrossRef]
29. Andersen, J.E.; Penner, R.C.; Reidys, C.M.; Waterman, M.S. Topological classification and enumeration of RNA structures by genus. *J. Math. Biol.* **2013**, *67*, 1261–1278. [CrossRef]
30. Pillsbury, M.; Orland, H.; Zee, A. Steepest descent calculation of RNA pseudoknots. *Phys. Rev. E* **2005**, *72*, 011911. [CrossRef] [PubMed]
31. Rubach, P.; Zajac, S.; Jastrzebski, B.; Sulkowska, J.I.; Sułkowski, P. Genus for biomolecules. *Nucleic Acids Res.* **2019**, *48*, D1129–D1135. [CrossRef]
32. Vernizzi, G.; Orland, H.; Zee, A. Enumeration of RNA structures by matrix models. *Phys. Rev. Lett.* **2005**, *94*, 168103. [CrossRef] [PubMed]
33. Vernizzi, G.; Ribeca, P.; Orl, H.; Zee, A. Topology of pseudoknotted homopolymers. *Phys. Rev. E* **2006**, *73*, 031902. [CrossRef] [PubMed]
34. Xu, X.; Chen, S.-J. Topological constraints of RNA pseudoknotted and loop-kissing motifs: Applications to three-dimensional structure prediction. *Nucleic Acids Res.* **2020**, *48*, 6503–6512. [CrossRef] [PubMed]
35. Zając, S.; Geary, C.; Andersen, E.S.; Dabrowski-Tumanski, P.; Sulkowska, J.I.; Sułkowski, P. Genus trace reveals the topological complexity and domain structure of biomolecules. *Sci. Rep.* **2018**, *8*, 17537. [CrossRef] [PubMed]
36. Antczak, M.; Popenda, M.; Zok, T.; Zurkowski, M.; Adamiak, R.W.; Szachniuk, M. New algorithms to represent complex pseudoknotted RNA structures in dot-bracket notation. *Bioinformatics* **2017**, *34*, 1304–1312. [CrossRef]
37. ten Dam, E.; Pleij, K.; Draper, D. Structural and functional aspects of RNA pseudoknots. *Biochemistry* **1992**, *31*, 11665–11676. [CrossRef]
38. 't Hooft, G. A planar diagram theory for strong interactions. *Nucl. Phys. B* **1974**, *72*, 461–473. [CrossRef]
39. Vernizzi, G.; Orland, H.; Zee, A. Classification and predictions of RNA pseudoknots based on topological invariants. *Phys. Rev. E* **2016**, *94*, 042410. [CrossRef]
40. Grothendieck, A. *Geometric Galois Action 1*; London Mathematical Society Lecture Note Series; Chapter Esquisse d'un Programme; Cambridge University Press: Cambridge, UK, 1997; Volume 242, pp. 5–48.
41. Zvonkin, A. Matrix integrals and map enumeration: An accessible introduction. *Math. Comput. Model.* **1997**, *26*, 281–304. [CrossRef]
42. Bon, M.; Vernizzi, G.; Orl, H.; Zee, A. Topological classification of RNA structures. *J. Mol. Biol.* **2008**, *379*, 900–911. [CrossRef] [PubMed]
43. Vernizzi, G.; Orland, H.; Zee, A. Prediction of RNA pseudoknots by Monte Carlo simulations. *arXiv* **2004**, arXiv:q-bio/0405014.
44. Bon, M.; Orl, H. Prediction of RNA secondary structures with pseudoknots. *Phys. A Stat. Mech. Appl.* **2010**, *389*, 2987–2992. [CrossRef]
45. Bon, M.; Micheletti, C.; Orland, H. McGenus: A Monte Carlo algorithm to predict RNA secondary structures with pseudoknots. *Nucleic Acids Res.* **2012**, *41*, 1895–1900. [CrossRef] [PubMed]
46. Bon, M.; Orland, H. TT2NE: A novel algorithm to predict RNA secondary structures with pseudoknots. *Nucleic Acids Res.* **2011**, *39*, e93. [CrossRef]
47. Cangiotti, N.; Grasso, S. Genus Comparisons in the Topological Analysis of RNA Structures. *arXiv* **2023**, arXiv:2304.07283.
48. Dash, K.C. *The Story of Econophysics*; Cambridge Scholars Publishing: Newcastle upon Tyne, UK, 2019.
49. Jovanovic, F.; Schinckus, C. *Econophysics and Financial Economics: An Emerging Dialogue*; Oxford University Press: Oxford, UK, 2017.
50. Mantegna, R.N.; Stanley, H.E. *Introduction to Econophysics: Correlations and Complexity in Finance*; Cambridge University Press: Cambridge UK, 1999.
51. Arioli, G.; Giovanni, V. What Is Really Quantum in Quantum Econophysics? *Philos. Sci.* **2021**, *88*, 665–685. [CrossRef]
52. Qadir, A. Quantum Economics. *Pak. Econ. Soc. Rev.* **1978**, *16*, 117–126.
53. Samuelson, P. A quantum theory model of economics: Is the co-ordinating entrepreneur just worth his profit? In *The Collected Scientific Papers of Paul A. Samuelson*; The MIT Press: Cambridge, MA, USA, 1999; Volume 4.
54. Shubik, M. Quantum economics, uncertainty and the optimal grid size. *Econ. Lett.* **1999**, *64*, 277–278. [CrossRef]
55. Haven, E. A discussion on embedding the Black–Scholes option pricing model in a quantum physics setting. *Phys. A Stat. Mech.* **2002**, *304*, 507–524. [CrossRef]
56. Ilinski, K. *Physics of Finance: Gauge Modelling in Non-Equilibrium Pricing*; John Wiley & Sons Inc.: Hoboken, NJ, USA, 2001.
57. Baaquie, B.E. *Quantum Finance—Path Integrals and Hamiltonians for Options and Interest Rates*; Cambridge University Press: Cambridge, UK, 2004.
58. Baaquie, B.E. A Common Market Measure for Libor and Pricing Caps, Floors and Swaps in a Field Theory of forward Interest Rates. *Int. J. Theor. Appl. Financ.* **2005**, *8*, 999–1018. [CrossRef]
59. Baaquie, B.E. Feynman perturbation expansion for the price of coupon bond options and swaptions in quantum finance. I. Theory. *Phys. Rev. E* **2007**, *75*, 016703. [CrossRef] [PubMed]
60. Baaquie, B.E. Action with Acceleration I: Euclidean Hamiltonian and Path Integral. *Int. J. Mod. Phys. A* **2013**, *28*, 1350137. [CrossRef]
61. Baaquie, B.E. Action with Acceleration II: Euclidean Hamiltonian and Jordan Blocks. *Int. J. Mod. Phys. A* **2013**, *28*, 1350138. [CrossRef]

62. Baaquie, B.E.; Liang, C. Feynman perturbation expansion for the price of coupon bond options and swaptions in quantum finance. II. Empirical. *Phys. Rev. E* **2007**, *75*, 016704. [CrossRef]
63. Baaquie, B.E. *Interest Rates and Coupon Bonds in Quantum Finance*; Cambridge University Press: Cambridge, UK, 2009.
64. Baaquie, B.E. *Quantum Field Theory for Economics and Finance*; Cambridge University Press: Cambridge, UK, 2018.
65. Bagarello, F. Stock markets and quantum dynamics: A second quantized description. *Phys. A Stat. Mech. Appl.* **2007**, *386*, 283–302. [CrossRef]
66. Guevara, H. Quantum econophysics. *arXiv* **2007**, arXiv:physics/0609245.
67. Maslov, V.P. Econophysics and Quantum Statistics. *Math. Notes* **2002**, *72*, 811–818. [CrossRef]
68. Paolinelli, G.; Arioli, G. A path integral based model for stocks and order dynamics. *Phys. A Stat. Mech.* **2018**, *510*, 387–399. [CrossRef]
69. Schinckus, C. A Methodological Call for a Quantum Econophysics. In Proceedings of the Quantum Interaction: 7th International Conference, QI 2013, Leicester, UK, 25–27 July 2013.
70. Baaquie, B.E. Price of coupon bond options in a quantum field theory of forward interest rates. *Phys. A Stat. Mech.* **2006**, *370*, 98–103. [CrossRef]
71. Hull, J.C. *Options, Futures and Other Derivatives*, 5th ed.; Prentice-Hall International: Old Bridge, NJ, USA, 2003.
72. Borinsky, M.; Kreimer, D. Feynman diagrams and their algebraic lattices. In *Resurgence, Physics and Numbers*; Edizioni della Normale: Pisa, Italy, 2017; pp. 92–107.
73. Connes, A.; Kreimer, D. Renormalization in quantum field theory and the Riemann-Hilbert problem. I. The Hopf algebra structure of graphs and the main theorem. *Commun. Math. Phys.* **2000**, *210*, 249–273. [CrossRef]
74. Amburg, N.; Itoyama, H.; Mironov, A.; Morozov, A.; Vasiliev, D.; Yoshioka, R. Correspondence between Feynman diagrams and operators in quantum field theory that emerges from tensor model. *Eur. Phys. J. C* **2020**, *80*, 471. [CrossRef]
75. Park, M.; Odom, R.I. Propagators and Feynman diagrams for laterally heterogeneous elastic media. *Geophys. J. Int.* **2005**, *160*, 289–301. [CrossRef]
76. Hasselmann, K. Feynman diagrams and interaction rules of wave-wave scattering processes. *Rev. Geophys.* **1966**, *4*, 1–32. [CrossRef]
77. Li, C.; Li, J.; Yang, Y. A Feynman Path Integral-like Method for Deriving Reaction—Diffusion Equations. *Polymers* **2022**, *14*, 5156. [CrossRef]
78. Sidler, D.; Hamm, P. Feynman diagram description of 2D-Raman-THz spectroscopy applied to water. *J. Chem. Phys.* **2019**, *150*, 044202. [CrossRef]
79. Enßlin, T.A.; Frommert, M.; Kitaura, F.S. Information field theory for cosmological perturbation reconstruction and nonlinear signal analysis. *Phys. Rev. D* **2009**, *80*, 105005. [CrossRef]
80. Enßlin, T.A. Information field theory. *AIP Conf. Proc.* **2013**, *1553*, 184–191.
81. Martin-Pereda, J.A.; Gonzalez-Marcos, A.P. Analysis of neuronal functions based on Feynman diagrams. In Proceedings of the Engineering in Medicine and Biology, 1999, 21st Annual Conference and the 1999 Annual Fall Meeting of the Biomedical Engineering Society] BMES/EMBS Conference, 1999, Proceedings of the First Joint, Atlanta, GA, USA, 13–16 October 1999.
82. Başar, E. *Brain Function and Oscillations. Volume I: Brain Oscillations. Principles and Approaches*; Springer: Berlin/Heidelberg, Germany, 1998.
83. Arno, L.; Desmond Kabus, D.; Dierckx, H. Analysis of complex excitation patterns using Feynman-like diagrams. *arXiv* **2023**, arXiv:2307.01508.

Disclaimer/Publisher's Note: The statements, opinions and data contained in all publications are solely those of the individual author(s) and contributor(s) and not of MDPI and/or the editor(s). MDPI and/or the editor(s) disclaim responsibility for any injury to people or property resulting from any ideas, methods, instructions or products referred to in the content.

MDPI AG
Grosspeteranlage 5
4052 Basel
Switzerland
Tel.: +41 61 683 77 34

Mathematics Editorial Office
E-mail: mathematics@mdpi.com
www.mdpi.com/journal/mathematics

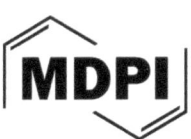

Disclaimer/Publisher's Note: The title and front matter of this reprint are at the discretion of the Guest Editors. The publisher is not responsible for their content or any associated concerns. The statements, opinions and data contained in all individual articles are solely those of the individual Editors and contributors and not of MDPI. MDPI disclaims responsibility for any injury to people or property resulting from any ideas, methods, instructions or products referred to in the content.

www.ingramcontent.com/pod-product-compliance
Lightning Source LLC
LaVergne TN
LVHW072350090526
838202LV00019B/2511